# The Fearful Dental Patient

## A Guide to Understanding and Managing

# The Fearful Dental Patient

## A Guide to Understanding and Managing

Editor

## Arthur A. Weiner, DMD

Professor, General Dentistry
Director, Behavioral Science II
Group Practice Coordinator, Undergraduate General Dental Clinic
Tufts University
Boston, MA

**WILEY-BLACKWELL**

A John Wiley & Sons, Inc., Publication

Edition first published 2011
© 2011 Blackwell Publishing Ltd.

Blackwell Publishing was acquired by John Wiley & Sons in February 2007. Blackwell's publishing program has been merged with Wiley's global Scientific, Technical, and Medical business to form Wiley-Blackwell.

*Editorial Office*
2121 State Avenue, Ames, Iowa 50014-8300, USA

For details of our global editorial offices, for customer services, and for information about how to apply for permission to reuse the copyright material in this book, please see our Website at www.wiley.com/wiley-blackwell.

*Library of Congress Cataloging-in-Publication Data*

The fearful dental patient : a guide to understanding and managing / [edited by] Arthur A. Weiner.
       p. ; cm.
   Includes bibliographical references and index.
   ISBN 978-0-8138-2084-2 (pbk. : alk. paper)
   1. Fear of dentists.  I. Weiner, Arthur A.
   [DNLM:  1. Dental Anxiety–prevention & control.  2. Dental Care–psychology.  WU 29 F288 2011]
   RK53.F43 2011
   616.85'225–dc22
                                      2010023257
A catalog record for this book is available from the U.S. Library of Congress.

Set in 9.5 on 12 pt Palatino by Toppan Best-set Premedia Limited

Printed and bound in Malaysia by Vivar Printing Sdn Bhd

1   2011

## Dedication

*I would like to dedicate this book to:*

My father and mother, Maxwell and Tillie, and my two sisters, Ann Charlotte and Janice Susan, whose combined sacrifices and love made it possible for me to attain the education and be the first in the family to get that all important sheepskin.

Uncle Fred Weiner, MD, who was always there with whatever help I needed, including words of encouragement and so many other little things that helped me along the way.

My lovely wife, Paula Sandra, to whom I truly owe everything. For 54 years of married bliss, constant encouragement, love, and support, no man could want more. For all the times she kept me on the straight and narrow, I could not love her any more than I already do. She is my heart and my soul, the most precious jewel any man could hope to find.

To my three children, Randy, Rickie, and Robyne, for all the joy and pride that they fill my days with, and for the wonderful grandchildren that they and their awesome spouses have blessed our days with. They have enriched our lives and truly made it all worthwhile.

Last, the wonderful young men and women, past and present, who make up the student body of the Tufts University School of Dental Medicine. For their kindness, support, and patience and their help with my many clinical research studies that have led up to this book, words of thanks are inadequate. As I have taught them, I also have learned much from them. They will always hold a special place in my heart.

# Contents

See the supporting companion website for this book: www.wiley.com/go/weiner

# Foreword

In *The Fearful Dental Patient: A Guide to Understanding and Managing,* Arthur Weiner and the contributors make the strong case that attending to the well-being of the apprehensive dental patient not only makes for a compliant and responsive patient, but yields an appreciative ambassador on behalf of the person-oriented dentist as well. Equally important, the authors make the case that when the clinician rises to the broader challenge of addressing the personal needs of his or her patients, as well as their oral health needs—that is, when the dentist acts as both a biologic and a behavioral change agent—then the dentist is rewarded with a greater sense of fulfillment that is accomplished in a clinical work environment that is less stressful. The dental practice becomes a kinder, gentler, and more productive place for the dentist as well as the patient!

Dr. Weiner's attention to this perspective on the dual role and responsibility of the dentist as a biobehavioral clinician is unique in a clinical dental text of this sort and represents a significant step forward in broadening what it means to be a dentist. But this advocacy is not simply for "touchy-feely" or "do-good" dentists and dentistry. A major accomplishment of *The Fearful Dental Patient: A Guide to Understanding and Managing* is that it provides the best available scientific basis for all the methods of assessing and managing fearful patients whose concerns about getting dental treatment can impair their oral health. These patients range from those who are mildly anxious to the most fearful, and, even phobic, patients. The authors apply a comprehensive approach to the very young, the elderly, and those burdened with physical and emotional disabilities that impact their lives.

But it is in the blending of underlying science and commonsense pragmatism that there emerges a powerful rationale for expanding the dentist's horizon about clinical practice: the basic science underlying the nature of fear, anxiety, and panic that the opening chapters present is sound; the clinical assessment measures recommended are similarly scientifically valid; the behavioral and pharmacologic methods offered to help the patient are evidence based as well as prudent; and the skills and methods are clearly presented, easy to learn, easy to apply, and proven in their patient acceptability and effectiveness.

Embedded throughout the text is the deep and necessary understanding that to effect changes in others—for dentists to serve as change agents, seeking to facilitate change in dental patient behaviors and negative thoughts and emotions—it is sometimes necessary for the dentist to consider changing as well. This change is reflected as increased knowledge and awareness, accompanied by acquisition of the modest tools of behavior change needed to alter the maladaptive ways in which some patients avoid dentists and their dentistry. This dual approach is truly unique, most welcome, and nothing less than an enlightened advance in our understanding of the complexities of how some patients became fearful, and how sometimes both patients and dentists are appropriate targets for change.

The organization of the text, including reliance on a number of superb clinician–teacher scientists, reveals the authors' understanding and familiarity with the need to acquire basic information about why something happens, and then to apply that understanding to the assessment of dental patients. Dr. Weiner and the contributors expand the acquisition of data about the patient from the expected clinical domains of restorative and surgical dentistry, which are well known and not covered here, to the domains of subjective experience as scientifically studied by clinicians and researchers in behavioral medicine and the behavioral sciences more generally. The dentist is thus guided to gathering in systematic fashion an individual database for each person that reveals what the dentist needs to know in order to establish a trusting, and, especially important, long-lasting dentist–patient relationship. A dentist–patient relationship built on valid information becomes the springboard for allowing the dentist to determine if the dentally related anxiety, fear, panic, and/or avoidance uncovered by the assessment process are of sufficient strength to warrant considering integrating behavioral and/or pharmacologic change methods (which form the bulk of this text) into a comprehensive treatment plan for the patient, whatever their clinical dental needs might be.

From his Preface to this book and throughout each of the chapters, it is clear that after more than a generation of clinical dental practice, dental teaching, and research Dr. Weiner has evolved as a careful dentist respectful of his profession's art and craft and attentive to its future. But it is also clear he is a dedicated teacher, seeking to impart to students and dentists that theirs is a profession of lifelong learning. This text expresses what he and the contributors have gleaned from abundant clinical experience and research, and which they now seek to share with readers, namely that dentistry reveals its better nature when dentists grasp an appreciation of what the patient is experiencing and make themselves knowledgeable about how best to manifest caring and management of those personal experiences when they interfere with maintaining oral health.

*Samuel F. Dworkin, DDS, PhD (Hon: DSci, DR Odont)*
Professor Emeritus, Department Oral Medicine

University of Washington, School of Dentistry

Professor Emeritus, Department of Psychiatry and Behavioral Sciences
School of Medicine, University of Washington

# Preface

As long as individuals have practiced the art and science of dentistry, fear and anxiety have been associated with dental treatment. Managing this fear and anxiety has been one of the most troublesome problems that the dental practitioner, as well as the profession at large, has had to face. In years past, dental professionals could afford largely to ignore the problem of dental anxiety. Practices could flourish based on technical virtuosity, while a fearful or anxious patient might be regarded as a burden rather than as a basis for concern.

In the past three decades or so, the advent of the field of behavioral medicine in psychology has brought with it a fresh perspective on a variety of emotional, psychological, and mental disorders, including those of personality, eating, depressive, somatoform, as well as anxiety/panic and posttraumatic stress, and their associated effects on dental care and its behavioral management. As a result of the great influence these disorders have, either individually or combined, on whether or not an individual will receive care, the dental profession has begun to devote increasing attention and involvement focusing on the potential effects and concerns that accompany these disorders. In particular, attention has been directed to those with fear, anxiety, and phobia, which are so often are associated with negative and aversive behavior in a dental patient. In recent years, issues of dentist–patient interaction and patient management have received considerable attention in the dental curriculum, and, at the same time, an increasing number of dental and behavioral clinicians and researchers have directed their efforts toward developing programs designed to increase knowledge and shed new light on this vexing problem of dental fear and anxiety. However, despite this increased attention, the problem of fear and anxiety remains as prevalent today as it did years ago. This is due in general to the lack of understanding of the basic principles of fear, anxiety, and phobias, and the various other disorders that often act in combination to initiate those negative behavioral manifestations that hinder the dental practitioner from successfully treating this segment of the population. In today's complex society, it is difficult to separate and treat only the physical needs of the patient while ignoring the emotional ones. Being a good dentist in today's world means not only producing a fine, accurate restoration; it must also include the understanding that a patient's behavior is crucial to the outcome of treatment. In dental school curricula, courses in the behavioral sciences are now required in order for these institutions to obtain full and complete accreditation, demonstrating the clear importance of this subject to the practice of dentistry. To this end, the practitioner must acquire as much knowledge and understanding as possible of these emotions, feelings, and behaviors and the combined role they play in all stage of dental care.

Since no text can completely cover all the complex psycho-physiological aspects of dental care, nor refer to all those dedicated clinicians and their contributions toward this phase of care, this text has been designed to present basic knowledge acquired through my own years of both private practice and academic research/teaching. It is also combined with the knowledge gained by other distinguished clinicians and academies through their individual and group experiences and studies, necessary to the successful understanding and behavioral management of the dentally anxious and fearful patient. Multiple approaches for various situations are demonstrated, which are practical, and, in many cases, simple, and can be utilized not only by the busy general practitioner, but by dental students, specialists, hygienists, and their staff. We hope the reader will be better able to make a correct assessment of a patient's combined psychological, emotional, and dental needs and to apply that information, and, if needed, the necessary behavioral and psychopharmacological techniques, to lead to the provision of optimal dental treatment. We hope this text, combined with continuous education courses, will act as an instrument to stimulate further and more detailed studies of this phenomenon of dental fear, at all levels of the dental profession.

*Arthur A. Weiner, DMD*

# Acknowledgments

Because I owe much to so many individuals who over the years have supported me and my unending quest to teach and help eliminate fear and anxiety in dentistry, I would need to author a text in itself to mention each and every individual. Please allow me to name a few to whom I am so indebted:

David V. Sheehan, MD, a most distinguished health provider, teacher, and talented psychiatrist, who introduced me to the research and study of fear and phobic disorders, and for 25 years, he has offered me support, guidance, and friendship. Much is owed to him by me that can never be repaid.

To Dean Lonnie Norris and Dr. Noshir Mehta for their unwavering support and the uninterrupted freedom to investigate and study the causes and management of dental fear, a subject very dear to my heart.

To Paul Stark, MS, ScD, and Carole Palmer, EdD, RD, LDN, for their generous help in critiquing the text and helping me to always stay organized and correct. They are two of our most valuable Tufts faculty members. Without their help and guidance, this text would not be as great as I believe it is.

To Dr. Phil Weinstein and Dr. Peter Milgrom of the University of Washington School of Dentistry for their many suggestions and support, not only in this text but in the early years when I first began to study and teach dental fear. Much gratitude is owed to them.

To Dr. Samuel Dworkin, a legend in the field of behavioral science in dentistry. Words of thanks are totally inadequate. His critique and advice on a large portion of this text was simply awesome and greatly appreciated.

To the wonderful women of the Hirsh Health Sciences Library, Gail Hendler, Amy Lapidow, Amy LaVertu, Jane Ichord, Eileen Moyer, Melissa Theroux, Tiffany Tawzer, Jamie Bears, Elizabeth Richardson, and Judy Rabinovitz. They all continuously made sure my reference material was readily available.

Last to my wonderful, talented, and capable senior dental student research assistants, Katharine Burton and Abigail Manter, and Alan Reid, my magnificent illustrator, who by the time this text will be published, will have graduated and brought grace, dignity, and honor to the title of Doctor of Dental Medicine. Knowing and working with them on this text and as their teacher has been an absolute joy and a privilege. May success and happiness follow them all their days.

*Arthur A. Weiner, DMD*

# About the Author

Dr. Weiner, a graduate of Boston College, received his degree of Doctor of Dental Medicine in 1958 from Tufts University School of Dental Medicine in Boston, Massachusetts. In 1962, he opened his practice of general dentistry after a brief tour of service with the U.S. Army Dental Corps. In 1967, he joined the faculty of Tufts Dental School, where he currently holds the title of Professor of General and Behavioral Dentistry. He is the Director of the Behavioral Sciences Course II, as well as a Clinic Group Practice Coordinator in the undergraduate student clinic. Dr. Weiner has lectured extensively in the United States as well as in France and Australia. His numerous clinical research papers have appeared in dental journals and have been cited in behavioral and psychological research journals on the subject of fear, anxiety, and phobias. He has also been published in *Acta Scandinavia Psychiatrica* for his work on the effects of exogenous and endogenous anxiety in dentistry. He has also authored a teaching manual titled "The Difficult Patient: A Guide to Understanding and Managing Dental Anxiety."

For his many contributions to dentistry, Dr. Weiner has been elected to Fellowship in the prestigious Pierre Fauchard International Dental Honor Organization, as well as in the American College of Dentists. He also holds Fellowships in the Academy of Dentistry International and Academy of General Dentistry. He is a member of the Omicron Kappa Upsilon National Dental Honor Society, and a past President of the local chapter at Tufts University. He resides in Ashland, Massachusetts, with his wife Paula of 54 years.

# Contributor List

**Laura Camacho-Castro, CD, DMD**
Associate Clinical Professor
Pediatric Dentistry
Tufts University School of Dental Medicine
Boston, MA

**Michael A. Gow, BDS (Gla), MSC Hyp (Lon)**
Clinical Director of Dental Anxiety Management
The Berkeley Clinic
Glasgow, Scotland, UK

**Ronald J. Kulich, PhD**
Associate Professor
Attending Psychologist
Tufts University School of Dental Medicine
Craniofacial Pain Center
and
Harvard Medical School
Massachusetts General Hospital
Pain Management Center

**Linda Maytan, DDS**
Executive Director, SUSTAIN
and
Department of Human Services
State Operated Systems
Faribault, MN

**Kathryn Ragalis, DMD, MS, RDH**
Associate Professor
Department of General Dentistry
Tufts University School of Dental Medicine
Boston, MA

**Morton Rosenberg, DMD**
Professor Oral and Maxillofacial Surgery
Head Division of Anesthesia and Pain Control
Tufts University School of Dental Medicine
Boston, MA
and
Associate Professor of Anesthesia
Tufts University School of Medicine
Boston, MA

**Samuel Shames, DMD**
Associate Professor General Dentistry
Director, Practice Management
Tufts University School of Dental Medicine
Boston, MA

**Gina M. Terenzi, DMD**
Assistant Professor
Director, Department of Public Health
General Practice Residency
Tufts University School of Dental Medicine
Boston, MA

**Michael Thompson, PhD**
Professor, Pharmacology
Department of General Dentistry
Tufts University School of General Dentistry
Boston, MA

**Kelly M. Wawrzyniak, MA, PsyD**
Massachusetts School of Professional Psychology
Tufts University School of Dental Medicine
Craniofacial Pain Center
Boston, MA

**Arthur A. Weiner, DMD**
Professor, General Dentistry
Director, Behavioral Science II
National Spokesperson for Fear, Anxiety, and Behavioral Management,
   Academy of General Dentistry
Group Practice Coordinator, Undergraduate General Dental Clinic
Tufts University
Boston, MA

# The Fearful Dental Patient

## A Guide to Understanding and Managing

# 1

# The basic principles of fear, anxiety, and phobia: past and present

Arthur A. Weiner

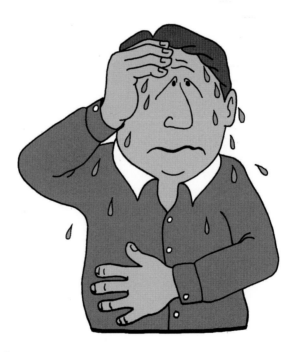

## INTRODUCTION

In 1621, Robert Burton wrote:

> Many lamentable effects this fear causeth in man, as to be red, pale, tremble, sweat; it makes sudden cold or heat to come all over the

*The Fearful Dental Patient: A Guide to Understanding and Managing.* Edited by Arthur A. Weiner
© 2011 Blackwell Publishing Ltd.

body, palpitations of the heart, syncope … it makes men amazed and astonished, they know nor what to do and where they are; it tortures them many days before, with continued affrights and suspicions. It hinders most honourable attempts and makes their hearts ake and be sad. They that live in fear are never resolute and secure, never merry but in continued pain. No greater misery, no rack, no torture unlike it, ever suspicious, anxious, solicitous, they are without reason or control, without judgment. …[1]

The word "fear" stems from the Old English word *fear*, meaning sudden calamity or danger. In Middle English, as in today's complex society, it denotes a normal, useful response to an active or imagined threat. For example, if an individual is confronted with an impending threat of fire, gunfire or very high winds, that fear can cause the individual to take life-saving actions. Fear can also sharpen one's wits, mobilize energies, and heighten reflexes. The physiological responses that emotional arousal causes are designed to prepare the body for the three Fs—"flight, fight, freeze."

Fear is the emotional response to a perceived threat or danger. It is composed of physiological changes, an inner feeling, an outer behavioral actions. Fear can cause a variety of physiological changes, such as pallor, pilomotor erection, pupillary dilation, tachycardia, cardio or pylorospasm, hyperperistalsis, hyper/hypogastrointestinal secretions, and increased flow of adrenalin. It can also cause a number of unpleasant feelings such as an inner feeling of terror, paleness, pounding heart, muscular tensions, dryness of the throat and mouth, sinking feeling in the stomach, nausea, vomiting, diarrhea, irritability, difficulty in breathing, sensations of faintness, loss of appetite, insomnia, and an urge to run and hide. Changes in external behavior may be reflected as a pattern of startle, withdrawal or avoidance, or fleeing. It can cause the individual to remain mute or motionless.

Fear may be divided into two types:[1–6]

- active or "real" fear = objective fear; and
- imagined or subjective fear.

*Objective* fear, or "real" fear, is that type of fear caused when a person is walking down a darkened street, and a large barking dog jumps out from behind the bushes. Immediately, a physiological chain reaction occurs, including an increase in the flow of adrenalin, muscle activity, and, the individual, without thought, takes flight. The heart rate has increased, breathing has increased, more sugar has been released into the blood stream, and all the necessary physiologic changes have occurred to preserve the integrity of the being.

*Subjective* or anticipated fear, the most common type of fear that affects most individuals, is the type of fear that Burton referred to back in 1621. The manifestations and feelings associated with it are unpleasant and do not disappear or resolve when the feared stimulus is removed, as in real objective fear. It afflicts individuals in varying degrees of intensity, and greatly influences their behavioral responses. For example, an individual might think that every time he or she visits the dentist, the dentist may slip and cut the tongue with the dental drill, or every time he or she rides in an automobile, he or she is at risk to hit the first telephone pole one encounters. When fear is learned as a response to a new situation, it is accompanied by a number of reactions that are either parts of the innate pattern of fear, or high in the innate hierarchy of response to fear. Fear can act as a cue to bring about responses that have previously been learned in other terrifying experiences, and can play a role in the development of varying degrees of anxiety, particularly affecting the outcome of dental care.

*Anxiety* is one of the most prevalent of all human emotions. It includes: (1) physical and mental awareness of being powerless; (2) presence of an impending threat; (3) a feeling of doom and danger that comes from within, the result of cognitive appraisal; and (4) an irresoluble doubt concerning the nature of the threat, the best means of reducing it, and one's subjective capacity to effectively utilize those means. How a person appraises a situation depends on two sets of factors: (1) those factors inherent in the stimulus object or event itself, and (2) interpersonal variables. With regard to the first, some individuals are conditioned to react negatively to dental care and the many facets associated with it. Second, one's ability to cope or manage a threatening situation governs the responses that will follow.

Both these factors are influenced by the individual's past history, personality, and ability to deal with threatening events. Fear is also differentiated from anxiety on the basis of one's ability to identify the threatening agent externally and to recognize the presence of behavior that will decrease or ameliorate the perceived danger. Anxiety can also be considered as an emotional state in which people feel uneasy, apprehensive, or fearful. People will often usually experience anxiety about events they cannot control or predict, or about events or situations they may consider threatening and harmful. There is a feeling of vulnerability, and severe anxiety can persist and eventually may even become disabling.

*Stress* is a word or term used to describe a change or disturbance in the psychophysiological equilibrium, and is most commonly associated with the response aspect. Stress is also a term most commonly used in association with the maladaptive aspects of response to the negative or aversive factors present.

All three—fear, anxiety, and stress—are negative or aversive states whose degree of severity of psycho-physiological symptoms is the result of the combination of the emotional response and the individual's appraisal of the threat at hand, which determine the degree and make-up of the behavior that will follow. For example, whether or not to keep the upcoming dental appointment, which most likely could or will involve receiving an injection and its accompanying pain. This behavior will also depend on the affect or influence within an individual who suffers from panic disorders, general anxiety, depression, and neuroticism. Persons with these disorders have been found to be associated with higher levels of dental fear, anxiety, and phobia.[7–9]

# MAJOR ETIOLOGICAL MODELS TO EXPLAIN ANXIETY[4–6,10–12,16]

Historically, three major etiological models have been postulated to explain anxiety, panic neurosis, and disorders:

- the psychological or psychosocial model;
- the behavioral model; and
- the biological model.

The *psychological* model considers anxiety the result of interplay between environmental stressors and internal conflicts, either past or present. The anxiety response is thought to be an action that attempts to adjust to the event or situation, to immobilize, ward off, and eventually avoid the anticipated overwhelming danger or threat. In the case of the dental visit, stress due to the thought of the associated pain, past experience, and encounter with the dental practitioner, weighted against the individual's need for dental care, sets up an inner conflict. The degree of past anxiety/fear experience often dictates the outcome by heightening the level of anxiety as the appointment nears, leading to avoidance.

The *behavioral* model holds that anxiety can occur even without conflict. Following the laws of learning theory, the anxiety response is believed to be acquired. It may take the form either as a classic conditioned response to trauma or stress, or as a demonstrable behavior that has been strengthened by operant conditioning, or both. These first two models are the two most associated with dental anxiety and dental phobia.

The *biological* model views anxiety and especially panic disorder as a genetic and/or metabolic disease that is similar to other metabolic disorders. Therefore, the fear/anxiety/panic manifested by patients at any given time during the cycle of visits may stem either from purely psychosocial/emotional factors or as the result of a medical disease process to which there is attached a genetic vulnerability, thought to be a chemical imbalance within the central nervous system.[9]

Anxiety bears two distinct components, *state* and *trait. State anxiety* is the individual's response to a specific object, event, or situation. It varies in intensity and fluctuates over time, increasing before dental treatment and decreasing afterwards. When anxiety occurs over a prolonged period and characterizes one aspect of the patient's everyday personality and behavior, it is called *trait anxiety*. It is part of the personality, involving the individual's predisposition to become anxious under a variety of circumstances. Patients who exhibit trait anxiety are also predisposed towards greater degrees of low pain threshold and pain intolerance. Corah in 1969 developed the Dental Anxiety Scale as a trait measure designed to assess a patient's tendencies to appraise a situation that might be dangerous and threatening such as dental treatment.[13] It is to this day still the most widely used scale to measure dental fear and anxiety. A recent study in the *British Dental Journal* by Fuentes and Gorenstein, examining the relationship between dental anxiety and trait anxiety, claimed that dental anxiety is specific and has its own features, and that its development is not necessarily associated with trait anxiety.[14,15]

As dental practitioners, we are interested in a patient's trait tendencies and how it affects the appraisal of a given situation that might be considered threatening, and its resulting effect on behavior and degree of sensitivity to pain and treatment. When those responses interfere with the ability to carry out everyday normal activities, such anxiety is said to be clinical, and the individual is usually referred for psychological intervention. When the patient is contemplating the aversive situation, and the current threat of pain, the practitioner can do much at this level to modify a patient's perception of anxiety. The more a practitioner can respond to a patient's current anxiety in a positive, compassionate and understanding manner, the less the patient is apt to consider the pain a threat. The practitioner's proficiency in history taking is the key to this. Methods on how to do this will be discussed in a following section.

The major difference between anxiety and fear is the immediacy of the etiological agent. For purposes of this discussion, the term fear is used to denote the emotional response of the individual within the dental office, reserving anxiety for those responses or reactions in anticipation of the dental visit.

# BEHAVIORAL INDICATORS OF ANXIETY[4,16–18]

Outward manifestations of anxiety can be noticed in an individual in one of two instances. First, the office receptionist can play an important role as the first member of the dental team, since he or she has the earliest opportunity to detect any possible signs of aversive and negative behavior in the reception area. Some of these patient behaviors may be *overtly visible*:

- heavy breathing;
- facial grimaces;
- pacing;
- frequent changes in sitting position;
- frequency of urination;
- excessive conversation;
- accelerated heat rate;
- sweating and moist palms;

- informing the dental practitioner of their fears; and
- knowledge of preexisting emotional disorders.

An awareness of and ability to recognize these behaviors in an individual permits office staff to speak with the patient and make an effort to determine the possible cause of these reactions. Gaining early knowledge of the causes permits both staff and practitioner to respond in a manner that might alleviate some doubts or anxieties about pending treatment. Such insight might also help determine whether the patient's anxiety stems from anticipation of treatment or from some other source, such as loss of employment, recent family tragedy, marriage problems, or a host of other factors. In addition, the presence of disorders such as depression, somatoform disorders, substance abuse, and posttraumatic stress disorder, all can affect the dental visit. Knowledge of these circumstances might persuade the practitioner to postpone the day's visit, allowing the patient to deal with the present calamity without the added stress of the dental visit. Such an action on the part of the dental practitioner allows the patient to see his or her practitioner as someone who has the capacity to be understanding and compassionate, as well as a fine dentist. The frequent use of self-reporting questionnaires can yield much information and aid in predicting a patient's levels of sensitivity to treatment, as well other anxiety-causing related events that might affect the dental visit.[13,19–25]

## Indirect indicators

Some overt behavior prior to dental treatment are symptomatic of anxiety over pending dental treatment. Taken individually, they may seem innocuous, but are obvious to the astute practitioner/staff. For example:

- frequent cancellations;
- frequent questioning;
- arriving late;
- multiple trips to the restroom;
- avoiding periodic check-ups;
- abnormal number of telephone calls;
- forgetting or missing appointments;
- multiple complaints;
- numerous different excuses; and
- unreasonable demands.

All these above actions are probably manifestations of anxiety/phobia to the dental situation. They may be the result of some personal past or present negative experience, or the result of some vicarious learning habits within the patient's environment. When they continuously appear in an individual's record, the practitioner must set aside a period of time to inquire about the cause of this behavior, and what can be done on the part of the practitioner/staff to ameliorate it. Understanding the root causes of such behavior allows the practitioner/staff to develop the means and behavioral modalities that will help assure treatment compliance and reduce existing stress on the part of all concerned. Sometimes, it may take only a brief explanation of upcoming procedures, a correction of false information, or the recognition of an underlying emotional disorder not yet successfully managed. Fear and anxiety is a multifaceted phenomenon, and the behaviors that practitioners and staff exhibit play an important role in a patient's levels of fear and avoidance of care.

## NATURE OF DENTAL ANXIETY

In order to identify and manage anxiety effectively, its nature must be clearly understood. Dental anxiety can be defined as a state of anxiety elicited by the provision of dental care. Anxiety is actually a multifaceted phenomenon that requires further analysis to guarantee its management. There are three characteristics essential in understanding dental anxiety: How fear and anxiety are manifested within the individual echelons of expression, timing, and severity.

(1) Echelons of expression;
   - biological;
   - psychological; and
     (a) association;
     (b) attribution; and
     (c) appraisal
   - sociological;
(2) timing; and
(3) severity.

## ECHELONS OF EXPRESSION

At the *biological* echelon, anxiety is closely related to those physiological processes that mediate arousal. These processes are governed by certain mechanisms and systems within the brain, especially those involving sub-cortical regions and their connections with the higher cortical areas. At this level, anxiety is manifested in numerous ways, which include sweating, muscle tension, increased heart rate, hyperventilation and fearful facial expressions.

At the *psychological* echelon, anxiety is the result of a learning process that involves three features:

(1) *Association* refers to a process of learning in which pain eventually becomes associated with dental treatment, so that the dental treatment

itself elicits a fearful/anxious reaction. This is a process of classic conditioning, whereby previously neutral stimuli (the needle, the sound of the drill, the sight of the instruments) become stimulants for arousal and anxiety through being paired with pain, one's own past experiences, or similar negative experiences of others.

(2)  *Attribution* is a process that occurs in response to a heightened biological arousal as discussed above. Here the patient must explain why such arousal has occurred, causing such unpleasant body symptoms and feelings. The individual may do so by attributing it to the fact that he or she is in the dental office, about to have a dental injection that is most likely to result in pain and discomfort. Therefore, the anxiety and accompanying unpleasant feelings must be due to this upcoming, potentially frightening experience.

(3)  *Appraisal* is the process by which we think about past dental care. It involves the reconstruction of negative experiences rather than positive happenings that account for the accrual of anxiety—the pain of the injection, the ouch of the drilling. It is that appraisal in the role of cognition and how we think that is a very important aspect of anxiety. Such a cognitive appraisal may result in cancellations and avoidance. These characteristics can begin to operate early in life, even before contact with dental treatment, through vicarious learning experiences with family or friends. Many times, a family history of negative dental experiences, or instances of poor direct care will produce significant dental anxiety and avoidance. Other contributing factors also include the following:

- Some people do not visit the dentist very often and therefore do not have the opportunity to learn a different response other than negative thoughts, pain, and anxiety.
- There is sometimes a failure on the part of the dental practitioner to share information concerning treatment, limiting the ability of the patient to have any false ideas or cognitions dispelled. The patient's knowledge frequently comes from his or her peers, who also may share negative associations about their dental experiences.
- Some individuals tend to remember the bad and negative experiences of dental treatment, often making it difficult to change memories and therefore modify aversive behavior.

Finally, it is also the process by which we think about past dental care, that sometimes causes us to form inaccurate or biased cognition about these past experiences, which then lead us to negative expectations about upcoming care. Such a cognitive appraisal may result in cancellations and avoidance. These characteristics can begin to operate early in life, even before direct contact with dental treatment, through vicarious learning experiences with family or friends. Often a family history of negative dental experiences, combined with a few instances of poor direct care, produce significant dental anxiety and avoidance. Psychological learning does not occur by itself; it has many root causes.

At the *sociological* echelon, anxiety is viewed as an outcome of interpersonal and social processes. For example, there is never a shortage of bad press concerning dentistry. One has only to pick up a newspaper or turn on the TV to see how often dentistry is at the core of a joke or portrayed as being painful and unpleasant. Although harmless by itself, this phenomenon demonstrates the generalized way in which dental anxiety is socially constructed. A less obvious example of the interpersonal process involves dental professionals themselves, in that they sometime unwittingly play a role in the development of dental anxiety through their behavior and attitude toward their patients. Anxious practitioners can create anxious patients, so the prevention of dental anxiety demands an awareness of one's own feelings, as well as those of the patient during treatment.

## TIMING OF DENTAL ANXIETY

The second characteristic associated with understanding the nature of anxiety is its timing. Frequently, dental anxiety is discussed only in term of its presence during treatment, but it also represents responses to situations that are sometimes somewhat vague, poorly defined and not immediately evident. This can be misleading because dental anxiety is often the result of a process that begins long before patients arrive in the reception room and continues long after they leave it. Therefore, the timing of dental anxiety can be also divided into three phases:

- pre-appointment;
- in-treatment phase; and
- posttreatment.

*Pre-appointment* anxiety refers to that anxiety that begins before the dental visit actually takes place. The thought and feelings of fear and anxiety are aroused within the individual in anticipation of the upcoming dental encounter. It is usually the most debilitating, since anxious patients often form inaccurate expectations about pain and discomfort before they receive treatment. During treatment, these evaluations do not differ from nonanxious patients, as both are capable of forming misconceptions of any facet of a visit. With this in mind, one can postulate that the identification and management of dental anxiety may need to occur before individuals begin treatment. Ideally, the collection of patient information should be an essential part of the initial appointment and history gathering. It should include past and present medical and dental history, both of the patient and patient's family. An early assessment of any problem behaviors or psychosocial factors should be sought. Specific questions can be asked, which can help identify the complex patient behaviors, such as obsessive compulsive disorders, somatoform disorders, and uncontrolled forms of depression. Some of this information can be found in the medical history of an individual. The amount, details, and worthiness of the information collected are directly proportional to the practitioner's skill in history taking, an important aspect in the success or failure of treatment.

*In-treatment* or current anxiety is anxiety that occurs in the dental office during treatment. It represents the current psychological and emotional state of the patient's thoughts and feelings, and the degree of negative behavior exhibited will be directly proportional to the degree of fear currently felt. For the dental practitioner, it is the easiest to treat and recognize. Such management, however, requires that patients be encouraged to express their anxiety and concerns early. The initial interview is an opportunity for patients to discuss any concerns they might have regarding current treatment, past experiences, concerns, fears, or anxieties that may have resulted from previous care. This information can be obtained through the use of questionnaires sent to patients prior to the initial visit. These questionnaires can serve as staring points in the collection of information, and will be discussed in detail in a subsequent section.

The practitioner should also inquire at the beginning of each of the subsequent visits, to see if prior concerns still exist and if the patient understands the procedure to be done this visit, with the purpose of alleviating any potential anticipatory anxiety due to a misunderstanding or erroneously interpreted information.

*Posttreatment* anxiety is that anxiety that occurs following treatment and, many times, after the patient has left the office. During this period, the patient makes a judgment, an appraisal, on whether or not the visit was painful, if the dentist responded to his or her emotional needs, if the anesthesia was effective, whether stated goals were achieved and whether the dentist and staff was caring. It is the fear/anxiety that results when the patient psychologically reconstructs and appraises the encounter. Without effective management, adequate explanations, and a demonstration of concern and empathy on the part of the practitioner, this appraisal can leave patients even more likely to be anxious about future care, bringing the whole process back full cycle to the before-treatment phase. Each time this cycle is completed without improvement, and without an effective method of understanding the patient's behavior and appropriately needed management, the greater is the chance for development of increased anxiety and initiation of continued avoidance.[5,6,16,18] The severity of a patient's anxiety and aversive behavior will always be directly proportional to the degree of initial fear experienced and the failure to use proper management techniques to lessen or ameliorate it.

## SEVERITY

The third characteristic associated with understanding the nature of dental fear/anxiety is the degree of severity the individual experiences in a given situation. The severity of a patient's behavioral response to treatment will always be at least equal to and sometimes greater than the degree of fear initially experienced.

## DIFFERENTIATING PSYCHOLOGICAL (EXOGENOUS) ANXIETY FROM MEDICAL (ENDOGENOUS) ANXIETY

It has been suggested in a number of recent and past studies that dentally anxious individuals are not a homogeneous group of patients.[26–31] In 1988 and 1990, Weiner and Sheehan suggested that we alter the current accepted view of anxiety-panic disorders as a single continuum of traumatically conditioned experiences and instead classify them into two separate clinical entities for purposes of patient management. This revised classification would divide anxiety and phobic disorders into two major groups, an exogenous (psychological) group and an endogenous (medical) group, according to the etiology of their symptom.[28–31] Within this system of two distinct entities, some individuals are thought to develop dental fear through aversive conditioning experiences (exogenous), while others appear to demonstrate a biological vulnerability to developing anxiety/ phobic disorders, such as panic disorders or dental phobia, potentiating their receptiveness to acquire multiphobic symptoms, including dental anxiety (endogenous). The importance of this distinction is that at any give time, a practitioner might have two individuals in the reception area, each professing to being dental phobic. Each may have similar symptoms, but different etiology. Failure to differentiate properly between the two could result in mismanagement, lack of proper treatment, and failure to identify a possible medical disorder requiring specialized care.

The *exogenous* group displays situation-related, anticipatory anxiety symptoms, such as moist palms, fluttery stomach, fine hand tremors, warm all-over feeling, shaky inside, and rapid heartbeat. These are symptoms seen when individuals are normally stressed or threatened. The etiology of the symptoms is found in the external environment. The degree to which an individual manifests fear and anxiety symptoms can be equated to the degree of stress felt in the initial encounter. When an individual is repeatedly stressed or harmed in a particular situation, the individual will often become conditioned to be fearful and anxious each time he or she is exposed to that situation. This form of anxiety or phobia is a normal reaction to stress occurring outside the confines of the body, and is termed exogenous anxiety.

The second or *endogenous* group, which is *nonsituation*-related, is characterized by a more severe cluster of symptoms that include lightheadedness, dizziness, difficulty in breathing, paraesthesia, hyperventilation, lump in the throat, chest pains, and varying or continuous levels of anxiety. This set of anxious or phobic symptoms appears related to some underlying core metabolic–biochemical disturbance within the central nervous system, to which there appears to be attached a genetic vulnerability. Due to the wide range of symptoms, an endogenous anxiety disorder is a great mimic of other illnesses. In endogenous anxiety-phobic disorders, the patient has attacks of anxiety that occur spontaneously, unexpectedly, and without provocation. The abruptness of these symptoms and the fact that they present themselves without warning or in the presence of any detectable stress, situation, or object, sets this form of anxiety clearly apart from the otherwise normal response to threat. The etiological factor responsible for the symptoms comes from within the individual's body—hence the term *endogenous*.

It is *not* a response to a situation-experienced stress event, but rather a disease process that does not respond alone to rest, relaxation, and behavior modification techniques. If stress were the major etiologic factor, one would find the age of onset of this disorder evenly distributed through all age groups, since stress affects all age groups and sexes evenly, but it is a random occurrence. With endogenous anxiety, one finds the onset of age of symptoms, in the majority of cases, in the late teens and early 20s. Such an age of onset distribution is a characteristic of a biological illness that permits a disease to favor one age group or sex over another. Approximately 75% of those afflicted are female.[32] In the natural history of the endogenous disorder, these unexpected attacks may later be complicated by limited or extensive phobic avoidance behavior.

# NATURAL HISTORY OF ENDOGENOUS ANXIETY[26–28,31,33–35]

This disorder, like many other medical disease processes, has a distinct pattern of symptom development that carries it from the mild phase of the disorder through to the very severe phase, which for the patient ends in almost complete avoidance of every situation or encounter. The patient almost always ends up housebound and withdrawn.

## Explanation of stages of disorder

### Stage I—Subpanic attack spells

The individual has a brief feeling of lightheadedness and/or dizziness, difficulty in breathing or floating sensation. The episodes are short lived and do not interfere with function. The individual cannot explain the feelings, but merely senses that some part of the body is racing out of control, briefly and often in the absence of marked cognitive anxiety. At this stage of the disorder, everyday psychosocial activities are not affected.

## Stage II—Polysymptomatic panic attacks

The spontaneous unexplained episodes increase in frequency and in the number of symptoms in the cluster. Spontaneous anxiety/panic attacks are clusters of many spells of a variety of symptoms occurring at once. The individual further feels the body racing out of control to a greater extent. These attacks are accompanied by mental panic and often associated with a flight response. At this stage, the patient begins to think of seeking medical advice and help.

## Stage III—Somatic overconcern (hypochondriasis)

In this stage of the disorder, the patient, after repeated and worsening spontaneous attacks, begins to seek medical help, usually choosing a physician who specializes in the most prominent symptom in the set of symptoms (e.g., lump in throat—ENT; chest pains—a cardiologist; difficulty in breathing—lung specialist). When the examinations reveal no abnormality, patients turn to a different specialist, but each time the examinations reveal no abnormalities. As each of the following examinations continues to prove negative, individuals may begin to think they are losing their mind and become preoccupied with their health and the seeking of specialized professional help. The patient begins to be treated as a hypochondriacal, hysterical person responding abnormally to everyday stress.

## Stage IV—Limited phobic avoidance

The panic attack and severe body symptoms are associated with the situation in which the attack occurs (e.g., shopping market, dental office, department store). Due to the severity of the attack, the individual associates the place as the source of anxiety and seeks relief by fleeing. This then begins a pattern of avoidance behavior. When relief occurs after fleeing, because these attacks only last between 2 and 30 min, this reinforces the association between the situation and the accompanying fear, and reinforces the phobia.

## Stage V—Social phobias

If the attacks persist or increase in intensity and frequency, the patient often progresses to a stage of social phobias. The patient avoids any of the many social events he or she may associate with a previous attack. In many cases, the individual now fears the symptoms more than the activity or place. By now, they have most probably developed the "what if it happens here" attitude: What if I go to the dentist, and "he or she may slip and cut my tongue, or the needle breaks, or I get into an accident on the way to the office?"

## Stage VI—Agoraphobia and polyphobic behavior

With the continuing increase in number and severity of attacks, the patient acquires numerous phobias. At this stage, the patient often becomes housebound and fears almost everything, and is considered to be exhibiting "agoraphobic" behavior, or fear of the marketplace and outside environment.

## Stage VII—Secondary depression

Inability to find a cause or relief from these symptom attacks, combined with the phobic restrictions and the inability to meet everyday demands, leads to pessimism and a secondary demoralization and depression. The individual becomes extremely dependent on a friend or a family member.

One must understand how the biological case of the endogenous disorder leads to the subsequent development of learned phobic avoidance. Endogenous anxiety/panic disorders and their associated symptoms reflect the core biochemical disturbance in the central nervous system. As the disorder progresses, extraneous situations in the environment also acquire by association the ability to bring on a panic attack as in Pavlovian or clinical conditioning.[4,6,18,36,37] At any stage in the course of the disorder, the spontaneous symptom attacks may cease, but the avoidance behavior and phobias can remain. They can continue to be nourished through other psychological mechanisms. For example, recalling a prior frightening panic attack, while seated in the dental reception room, may evoke anxiety anticipatory to this extraneous situation, which developed as a result of its association to the original attack. The anxiety symptoms and phobia (dental, in this case) are initially triggered and nourished from within by the core biochemical disturbance, and further reinforced from outside by various environmental factors. Eventually, the spontaneous symptom attacks may abate or make up only a relatively small part of the overall picture. The majority of the symptoms are of the anticipatory type. Individuals who fear leaving the home or driving cannot get to the dental office. If as explained above, a spontaneous attack occurred in the dental office, anticipatory anxiety will reinforce avoidance of the dental encounter. The patient is a dental phobic—but a phobic secondary to a medical illness process and not a prior traumatic or prior external negative experience (see Table 1.1).

Understanding the differentiation between these two subtypes of anxiety/panic is crucial in determining the proper treatment modalities these two distinct subtypes require. Keeping these principles in mind, it becomes important to see how they might apply to this particular example of a possible future scenario within the dental office. A practitioner may

**Table 1.1**  Diagnostic criteria of endogenous and nonendogenous anxiety[4,30,31,34,35]

| Anxiety disorder | Symptoms | Pattern of attacks |
|---|---|---|
| Endogenous anxiety | Spontaneous, autonomous, clonic, phasic episodes of the following (one or two in the case of a minor attack, three or more in a major attack). | Minimum duration: Symptom attack must persistently recur over a period of at least 1 month |
| | Skipping or racing heart<br>Dizzy spells or faintness<br>Difficulty getting a breath<br>Hyperventilation<br>Choking sensation<br>Tingling or numbness<br>Nausea or vomiting<br>Sudden unexpected panic or anxiety feelings that occur with little or no provocation<br>Hot flushes or cold chills<br>Shaking or trembling<br>Derealization or depersonalization<br>Chest pain, pressure or discomfort<br>Feeling of losing control<br>Skipping or racing heart<br>Dizzy spells or faintness<br>Difficulty getting a breath | Frequency: Within a 3-month period, there must be at least three discrete major or minor attacks for a diagnosis of major or minor endogenous anxiety respectively.<br><br>Attacks must occur in the absence of any psychotic disorder or medical illness or life-threatening danger that could explain the symptom. |
| | Hyperventilation<br>Choking sensation<br>Tingling or numbness<br>Nausea or vomiting<br>Sudden unexpected panic or anxiety feelings that occur with little or no provocation<br>Hot flushes or cold chills | |
| | Shaking or trembling<br>Derealization or depersonalization<br>Chest pain, pressure or discomfort<br>Feeling of losing control<br>Hypochondriasis<br>Bouts of diarrhea<br>Sweating episodes | |
| Nonendogenous | No spontaneous panic or anxiety attacks or history of the same<br>Tension and symptoms of anxiety occur in response to immediate clear-cut, identifiable environmental special stimuli | The onset of each attack is neither very sudden nor of the unexpected; it is related to the immediacy of a triggering stimulus. In the case of symptoms involving motor function sensory perception, or senses, the symptom may occur along, with no overt anxiety. |

Source: Weiner A and Sheehan D. 1988. Differentiating anxiety-panic disorders from psychologic dental anxiety. *Dent Clin North Am* 32(4):823–40. Reprinted with permission from Elsevier Publishing. All rights reserved.

have two individuals in the reception area, each professing to be severely anxious and phobic, and at times engulfed with sheer panic. After an initial interview, the practitioner determines that each of the individuals actually differ and required a different mode of treatment. The individual who claims that past dental trauma and negative attitude of a past practitioner are responsible for current behavior requires behavioral modalities. These could include some form of conscious inhalation or IV therapy, as well as applicable behavioral modalities combined with a complete review and evaluation of past and present medical/dental history. Clues obtained from a patient's history may provide additional information, which could be valuable in determining the correct behavioral modality needed to ensure treatment compliance. The patient's history may reveal hidden emotional disorders, or goals that are unreasonable and require outside psychological intervention before dental care. Certain fears individuals harbor that occur outside of the dental setting in the external environment, may also cause disruptive behavior and avoidance of dentistry. For example, the aquaphobic who fears water, might fear the water spray, or the claustrophobic, the rubber dam. Knowing that these items are associated with dental treatment might cause these individuals to avoid care. Having this knowledge permits the practitioner to devise a strategy to help the patient overcome the fear of this part of dental treatment.

The second individual who also claims to be severely anxious and phobic, but cannot recall any negative thought or actual occurrence of prior trauma or excessive pain, has a different etiology. This patient, upon questioning, states that he or she experiences unexplained, out of the blue, episodes of spontaneous attacks of anxiety and panic. Past history shows that such episodes occur frequently, and that one such attack previously occurred in a dental office. The patient claimed that the symptoms and feelings were quite terrible, and not being able to fully explain them assumed that anticipation of the dental visit was the responsible factor, thus leading to avoidance and fear of a further dental encounter. In this patient, the discriminating diagnostic factor is a history of unexplained, spontaneous attacks, and an inability to attach a precise cause to the fear and anxiety that engulfs him or her. To attempt to treat this patient without realizing the emotional, psychiatric, and medical aspects of this disease process would only result in frustration on the part of the dental practitioner, and unexplained multiple broken appointments, all due to this undiagnosed endogenous panic disorder.

Diagnosis and differentiation are limited to clinical observation and questioning. To date, no specific laboratory test exists. The discriminating diagnostic factor remains the presence or absence of spontaneous attacks of anxiety/phobia symptoms that occur without provocation or expectation at any time and in the absence of any visible etiologic agent. When symptoms of a possible endogenous anxiety disorder are recognized by a dental practitioner, psychiatric intervention must be sought. To do otherwise would result in frustration and an inability to perform dental treatment, not to mention the fact that a medical condition is not being referred for proper care. It may be necessary and proper to confer with the individual's primary care physician to present your findings, permitting him or her to make the suggestion of referral to a psychiatrist for specialized intervention.

## Case example 1

A young female of 28 years of age was referred from a local nursing service. The young woman, a registered nurse, was increasingly avoiding her duties with numerous excuses. Her supervisor was increasingly concerned, especially since she complained of a severe toothache as her last excuse. On examination, the young woman confessed she did not have a toothache, but rather suffered from severe attacks of panic, which caused her to flee from wherever she was at that moment. They occurred without reason at different times, and she was fearful that something was terribly wrong with her. She dreaded that such an attack might occur while attending a patient, or in front of her colleagues, causing her embarrassment and perhaps loss of her job. Her medical history was uneventful, and visits to her physicians produced no medical reasons for her panic attacks.

It was explained to her that there was a possibility that she might have some sort of chemical imbalance within her central nervous system that often was associated with panic symptoms like she was feeling. She was referred to the Psychosomatic Medicine Clinic of Massachusetts General Hospital for diagnosis and treatment. She was treated with Nardil (phenelzine antidepressant),[38–40] an MAOI inhibitor, a past drug of choice, and, after a period of time, with behavior modification. I was notified that she had been diagnosed as having an endogenous panic disorder characterized by spontaneous attacks of anxiety that occurred without reason or cause, and that her panic symptoms had abated. She was able to return to a very normal routine existence. Although this disorder mainly affects woman, we have seen cases involving men at the Tufts University Dental Clinic.

## Case example 2

This individual, a 42-year-old white male, was a registered pharmacist who was employed in a local hospital. On inquiring into his reasons for lack of dental care, he stated he found it impossible to travel into Boston proper, because every time he seemed to stray from home, he developed panic attacks that always came "out of nowhere," especially when he traveled over the main bridge into Boston or through the tunnel that led into the city. He also complained of these severe panic attacks, which began some 12 years ago and would occur at any time of the day. He stated he had sought treatment from his physician, had been given a variety of tranquilizers, and had even seen a psychologist, but nothing had helped. He feared losing employment every time he had to make up some excuse for not coming to work. His dentition showed a number of teeth badly decayed, with signs of poor oral home care habits.

He was asked to reply to a written fear/anxiety questionnaire routinely used at Tufts for those individuals who during initial consult, expressed some concerns regarding dental treatment. When completed, it was noted that almost every response was either a 4 or 5 on a Likert scale of 1–5, with 4 representing severely fearful and 5 total avoidance. When asked whether or not he still experienced spontaneous attacks of anxiety that appeared out of the blue, without any obvious cause, he answered an emphatic "yes." He also explained that these attacks appeared more frequently and severely the older he got. It was suggested that he might be suffering from a possible chemical imbalance within his central nervous system, which might be the cause of the symptoms, and that they might respond to certain specific medications. He was provided with some reading material and referred to the Psychosomatic Medicine Clinic at Massachusetts General Hospital for diagnosis and treatment by a psychiatrist. He was assured that he was not losing his mind, and that the reason for a psychiatric referral was that a psychiatrist was the best qualified and most knowledgeable physician to treat this particular disorder. It is extremely important to reassure the individual that this referral to a psychiatrist is like any other medical referral and in no way means that the individual is suffering from some mental disorder. There has always been some sort of social stigma attached to seeing a psychiatrist that can cause patients to avoid seeking help.

The individual was seen 1 month after beginning treatment, and he stated it was the first time he could remember having a whole day free of anxiety. He was being treated with and SSRI,[41–44] and some behavioral desensitizing modalities. As time passed, his panic attacks subsided, and he was able to lead as he described "a normal life," including completing needed dental care.

These examples must serve as reminders that fear and avoidance of dental care is not rooted just in prior trauma, negative vicarious learning habits, or fear of pain, but is rather the result of many varied factors, components and causes, some of which in the beginning have nothing to do with dentistry. It is for this reason that the student, practicing dentist, hygienist, and clinical researchers must conduct detailed initial examination and consultations to make sure they gain both the medical and psychological information needed to ensure treatment success.

# PHOBIAS[1,2,5–7,16–18,45–48]

Phobias are a particular kind of fear. The term derives from the word "phobos," which in Greek refers to flight, terror, and the deity of the same name who could provoke panic and fear in one's enemies. A phobia can be defined as "a morbid fear out of proportion to the apparent stimulus, fear which is inappropriate and unreasoning." In 1962, Errera[46] defined it as "a persisting fear of an object, situation or idea which does not ordinarily justify fear."

A phobia[1,2,] may also be defined as an irrational fear of a particular object or situation. The Diagnostic and Statistical Manual of Mental Disorders (DSM-III and IV)[33–35] describes it "as a marked and persistent fear that is excessive and unreasonable." It is a specific fear triggered by a stimulus that is disproportionately small, compared with the severity of the reaction. Phobic disorders are variants of anxiety disorders in which the phobia predominates. Phobias cannot be explained or reasoned away; they are beyond voluntary control and eventually leads to total avoidance of the feared stimulus. A phobia can become so intense that it becomes an unreasonable morbid fear producing severe physiologic reactions that interfere with everyday functions. Phobias can cause individuals to manifest shame and helplessness, and to become chronic avoiders, constantly making up excuses such as not feeling well, or my "car is not working," in order to help them avoid an anticipated encounter with their feared stimulus. Phobic individuals are usually aware that their fear is unrealistic compared with the reactions of others to the same object.

Almost all phobias are learned. They develop over a period of time as acts of avoidance, as a release valve, *protecting* the individual from their feared stimulus, and, of greater importance, protecting them from the very unpleasant body feelings that are associated with them. They often manifest shame of their fear symptoms to avoid ridicule. Phobias involve three components: (1) a subjective inner state felt by the individuals, (2) the outer aspect seen by others, and (3) the accompanying autonomic physiological symptoms associated with these phobias. When there is a sudden, overwhelming surge of these symptoms, individuals often refer this sudden change as a *panic* attack.

In phobia, the origin of the fear may sometimes be obscure and stem from childhood. The strong fear involved in phobias can sometimes be expected to transfer to new cues in a number of ways. One example is known as *stimulus association*.[17] When an individual learns to fear a particular situation, he or she tends to fear similar ones. Stimuli similar to the original traumatic one may elicit a much stronger fear response called a "gradient of generalization." If the initial stimulus is sufficiently terrifying, such as a needle breaking or causing excessive bleeding during a vaccination in the arm, the individual may develop a morbid fear to all kinds of injections, especially one within the oral cavity.

## CAUSES OF PHOBIAS[1,2,6,9,11,12,37,45–48]

(1)   According to Burton,[1] phobias are usually the result of a social inheritance, some member of the family possessing the phobia and passing

it along from generation to generation. For example, Kleinknecht, Klepac, and Alexander noted in 1978 that the negative and aversive attitudes exhibited by some individuals toward dental treatment were actually derived from the negative attitudes of others—a result of social learning.

(2)   *Prior traumatic experience*: In 1971, Lautch[46] demonstrated that prior dental trauma and length of duration of pain were the prime etiological factors in the development of severe dental phobia.

(3)   *Vicarious learning*: People sometimes observe the actions of others and tend to mimic and adapt the behavior learned from the experience of others, a process known as vicarious learning. Unintentional or informal observation often reveals that fears and phobias may be acquired by someone who observes the pain and fear reactions in another person confronting an aversive stimulus, such as receiving a dental injection or undergoing an extraction of a tooth. In 1962, Berger[36] demonstrated that in experiments of vicarious classical conditioning, one individual (the Observer) witnessing another (the Model) undergoing an aversive conditioning procedure (e.g., drilling a tooth) will also begin to show emotional responses to the conditioned stimulus (drilling) alone, even without having experienced the *un*conditioned stimulus directly. This is a clear demonstration of classic vicarious learning. Modeling is a technique used by pedodontists to help children overcome their fear of dental treatment, and is an extremely important and valuable tool in overcoming and managing childhood fears. This may have important bearing on whether or not a parent or another sibling should be present in the dental operatory without first having knowledge of the behavior of the one who would be the model. Anxious parents have been known to exert aversive and negative influence on a child's behavior within the treatment room. On the other hand, Bandura,[49] back in 1967, postulated that modeling not only could be responsible for the acquisition of new aversive behaviors, but could also have an opposite effect, causing individuals to be relieved to know they are not the only ones affected by the same fear, thereby lessening their adverse own interpretation of how bad their own experience really is.

(4)   Cultural, gender, age and economic influences

- *Culture*: Great differences exist among different cultures and societies. These differences are greatly responsible for the variation in responses and development of varying degrees of phobias, especially to dental treatment. What is accepted in one culture may not be in another. With regards to dentistry, the many different expressions of fear by different cultures are seen in their different, behaviors, emotions, attitudes, and response to fear related stimuli, as well as to certain methods of dental care, as reported by Kiyak and by Lipton and Marback.[50,51] Some groups go about to dramatizing their responses to treatment with a variety of body movements and degrees of more vocalizations, while others tend to be stoic and complain less. Earlier studies noting these variations and responses have for the most part endured, including two such studies, one by Zola,[53] that found that different cultures seem to apply different grades of approval when it comes to responding to fear and fear-related events, while Zborowski,[54] arranged the behavioral responses to fear related treatment into five different groups: (1) bodily movement, (2) vocal responses, (3) verbal responses, (4) social responses, and (5) the absence of any response.

- *Gender* also has been found to affect the response to fear of dental treatment, as well as the response to and acceptance of often needed specialized care. In a study by Liddell and Locker,[52] women seemed to demonstrate less acceptance of discomfort, responding to it more negatively than males, as well as a desire to maintain greater control during the dental visit. My own experience has shown that a greater percentage of males versus females often presented higher levels of negative behavior to fear of treatment discomfort, which seemingly differs slightly with this study. This is purely my own clinical observation and may be reflective of the type of dental practice which by reputation was almost entirely composed of the fearful, phobic individuals.

- *Socioeconomic* factors also often play a role in predicting the response to fear and anxiety of treatment. Those on the lower economical scale tend to be unable to seek care as frequently as the well-to-do, the result often being higher decay rates, diminished opportunities to receive restorative procedures, failure to learn the positive aspects of treatment, and greater numbers of tooth extractions. In consequence, according to Riley, Gilbert, and Heft,[55] they have greater fear-related experiences, and higher levels of avoidance, than those in the higher socioeconomic scale. Pau et al suggested in 2003 that the combination of age and economic status played a role in the degree of fear and associated negative behaviors accompanying treatment. He concluded that younger and less socioeconomically advantaged individuals responded more strongly, both verbally and behaviorally, to both fear of treatment due to lack of regular attendance, and had a lessened ability to learn the positive side of treatment, demonstrating a greater degree of avoidance than those individuals who were older and more economically advantaged.[56]

A person's fear and emotional–behavioral response to treatment may result from a combination of any or all of the factors above, modified by whatever particular cultural and social influences are in play. While different factors may be present in different ethnic groups, affecting the response to the fear of treatment, little difference exists in their description of those responses and attitudes to that unpleasant sensation of discomfort. On the other hand, gender, age, and ethnic background of the office staff can play a role in a patient's response to treatment, including response to pain.

In a further study, Riley et al.[57] noted that patients' attitudes about past experiences, age, and their inability sometimes to communicate their perceptions and concerns to their dentist, often results in their receiving less care and being at greater risk for dental disease. Again, the response to fear sometimes tends to run in families, while cultural influences can affect the popularity of certain reported phobias. For example, in earlier years, Western societies feared witches, demons, and sorcery. Today, common fears are heart disease, cancer, flying, or atomic war.

It is for all of these reasons that it becomes essential that practitioners know as much as possible about their patients' past, including not just medical, dental, and psychological histories, experiences, but social and cultural influences, parental influences, and much more. Many phobias have remained unchanged throughout the ages, despite the many advances in science and technology, dentistry being one of them.

Dental phobia is essentially the same as severe ordinary fear, only it is expressed and felt much stronger by some people who usually know what will happen when he or she goes to the dentist or encounters their phobic stimulus and remembers past experiences. If those are negative, patients can become so terrified as actually to feel unwell just from the thought of a recurrence. To avoid the terrible feelings and symptoms often felt, self-control takes over, and an appointment is missed.

This often leaves practitioners bewildered and frustrated. In my own experience over the years, the simple and truthful answer to why the individual continue to miss appointments may lie in the practitioner's failure to take the extra initial time to secure a complete past and present medical, psychological, social, and dental history, which might reveal why the patient is fearful. Unfortunately, a simple missed piece of information might be the missing link that would enable a practitioner to devise a method that would help the patient develop a coping strategy to deal with their high level of fear. In taking a thorough history, the practitioner helps to lessen and remove the barriers to treatment, as well as helping to build a trusting and a positive patient–dentist relationship.

## SUMMARY

In today's practice of dentistry, many of the efforts that are directed toward the lessening and amelioration of dental fear center around procedures and modalities that assume that dental treatment and its component parts are the cause of fear and anxiety. In fact, fear and anxiety have many faces and occur differently for different individuals. We live in a complex and multifaceted world where a multitude of variables exist, and their interplay contribute to the different levels of anxiety and fear each of us experiences at different times and in different situations. Many of these variables have no direct relationship to dental care, but nevertheless, they can directly affect the dental visit. An example of this is the endogenous cluster of body and psychological symptoms in agoraphobia disorder that are the result of a chemical imbalance within the central nervous system. These individuals do not respond to the accepted behavioral modalities available to practitioners, first, because of failure of recognition on the part of the dental practitioner, and, second, because such patients need a totally different approach and care unfamiliar to the practitioner. Hence, they should be referred to a medical specialist (psychiatrist) for specific psychopharmacological intervention and behavioral training.

The advent of the behavioral sciences in the past three to four decades in the fields of medicine and dentistry has brought with it new insights and perceptions regarding the emotions of fear and anxiety. This has resulted in the formation of newer and simpler modalities designed to lessen and or ameliorate fear.

Practitioners at all levels must make sure that complete past and present medical, dental, and psychological histories become an essential component of the examination process. Many patients bring with them some form of an emotional disorder or negatively learned cognitions and their associated behavior. These are often hidden, but at some time during the treatment phase, surface and can directly affect treatment. With proper diagnosis and specific management plans, which may need to involve both behavioral and psychopharmacological modalities, patients can be helped to overcome their fears, especially the fear of dentistry.

## NOTE

Portions of this chapter is reprinted from *Quintessence International Digest* (1980), 11(9):119–23 and (1982), 13(9):981–986, with both the permission of the publisher and copyright holder, Quintessence Publishing Co. Hanover Park, IL, and of the author, Arthur Weiner.

## REFERENCES

1. Burton R. 1969. Chapter 1. In: Marks IM (ed.), *Fears and Phobias*, Vol. 5. New York: Academic Press, pp. 1–4.
2. Weiner AA. 1980. The basic principles of fear, anxiety and phobia as they relate to the dental visit. *Quintessence Int Dent Dig* 9:119–23.
3. Weiner AA. 1980. The theory and management of anxiety and phobic disorders as they relate to the dental visit. *Quintessence Int Dent Dig* 3(2):5–13.

4.  Weiner AA. 1994. *The Difficult Patient: A Guide to Understanding and Managing Dental Anxiety*, 3rd edn. Randolph, MA: Reniew Publications Co.
5.  1Eli I. 1992. *Oral Psychophysiology: Stress, Pain, and Behavior in Dental Care*. Boca Raton, FL: CRC Press.
6.  Mostofsky DI, Forgione AG, and Giddon DB. 2006. *Behavioral Dentistry*, Vol. 1, 1st edn. Oxford, UK: Blackwell-Munksgaard.
7.  Berggren U and Meynert MG. 1984. Dental fear and avoidance: Causes, symptoms and consequences. *J Am Dent Assoc* 109:247.
8.  Schuurs A, Duivenvooden H, Kakkes P, et al. 1988. Personality traits of persons suffering from extreme dental anxiety. *Community Dent Oral Epidemiol* 16:38.
9.  Sheehan DV. 1982. Panic attacks and phobias. *N Engl J Med* 308:156–8.
10. Locker D and Lidell A. 1991. Correlates of dental anxiety among older adults. *J Dent Res* 70:198.
11. Kleinknecht RA and Bernstein BD. 1978. Assessment of dental fears. *Behav Ther* 9(6):626–34.
12. Bernstein DA, Kleinknecht RA, and Alexander LD. 1979. Antecedents of dental fear. *J Public Health Dent* 39:113–24.
13. Corah NL. 1969. Development of a dental anxiety scale. *J Dent Res* 48(4):596.
14. Fuentes D, Gorenstein C, and Hu LW. 2009. Dental anxiety and trait anxiety: An investigation of their relationship. *Br Dent J* 10:253.
15. Tullman GM, Tullman MJ, and Rigers BJ. 1979. Anxiety in dental patients: A study of three phases of state anxiety in three groups. *Psychol Rep* 45:497.
16. Dworkin SF, Ferrence TP, and Giddon DB. 1978. *Behavioral Science in Dental Practice*, Vol. 1. St. Louis, MO: CV Mosby.
17. Miller N and Dollard J. 1950. *Personality and Psychotherapy*, Vol. 1, 1st edn. New York: McGraw-Hill, pp. 76–84, 161.
18. Milgrom P, Weinatein P, Kleinknecht R, et al. 1995. *Treating Fearful Dental Patients: A Patient Management Handbook*, 2nd edn. Seattle: University of Washington.
19. Heaton LJ, Carlson CR, and Smith TA. 2007. Predicting anxiety during treatment using patients' self reports. *J Am Dent Assoc* 138:168–95.
20. Corah N, Ziel MA, and O'Shea RM. 1986. Development of an interval scale of anxiety. *Anesth Prog* 33:220–4.
21. Daily YM, Humphris GN, and Lennon MA. 2001. The use of dental anxiety questionnaires: A survey of a group of UK dental practitioners. *Br Dent J* 190(8):450–3.
22. Klages U, Kianifard S, Ulusoy O, et al. 2006. Anxiety sensitivity as a predictor of pain in patients undergoing resorative dental procedures. *Community Dent Oral Epidemiol* 34:139–45.
23. Klages U, Sadjadi Z, Rust G, et al. 2008. Development of a questionnaire measuring treatment concerns in regular dental patients. *Community Dent Oral Epidemiol* 36:219–27.

24. Zvolensky MJ, Eifert GH, and Lejuez CW. 2000. Assessing the perceived predictability of anxiety related events: A report on the predictability index. *Behav Res Ther* 31:201–18.

25. Weiner AA. 1988. Dental anxiety: An efficient means of identification. *J Amer Analg Soc* 22(2):14–7.

26. Sheehan DV and Sheehan KH. 1982. The classification of anxiety and hysterical disorders. Part I: A historical review and empirical delineation. *J Clin Psychopharmacol* 2:235–44.

27. Sheehan DV and Sheehan KH. 1982. The classification of anxiety and hysterical states. Part II: Towards a more heuristic classification. *J Clin Psychopharmacol* 2:386–93.

28. Sheehan DV and Sheehan KH. 1982. The classification of phobic disorders. *Int J Psychiatr Med* 12:243–66.

29. Lidell A and Grosse V. 1998. Characteristic of early unpleasant dental experiences. *J Behav Ther Exp Psychiatry* 29:227–37.

30. Roy-Byrne P, Milgrom P, Tay K-M, et al. 1994. Psychopathology and psychiatric diagnosis in subjects with dental phobia. *J Anxiety Disord* 8:19–31.

31. Weiner AA and Sheehan DV. 1988. Differentiating anxiety-panic disorders from psychological dental anxiety. *Dent Clin North Am* 32(4): 823–40.

32. Crow R. 1985. The genetics of panic disorder and agoraphobia. *Psychiatr Development* 2:171–86.

33. American Psychiatric Association Task Force on Nomenclature and Statistics, American Psychiatric Association. Committee on Nomenclature and Statistics. 1980. *Diagnostic and Statistical Manual of Mental Disorders*, 3rd edn. Washington, DC: American Psychiatric Association.

34. American Psychiatric Association. 1987. *Diagnostic Criteria from DSM-III-R*. Washington, DC: American Psychiatric Association.

35. American Psychiatric Association. 2004. *Diagnostic and Statistical Manual of Mental Disorders: DSM-IVTR Guide Book*, 4th edn., text rev. Washington, DC: American Psychiatric Association, pp. 231–4.

36. Berger SM. 1962. Conditioning through vicarious instigation. *Psychol Rev* 69:450–66.

37. Berggren U and Meynert G. 1984. Dental fear and avoidance: Causes, symptoms and consequences. *J Am Dent Assoc* 109:247.

38. Sheehan DV, Ballenger J, and Jaconson G. 1980. Treatment of endogenous anxiety with phobic, hysterical and hypo-chondriacal symptoms. *Arch Gen Psychiatry* 37(1): 51–9.

39. Sheehan DV. 1984. Delineation of anxiety and phobic disorders responsive to monoamine oxidase inhibitors: Implications for classification. *J Clin Psychiatry* 45(7 Pt 2):29–36.

40. Sheehan DV. 1985. Monoamine oxidase inhibitors and alprazolam in the treatment of panic disorder and agoraphobia. *Psychiatr Clin North Am* 8(1):49–62.

41. Ashok R and Sheehan DV. 1999. The use of selective serotonin reuptake inhibitors in panic disorder. *Home Health Care Consultant* 6(4):15–9.
42. Sheehan DV, Harnett-Sheehan K, and Raj BA. 1996. The role of SSRIs in panic disorders. *J Clin Psychiatry* 57(10 Suppl Rev):51 (discussion), 59–60 (review).
43. Barlow DH. 2002. *Anxiety and Its Disorders: The Nature and Treatment of Anxiety and Panic.* New York: Guilford Press.
44. Sheehan DV. 1999. Current concepts in the treatment of panic disorder. *J Clin Psychiatry* 60(Suppl 18):16–1.
45. Laughlin HP. 1956. *The Neuroses in Clinical Practice.* Philadelphia, PA: Saunders.
46. Lautch H. 1971. Dental phobia. *Br J Psychiatry* 119:151.
47. Errera P. 1962. Some historical aspects of the concepts of phobias. *Psychiatr Q* 36:325–36.
48. Beck T and Emery G. 1985. *Anxiety Disorders and Phobia.* New York: Basic Books.
49. Bandura A, Grus J, and Menlove FL. 1967. Vicarious extinction of avoidance behavior. *J Pers Soc Psychol* 5:16–23.
50. Kiyak HA. 1981. Dental beliefs behaviors and health status among Pacific Asians and Caucasians. *Community Dent Oral Epidemiol* 9:10–3.
51. Lipton JA and Marback JJ. 1984. Ethnicity and the pain experience. *Soc Sci Med* 19:1279–98.
52. Liddell A and Locker D. 1997. Gender and age difference in attitude to pain and dental control. *Community Dent Oral Epidemiol* 25:314–8.
53. Zola K. 1966. Culture and symptoms: An analysis of patients presenting complaints. *Am Soc Rev* 31:615–9.
54. Zbrorowski M. 1952. Cultural components in response to pain. *J Soc Issues* 8:16–20.
55. Riley JL, Gilbert GH, and Heft MW. 2003. Socioeconomic and demographics disparities in symptoms of oral pain. *J Public Health Dent* 63:166–73.
56. Pau A, Croucher R, and Marcenes W. 2003. Prevalence estimates and associated factors for dental pain: a review. *Oral Health Prev Dent* 1:209–20.
57. Riley JL, Gilbert GH, and Heft MW. 2004. Oral attitudes and communication with laypersons about Orofacial pain among middle-aged and older patients. *Pain* 107:116–24.

# Determinants associated with creating fearful dental patients

## Arthur A. Weiner

## INTRODUCTION

The dental experience is a multifaceted combination of physical, emotional, psychological, cognitive, socioeconomic, and vicariously learned factors and situations. These cues are in some manner or form the cause of a biological, psychological, and emotional response, which can include behavior that impedes dental care. A patient's response to these cues is directly proportional to the degree of severity of a patient's initial encounter with the fear-evoking cue or stimulus. In turn, these responses are affected by other etiological factors that combine to influence not only the behaviors of everyday life, but also one's response to needed dental care. These factors influence both one's physiological and psychological responses to the dental encounter, and the great variety of behavioral reactions associated with dental treatment or lack of it. How do these many determinants responsible for a person's fear, avoidance, or delay of treatment affect the chairside practitioner's efforts to overcome the poor dental health of some of his or her patients? To answer this question, and to begin to develop a successful chairside dental fear amelioration program, it is important to examine each of these causative factors and the clinical findings associated with them. Over the years, my own technique has been to study the findings of each of the factors listed below, and to investigate clinically how they affect clinical care and impede a practitioner's ability to perform treatment. The objective is to find a characteristic most common to the etiological factor in each determinant (e.g., pain-related fear from

*The Fearful Dental Patient: A Guide to Understanding and Managing.* Edited by Arthur A. Weiner
© 2011 Blackwell Publishing Ltd.

prior trauma). The greater goal is to combine these common findings to fit individual patients' needs as the practitioner collects past and present history pertinent to successful patient management and positive treatment outcome. Granted, practitioners often tend to ask questions that are not necessary, which may cause individuals to hold back information they might otherwise have provided had the questions had been properly designed, but a simple effort to help gather sufficient information about a patient will play an important role in helping to overcome his or her fear of treatment and ensure treatment compliance and success. It is my goal that in following this theme, this text will be more beneficial to the practicing chairside clinician.

## PREVALENCE OF DENTAL FEAR

The problem of fear of dental treatment as it existed in the past, and as it exists today, has changed little, despite the advances in dental procedures, equipment, and anesthetic technology. Numerous studies over the years, have documented this phenomenon, claiming that 3%–5% of the population suffer from dental phobia, while some 40% of the adult population have been reported to suffer from fear of dental treatment.[1-4]

As far back as 1978, Kleinknecht[5] concluded that one could use the number of missed and cancelled dental appointments to calculate the prevalence of fear of dental treatment. Gatchell et al. noted in 1982 that the prevalence of dental fear and avoidance of routine dental care reached almost as high as 50%–70%.[6] In 2001, Lockeret et al.,[7] in a discussion of psychological disorders in a young adult population, mentioned that epidemiological studies suggest that between percent(20%) of that segment of the population have levels of fear and anxiety regarding dental treatment that can be problematic. Cohen, Fiske, and Newton[8,9] noted in 2000 the prevalence of dental fear and anxiety in the United Kingdom, indicating that studies found about one-third of the adult population to be dentally anxious. Milgrom et al. in 1985, also noted the extent of dental fear and its effect on dental treatment.[10] In 1988, Domoto et al found that 80% of Japanese college students claimed to fear dental treatment in varying degrees, while 6% to 14% stated they were terrified of going to the dentist.[11] The same range has been found in other studies involved in examining the prevalence of dental fear and anxiety.

As dental practitioners, we are faced with a phenomenon that knows no limit and affects almost everyone, causing stress to the practitioner and possibly having widespread general and oral health consequences. Therefore, our search for the answer to the best way to lessen fear should begin with when and how an individual develops a fear. Since no one is born fearful, it follows that fear of dental treatment must be either learned as the result of a direct experience with dental care, or from an external source within the psychosocial environment. Two common concepts must be considered in discussing the development of the dentally fearful individual:

- the role of direct conditioning; and
- the development of the approach-avoidance conflict.

## DIRECT CONDITIONING

This method is most likely to cause an individual to develop fear of direct trauma or an accidental slipping of the drill. Such an incident may result in intense pain, or a negative interpersonal interaction between the patient and the dentist. Either way, the patient comes to regard dentistry or some aspect of it as being either unpleasant and perhaps even terrifying. This experience then acts as the initial stimulus triggering a specific emotional response, namely fear. If the dental practitioner fails to respond to the adverse emotional and behavioral response and discomfort caused by this incident, the patient may then appraise the event in a negative manner, thus initiating the development of a negative conditioning factor, resulting in the patient's avoiding the unpleasant experience and dental care. A new habit is created that may negatively affect the patient's oral and general health in the future. Milgrom and Weinstein et al.[10] present the development of fear and avoidance of dental treatment in a slightly different manner. They illustrate how direct experiences through simple conditioning can lead to fear and avoidance of dental care.

(The following paragraph has been printed with the express written permission of the authors, Dr. Philip Weinstein, a co-author of *Treating Fearful Dental Patients: A Patient Management Handbook*.)[10]

*Simple conditioning*[12] results from the formation of an association between a conditioned stimulus (CS)—the dentist—and a response from an unconditioned stimulus (US)—cut lip from the dental drill. The original response to the unconditioned stimulus (cut lip) is called a unconditioned response (UR). The learned response to the conditioned stimulus (the dentist) is called a conditioned response (CR). The strong emotional component expressed as fear and avoidance that develops is called a conditioned emotional response (CER). The conditioned response (CR) results by associating a conditioned stimulus (CS) the dentist with an unconditioned stimulus (US) the cut lip. The (CER) that follows is developed by associating the pain and discomfort with a second stimulus, which serves to cause the patient to avoid similar encounters again. That stimulus could be the drill, the needle or the dentist's attitude. Continued anticipation of a dental encounter accompanied with continued fear and avoidance of the CS serve to reinforce and strengthen the CER, namely in the form of heightened fear and avoidance. The CER may also be strengthened if the patient's thought of the dentist elicits a strong emotional response. There are many other factors that play a role in determining the strength of the conditioned emotional response. They can include:

- attitude of the staff personality traits of the patient as well as the practitioner.
- the manner in which the patient perceives the dentist, the accuracy of that perception, as well as other factors that will be examined as common determinants of dental fear and anxiety.

# THE APPROACH–AVOIDANCE CONFLICT THEORY

This is a concept that evolves from the above explanation of simple conditioning. It explains the vicious cycle of stress and avoidance of treatment that afflict some individuals. It is a continuous cycle, magnified by past memories of trauma, negative experiences, and defensive actions developed to avoid a repetition of terrifying situations. It was first postulated in 1950 by Miller and Dollard.[13] Simply expressed, an approach–avoidance conflict exists when a person has two competing tendencies—for example, one may be aware that good oral health is a necessity, and, in order to achieve this, regular dental care is required; on the other hand past dental experiences and memories of pain and discomfort cause the patient to be fearful of a reoccurrence and creates an urge to avoid another painful experience. The two competing tendencies—one to approach, one to avoid—leaves the individual in a state of conflict. The approach tendency predominates when the patient makes an appointment with the dentist some weeks in the future. However, as the appointment time nears and the thoughts of past traumatic experiences surface along with vicariously learned negative images of dentistry, and negative personal behavior of the dentist are recalled, fear and anxiety reign supreme, and the avoidance tendency predominates. The result is often a broken appointment, a bewildered practitioner not knowing what he or she may have done, and a large block of unused time. The practitioner needs to change this avoidance pattern by taking the time to set up an appointment solely for the purpose of consulting with the patient. The intent is to learn what went wrong and to attempt to establish rapport, trust, and a positive cycle of treatment once again. This is the time to examine, discuss, and evaluate. Each participant can evaluate the other, without the presence of impending treatment or fee. A dental practitioner can improve rapport and trust by expressing concern and encouraging a patient's positive awareness and desire for a well cared-for dentition. Often when the practitioner fails in creating a positive patient-dentist relationship and lacks a total understanding of his or her patient, a mid-treatment crisis is invited, and a time-out is needed. Such changes may be just what is needed to lower the avoidance level. I believe this is one of the first important steps a practitioner can take in beginning to recognize and understand how to lessen fear and promote mutual understanding.

## Clinical chairside consideration

Learn to recognize warning signs and become aware of reasons for

- developing negative behaviors;
- lack of trust;
- frequent questioning;
- increased criticism of ongoing treatment; and
- apparent dissatisfaction.

When they appear the practitioner must reestablish a positive and caring cycle of treatment by pausing to determine the reasons for this new developing patient behavior. A "time-out" is required to establish an understanding of the reasons for this developing negative behavior, pointing out to the patient the practitioner's awareness of this change in behavior and how that is affecting care, in a statement like "I do not know if you notice, but I sense a change in your measure of trust and understanding of what our goals were when we both undertook this particular treatment plan. Is there something I neglected to explain fully or that you do not completely understand? I suggest we pause for a moment and discuss what may be bothering you. I am sure it is a very simple thing and a moment of discussion will put you at ease and we can continue. Agreed?" (Figure 2.1).

## Chairside implications

- Failure to recognize the hidden signs of unrealistic demands/ expectations or subtle signs of possible emotional and psychological disorders due to incomplete pre treatment history gathering, combined with a lack of knowledge of behavioral modalities to manage them, invites potential failure.

# EXPLORING THE LITERATURE CATALOGING THE COMMON FINDINGS OF EACH OF THE DETERMINANTS OF DENTAL FEAR

*Pain-related fear and anxiety* is an everyday reality within the dental office. There are many stimuli within the dental environment that can act to trigger fear of pain, such as the sound of the drill or the sight of dental instruments, the needle and the dentist. Fear is also influenced by thoughts of past negative and aversive experiences, as well as a host of physical, psychological, emotional, and sociodemographic factors that predispose individuals to experience pain.[14,15] Fear of pain that is associated with dental treatment has been identified as a major element of

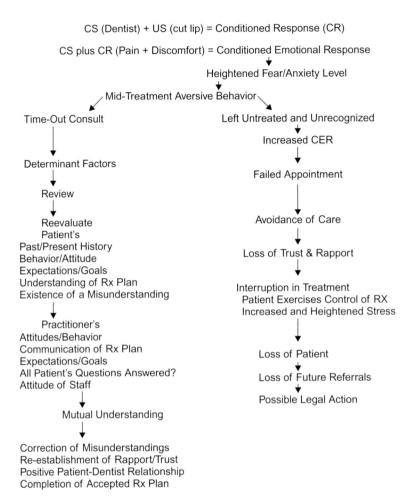

CS (Dentist) + US (cut lip) = Conditioned Response (CR)

CS plus CR (Pain + Discomfort) = Conditioned Emotional Response

Heightened Fear/Anxiety Level

Mid-Treatment Aversive Behavior

Time-Out Consult

Left Untreated and Unrecognized

Increased CER

Determinant Factors

Failed Appointment

Review

Reevaluate
Patient's
Past/Present History
Behavior/Attitude
Expectations/Goals
Understanding of Rx Plan
Existence of a Misunderstanding

Avoidance of Care

Loss of Trust & Rapport

Interruption in Treatment
Patient Exercises Control of RX
Increased and Heightened Stress

Practitioner's
Attitudes/Behavior
Communication of Rx Plan
Expectations/Goals
All Patient's Questions Answered?
Attitude of Staff

Loss of Patient

Loss of Future Referrals

Possible Legal Action

Mutual Understanding

Correction of Misunderstandings
Re-establishment of Rapport/Trust
Positive Patient-Dentist Relationship
Completion of Accepted Rx Plan

**Figure 2.1**   Chairside model to eliminate fear—one to ameliorate fear, the other to maintain and enhance the negative effect of it.

dental anxiety, and the anticipation of that pain a major obstacle to seeking treatment.[2,16–19]

*Pain* has been described in the literature in 1967 by Mersky and Spear[20] as "an unpleasant experience which we primarily associate with tissue damage or describe it in terms of tissue damage or both." In 1979, the definition was modified by an international group of pain experts to include " an unpleasant sensory and emotional experience associated with actual or potential tissue damage."[21] These definitions seem to imply that the presence of pain means an individual is having a negative or aversive experience that is related to or is perceived to being related to body damage. Dworkin[22] broadens the definition of pain to "that which the individual decides hurts." The key words in this definition are:

(1)  *the individual,* implying long + term developmental, personality, or character logical traits of the patient that combine to contribute to the patient's current fear related pain behavior.
(2)  *Decides* refers to momentary and additional immediate factors that determine the current state of the individual, leading to a decision either to report or to withhold a pain response.
(3)  *Hurts* suggest a quality and quantity of the sensation perceived as and responded to as pain, including its duration, location, and nature.

This definition by Dworkin expresses what the average dental practitioner seems to wonder about when his or her patient says "it hurts" or "I put off coming because I fear the pain that I expect is part and parcel of the cure." What factors, either physiological or psychosocial, are responsible and are in play at this moment, that have produced this negative feeling of pain and/or anticipation of it? What can I, the practitioner, do now and in the future to both anticipate and prevent this barrier to dental care? This is what has so often filled my chairside thoughts as well many others dentists, I am sure.

Several concepts have been suggested to explain fear and anxiety related pain in dentistry. Mower's two-factor theory, developed in 1939[23] and modified by Milgrom and Weinstein in 1985,[10] explains how a patient develops a conditioned emotional response to a particular dental stimulus such as the sound of the drill, and learns to avoid and strengthen that response by avoiding encounters with the initial dental stimulus. Davey's model[24,25] presents a wider and more diverse approach to the learning of fear of pain. It has a twofold explanation in which dental events may inhibit or prevent future fear of pain. Another model is called "latent inhibition," which states that if an individual experiences many years of treatment without experiencing a negative event, the many positive experiences may moderate a conditioned response, such as pain. The positive relationship developed over the years is too strong to permit a strong emotional response by another unconditioned stimulus, such as cut lip, the result of the drill slipping. A third model, or "the expectancy model," put forth by Reiss and McNally[26] in 1985, and is founded on two components to fear. One is that expectations of loss of emotional control happen in certain situations, and the other is anxiety sensitivity, a belief that these expected experiences pose a danger and are threatening. Combined, these two components act to influence the behavioral response, especially the avoidance factor. A more detailed view of these three concepts may be found in Mostofsky, Forgione, and Giddon's *Behavioral Dentistry.*[27]

## Anxiety sensitivity—a predictor of pain-related fear

Anxiety sensitivity refers to the presence or absence of fear and anxiety-related symptoms and the belief that these symptoms possess negative somatic or psychosocial consequences. It represents a psychological dimension that serves to intensify the anxious and fearful response to potentially anxiety-evoking stimuli. For example, if an individual perceives that certain aroused bodily feelings are signs of a potential threat or harm, this heightened state of anxiety sensitivity will be likely to result in increased degrees of anxiety. If the individual lacks a method of coping or control, he or she may be at risk of panic.[28] This could result in avoidance of the perceived potential threat.

*Predictability and controllability* are believed to be critical components in the development and continuation of fear and anxiety, with unpredictability being associated with heightened levels of anxious and fearful responses. Being able to predict negative events and situations in the dental environment has been recognized as a central means in determining the development and maintenance of an individual's level of susceptibility to fear, anxiety, and panic regarding dental treatment, according to Zvolensky et al.[29] Asmundson[30] hypothesized in 1999 that anxiety sensitivity may increase the risk of developing high levels of pain-related fear, because many individuals may be more likely to fear the painful consequences associated with dental care. Several studies have evaluated anxiety sensitivity as a predictor of pain-related fear and anxiety, but it is not within the scope of this text to detail each study, though I shall list some of them.[31–37] Overall, these findings reiterate the importance of anxiety sensitivity in understanding pain-related fear and anxiety. They suggest that anxious and fearful response levels can be predicted with greater accuracy when more information is available about the anxiety sensitivity-causing event, such as the patient not knowing how long anesthesia will last during an extraction, the time involved in a crown preparation, or the length a particular procedure may last. This lack of information could result in increased anxiety sensitivity and subsequent increased levels of pain response and avoidance.

## Common findings in the literature suggest a direct relationship between:

- predictable levels of anxiety sensitivity;
- the amount and quality of treatment information provided; and
- the manner in which it affects the patient's perception and response to the anticipated threat.

In 2002, Maggirias and Locker[38] suggested that pain was more likely to be reported by those with prior fear-related painful experiences; furthermore, those who were anxious about dental treatment expected treatment to be painful and thought they had little control over treatment. They suggested that pain and fear-related response to pain are as much a cognitive and emotional construct as a physiological experience. These cognitive processes responsible for generating and maintaining these beliefs must be considered, as well as the sensory pain experiences that occur during treatment. Also, subjects who feel they have no control over what happens during treatment are more likely to report pain and pain-related fear. Maggirias and Locker also theorized that some individuals are more successful in conveying their concerns regarding fear of pain and pain itself to their dentist, thus enabling the dentist to modify his or her clinical or interpersonal approach to minimize the possibility of pain or the perception of pain. In 2006, a study by Klages et al. found that dentally fearful patients disposed to high anxiety sensitivity amplify pain anticipations when exposed to a stressful situation, such as dental treatment, and, furthermore, that when dentally fearful individuals are undergoing dental treatment, their beliefs about negative bodily arousal may negatively influence their cognitive evaluation of treatment related pain.[39] Therefore, providing pretreatment information might help lessen the negative anticipation individuals have of fear-related pain.

## Common findings in the literature

- Patients should be encouraged to express their concerns regarding pain.
- Dentists should be encouraged to respond and modify their clinical and behavioral approaches to meet the immediate needs and goals of the patient.
- Improved patient-dentist communication will reduce anxiety sensitivity and transfer *some degree of control to the patient.*

This suggests that the dentist has the ability to influence the patient's perception of pain by the use of interpersonal and behavioral strategies. Various studies support this approach.[40–43]

## Clinical chairside implications

- Increased information = enhances predictability = decreased fear = lessened pain response.
- Uninformed patients = unpredictability = heightened levels of anxiety and fear = failed/missed appointments = uncompleted treatment.

A well-informed patient, more knowledgeable about what is to be done, how it will feel, and how long the event will take, can better cognitively appraise the potential threat and formulate different methods to cope emotionally with the negative experience. However, the interpretation of situations and information will vary from individual to individual, so practitioners will have to determine whether more or less information will be beneficial.

## PATIENT CONTROL

The second component that determines the level of anxiety sensitivity and therefore the level of fear-related response is whether or not the individual has or perceives the ability to control the present event. In truth, while patients are in the dental chair undergoing a given procedure, real control is always in the hands of the dental practitioner but it is the degree of control that a patient *perceives* he or she has over the impending dental treatment that determines the level of anxiety sensitivity and therefore the level of fear related discomfort or stress. Patients benefit from a combination of knowing what, why and how a procedure will be done as well as how it will feel. When this occurs, they are more likely to avoid anticipation of the unexpected, and are better able to predict what will occur. This provides the patient with a perception of control, which Feldner and Hekmat[44] have shown to exert a direct influence on pain tolerance and its endurance. Control exercises a direct influence on the cognitive appraisal of any potential threat, giving credence to the theory that if one can help a patient perceive a degree of control during treatment, then autonomic body arousal might be lessened when a painful stimulus is encountered.

Patients with a high desire for control are usually associated with Type A behavior, higher education levels, and stronger achievement behavior; they come to the dental appointment with low felt control, expecting greater pain and distress than do other patients. Increasing such an individual's perceived control can result in lower levels of pain within this subgroup.

In the presence of aversive stimuli such as the drill or dental needle, the difference between perceiving control and feeling an inadequate level of control puts patients at risk for negative experiences. That difference can exacerbate aversive reactions during stressful dental procedures. Practitioner who provides control-enhancing coping strategies can be particularly effective in lessening the fearful response.[45] This greatly improves the ability of the dentist and the patient to develop specialized coping strategies, should they be required.

Still, it is important to remember that not all patients will need to have control within the dental setting. Some people believe that whatever life's events confront them, they are governed by external forces outside of their ability to control and therefore are resigned to accept whatever negative experiences might confront them, such as the pain of dental treatment. Individual past experiences, and individual differences in physiology and sensitivity to pain, will also influence the specific appraisal of dental treatment as threatening, and therefore play a role in affecting pretreatment anxiety sensitivity.

## Common findings in the literature

There are two dimensions to patient's dental stress:

- desired control
- perceived control(actual felt control) during dental procedures.

The greater the difference between high desire for control and actual felt control perceived, the greater likelihood of a perception of harm and distress by the patient, leading to greater aversive responses during treatment. Desired control may reflect the patient's level of threat, whereas felt control is a reflection of the patient's ability and confidence in his or her individual coping skills. The ability of the individual to utilize coping strategies may be a predictor of the levels of fear and avoidance that will accompany that patient during treatment.

## Clinical chairside implications

Autonomic bodily arousal and heightened anticipation of pain-related fear can be lessened by:

- *strategies and coping modalities* that permit increased perception of felt control by the individual during dental treatment.
- It is the *dental practitioner's responsibility* to acquire these skills.

# GENDER, AGE, SOCIOECONOMIC, LIFE STATUS DETERMINANTS OF DENTAL FEAR

## Gender and age

Gender and age are two of the most commonly reported factors in the literature that are associated with differences in levels of dental fear in response to dental care.[46–50] Gender and age have frequently demonstrated a relationship with dental fear and anxiety, which more frequently reported in females than males. In 2007, Heft et al.[51] found women were more likely to report general dental fear and general fear of dental related pain more than men, but men and women did not differ in their willingness to express their fearful feelings. However, regarding the fear of treatment or a particular aversive dental stimulus associated with dentistry, both men and women preferred using a more socially acceptable term like "dread," rather than words like frightened or fearful. Eli et al.[52] concluded in 2000 that females remembered more pain after treatment than males, while Locker[53] reported in 2003 that women often reported more negative dental experiences than males.

*Gender, age, dental fear and anxiety are consistently reported more frequently in women.* Domoto et al.[46] in their study of Japanese-Americans, found that fear and anxiety did not vary with age, while Locker and Liddell[54] in their study of correlates of dental anxiety among adults age 50 and over suggested that age is the only demographic variant that is associated with dental anxiety, with less dental anxiety existing among older adults than in younger ones. However, in some cases, younger individuals may carry their anxieties through adulthood and into old age. The relationship between age and dental fear/anxiety can also be explained in that dental anxiety declines with age, because with increasing age, there is a greater susceptibility to more serious ailments with more complicated treatments, permitting fear of dental treatment to have less value or intimidation in the scale of fearful experiences.

Liddell and Locker [55] found in 1997 that women showed greater anxiety about pain, but the painful experience was more important to men than women. They also concluded that the tolerance of pain was a greater and more significant predictor of dental anxiety and most probably the result of differences in the perception and meaning of the painful experience. Women demonstrate a greater disadvantage than men in their perceived ability to cope with the dental encounter. In women, there is a greater desire for control, but a lower ability of actual control is apt to be a contributor to increased dental fear and anxiety.

*Communication*: Gender differences also exists in healthcare provider–patient communication. These differences may emanate from numerous sources, including differences in male and female communication styles, and the way they accommodate the others within the interaction. These variations in styles include:

- differences in tone;
- conversation;
- facial expressions;
- gestures;
- mannerisms; and
- patience in listening and question and answer techniques.

Women generally talk to build rapport and community, whereas men may use talk to establish status and independence.[56] A practitioner's choice of wording uses in questions may negatively affect the flavor of a patient-dentist consultation, and heighten the expression of dental fear response as a result of embarrassment. Embarrassment can be a complex manifestation of dental anxiety for many people and a cause of avoidance and anxiety. Patients are more apt to recognize and acknowledge their dental fear and anxiety when questions are presented in a manner that does not threaten or diminish them, according to Moore, Brodsgaard, and Rosenberg[57] as well as a study by Brener et al in 2004.[58] In a survey on drug abuse, Fendrich et al.[59] concluded that study subjects who reported drug use behaviors felt more comfortable when asked how most people would respond to the questions rather than how "you" would respond. Subtle wording change can affect an individual's response to questions, which may affect the quality and quantity of the information supplied.

## Common findings in the literature

The most important contributors to dental fear and anxiety are:

- *Fear* of pain.
- *Females* are more likely to report fear.
- *Women and older subjects* report higher anxiety levels and demonstrate different attitudes to pain and control than men.
- *Women* have a greater desire for control but a lower perceived capability of actual control.[55]
- *Fear and anxiety* is more prevalent in relatively younger patients than older patients.
- *Men and women* are more willing to verbalize and express their fears if presented with less threatening synonyms.

## Clinical chairside implications

Data suggest that:

- The manner in which questions are posed may greatly affect a practitioner's ability to recognize the true degree of dental fear in an individual.
- Practitioners, in their attempt to collect information, should use less threatening and embarrassing words and phrases combined with more compassionate behaviors when posing questions. This approach should encourage individuals to express and cope with their fear of treatment, rather than to be made to feel foolish and incapable of dealing with their anxieties.
- "Dread" to some is a more socially acceptable term than "fear," and its use, as well as other less threatening terms, may more easily permit individuals, especially men, to admit to their fear and anxiety over various past dental experiences and present concerns.

## Determinants of early age of onset versus late onset of dental fear

One of the issues that may affect the origins of dental fear and anxiety is that age of onset. The age of onset with its respect to dental fear and anxiety is usually viewed as phenomenon originating in childhood. However, in 1987, Ost[60] found that 20% of the subjects studied acquired fear after the age of 14, and Milgrom et al.,[61] found that 33% of their study subjects claimed to have developed fear and anxiety during their adolescence and adult years. Locker and Liddell[62], in their study of adults over 18 years of age, found that of those reporting dental anxiety, 50% reported their onset of fear in childhood, and that a family history of dental fear and anxiety was predictive of child onset only. The data suggested that child-onset fear was more severe than for adolescent-onset and adult-onset subjects. This may be due to the fact that child-onset patients reported greater levels of fear of stimuli associated with invasive procedures, such as extractions and restorations. Furthermore, they suggested that their data was consistent with the classification of dental fear/anxiety as suggested by Weiner and Sheehan in 1990, involving at least two different paths to dental anxiety.[63] The first pathway included conditioning events, such as prior trauma or negative vicariously learned habits and was associated with early onset of anxiety, the result of exogenous stimuli within the external environment. A second pathway, representative of late-onset cases, was more apt to be characterized by genetic factors, such as high levels of general fearfulness and trait anxiety, chemical imbalances within the central nervous system, and accompanying symptomatology, and relatively few direct negative conditioning events. Early onset was associated with individuals who were nervous, vulnerable, sensitive, and more prone to worry, therefore more likely to develop dental fear before age 18.

In addition, early onset of dental fear seems to be related to poor dental health service use behavior, personality factors, and specific beliefs about health professionals. Late-onset dental fear (18–26 years of age) is most strongly related to aversive conditioning experiences, past negative experiences (i.e., caries and tooth loss, trauma, negative attitude of practitioner), characteristics and frequency of dental treatment, an external sense of control, and ability to avoid care due to one's cognitions and beliefs. Caries before age 15 and tooth loss between ages 18 and 26 play an important role in the development of dental fear in adulthood. Rachmann[64] suggested in 1991 that three types of conditioning may play a role in acquiring dental fear:

- direct experience;
- modeling; and
- threatening information.

Child-onset individuals were more fearful of direct pain-related procedures, while adolescent and adult individuals responded more negatively to dentists' behavior and attitude. Genetic and environmental risks factors also play a role as determinants of dental fear at different stages in an individual's life span. According to Ooterink, De Jongh, and Hoogstraten (2009), a heightened fear buildup of anxiety occurs in childhood and adolescence until the middle twenties, followed by a stable adulthood and a decrease in fear and anxiety in the older ages.[65]

## Common findings in the literature

Different age of onset of dental fear-anxiety is associated with different modes of acquisition.

- *Childhood* age of onset is associated with a frightening experience, modeling, vicarious learning, and with a parent or sibling who was anxious about dental treatment.
- *Young adulthood* up to 18 years age of is associated with negative dental conditioning experiences, such as a traumatic experience, high trait anxiety, and a failure to adopt routine dental healthcare practices.
- *Late adult*-onset dental anxiety–dental fear individuals are more likely to suffer from severe fears and symptoms possibly indicative of emotional psychiatric disorders.[66]
- Among *older adults*, the decrease in fear can be explained by older adults' tendency to use emotional coping skills acquired over their lifespan, learned either through the experience of confronting more serious health situations or by the intentional avoidance of potentially negative interactions.
- *Adult onset* patients, because of their psychological and personality characteristics, attitudes, past experiences, hostility toward dentists, set ways, and past vicarious conditioning (phenotype), may be more difficult for practitioners to manage as an age group.

## Clinical chairside implications

- Dentists should continuously emphasize the need for regular check-ups in the young adulthood. This facilitates familiarization with the dental environment, and, through education, helps to lessen future potential fear and anxiety.
- This preventative approach may reduce the incidence of dental anxiety in psychologically vulnerable individuals, who have had past negative experiences, negative cognitions, and beliefs.
- Older adults who report low or less fear must still be monitored with care due the significant physiological decline and multiple chronic disease processes associated with old age. Even moderate levels of anxiety can result in serious iatrogenic consequences.
- Dental practitioners most probably will require additional training in behavior management skills and application of behavioral techniques, for late-onset fearful dental patients.

## Socioeconomic and cultural determinants

Sohn, and Ismail,[67] in a 2005 study using the Corah Dental Anxiety Scale[68] to measure respondents' dental anxiety, after accounting for sociodemographic factors such as sex, age, and income, found that dental insurance status and perceived oral health status were significantly associated with frequency of visits. Among those who had dental insurance, not all the respondents who were fearful of dental treatment visited on a regular basis. Therefore, the presence of dental insurance is not always a guarantor of increased use by the individual, when negative or conflicting factors are in play.

Language and communication problems can lead to misunderstandings, which can lead to heightened levels of concerns about dental treatment. Members of ethnic minority groups often cite language and communication difficulties as considerable obstacles to dental care. Physical disabilities and lack of access with inability to gain entrance into dental premises are also a concern, especially to those individuals with special dental health needs. Another possible determinant of dental fear may be found in the influence of genetics[69] on fear and anxiety, including the role of the proopiomelanocortin gene, hormones derived from that gene called melanocortins, and the five receptors that are activated by melanocortin genes.[70] Recent research indicates that the melanocortinergic pathway is involved in anxiety-like behavior,[71] and that the melanocortin-4-receptor (MC4R) has been implicated in anxiety. The melanocortin-1 receptor (MC1R) is believed to be found in the tissues of fair skin and red hair in about 5% percent of whites,[72] and in the brain pathways that process pain, anxiety, and fear. MC1R has previously been demonstrated to reduce sensitivity to general and cutaneous local anesthesia.[73,74] In 2009, Binkley et al. studied the variations associated with red hair color and fear and anxiety to dental pain and avoidance.[75] Their study suggested that MC1R gene variants and their phenotype, red hair color, are associated with some individuals in increased dental care-related anxiety, fear of dental pain, and avoidance of dental treatment.

## Clinical chairside implications

- Dental practitioners and students alike should evaluate their patients for the existence of all possible determinants of dental fear.
- Although past[63] and recent[70] research has indicated some hereditary and genetic effects on levels of dental fear and anxiety, practitioners would be better served by attending to the history of the patient—the phenotype, accurately described—versus the still too elusive genotype.

Becoming more knowledgeable about the use of appropriate modalities to manage the many aversive behaviors associated with these negative emotions will better enable the practitioner to immediately be able to respond to negative and aversive behaviors when they are encountered.

# PRACTITIONERS' DETERMINANTS OF DENTAL FEAR

In past years, the majority of clinical investigations have been centered around dentists' provider communication, the dentist-patient relationship and those behaviors that effect treatment. These studies have mostly been concerned with the patients' viewpoint rather than the dentists' assessment, of his or her satisfaction with the patient encounter and its effect on treatment and stress.[76–79] Far less has been done to elicit information about the dental practitioners' understanding of the emotions of fear and anxiety, their perceptions and beliefs of the causes of stress and their up to date understanding of behavioral science and its everyday application.

In 1995, Weiner and Weinstein[80] studied the dentists' knowledge, attitude and assessment practices in relation to fearful dental patients. In their two-part questionnaire[80] (see Figure 2.2), the first part addresses the dentists' knowledge of behavioral science and behavioral techniques, and the second part is concerned with the dentists' attitude and its effect on patient assessment and management. Answers to the questions concerning dentists' attitude demonstrated that a majority of dentists responded to feeling more stress than would be desired when treating fearful patients, while a third of the responding dentist reported avoiding such patients. More than 97% rated such patients as uncooperative and disruptive, and having to spend greater time with them while earning less income in return. With regards to fear assessment questionnaires, the vast majority claimed never to have used them, as well as never having using questionnaires that would provide feedback concerning levels of patient satisfaction or dissatisfaction. If fear and anxiety is such a continuous barrier to treatment, one has to ask why so many respondents fail to use methods that would enable them to gain insight into the specific barriers that hinder patients from seeking care. The only reasonable answer is the practitioners' lack of both knowledge and use of these methods. A number of cost-effective, behavioral management modalities such as minimizing cues to anxiety, building positive associations, relaxation, providing positive attributes to negative experiences and more, are all available to practitioners and will be discussed in a future chapter.

A majority of the respondents also believed that more courses and lectures were needed to help practitioners understand, develop, and use effective behavioral management modalities. In 1993, Tay et al.[81] concluded that dentists who had received behavioral science instruction, made greater efforts to address fear and anxiety during patients' initial consult, had less stress in their practice, were more successful in treating the fearful the patient, and noted less cancellation of appointments. Milgrom and Cullen[82] perceived patient noncompliance as also one of the most frequent source of practitioner frustration. They reported frustrating patients did not accept responsibility for their own health or comply with treatment recommendations. Spending too much time with a patient was the second

**Dental practitioners' fear/anxiety attitude, knowledge, and management approach questionnaire**

Age ____ Gender ____ Year of graduation ____

Type of practice: General ____ Periodontics ____ Endodontics ____

Orthodontics ____ Other ____

Below is a list of questions designed to assess the attitudes, knowledge, skills, and everyday dental management approach to the very fearful/anxious patient. It is hoped that the information obtained will lead to the development and presentation of precise and needed patient-management courses to help practitioners deal with this complex, frustrating everyday problem that adds undesired stress to all concerned.

Please check Yes or No for each question

1. Do you understand the basic principle of behavioral science and management?                                                                    Yes___No___
2. Have you ever attended a course in dental behavioral science?                     Yes___No___
3. Do you understand fully the basic principle of fear/anxiety and their characteristics as applied to dental practice?                                        Yes___No___
4. Do you use behavioral assessment techniques and treatment strategies in everyday practice?                                                              Yes___No___
5. If so, which ones: Assessment questionnaire___Modeling___Minimizing cues___Building positive associations___Providing information___Distraction___ Refractory analysis___Alternative attributes___Nitrous oxide___Coping___
6. Do you believe more courses and lectures should be presented at various local, state, and national meetings to help practitioners develop behavior-management skills?                                                                   Yes___No___

Please circle one of the numbers to the right that best reflects your attitude and patient-management practices regarding treatment of very anxious patients.
(1) Never (2) A little (3) Somewhat (4) Ofter (5) Always

| | |
|---|---|
| 1 I find it stressful to treat very anxious patients | 1 2 3 4 5 |
| 2. I am unclear about methods that rely on behavioral modes of intervention | 1 2 3 4 5 |
| 3. I try to avoid treating very anxious patients | 1 2 3 4 5 |
| 4. Anxious patients are usually uncooperative and disruptive | 1 2 3 4 5 |
| 5. Treating very anxious patients requires more time and involves loss of income | 1 2 3 4 5 |
| 6. I schedule very anxious patients further apart than less anxious patients | 1 2 3 4 5 |
| 7. Anxious patients complain more | 1 2 3 4 5 |
| 8. Knowing how to treat very anxious patients has been beneficial to my practice | 1 2 3 4 5 |
| 9. I use assessment questionnaires to elicit patient information: | |
| a. During the anticipatory phase of treatment | 1 2 3 4 5 |
| b. Here-and-now phase of treatment | 1 2 3 4 5 |
| c. Refractory (posttreatment) phase | 1 2 3 4 5 |
| 10. Anxious patients require more explanation, which I find annoying | 1 2 3 4 5 |
| 11. I charge higher fees to treat very anxious patients | 1 2 3 4 5 |
| 12. I take patients' fears personally and respond with anger and frustration | 1 2 3 4 5 |
| 13. Being very anxious regarding dental treatment is expected and I treat it as if it does not exist | 1 2 3 4 5 |
| 14. I provide information regarding treatment and expectation to allay patient anxiety each visit | 1 2 3 4 5 |
| 15. My staff uses a prescribed assessment checklist to monitor and inform me of each patient's reception-room behavior | 1 2 3 4 5 |

**Figure 2.2** Two part questionnaire dentists asked to respond to.
Note: One hundred fifty-three dentists responded to this two-part questionnaire about fearful patients. Reprinted with permission from *General Dentistry* 43(2):164–168, 1995, copyright Academy of General Dentistry, all rights reserved.

most frequent source of stress; this may be the result of a practitioner's inability to deal with these and other issues, such as patient manipulation, patients trying to dictate treatment, or offering too many complaints. Moore and Brodsgaard,[79] in their study of Danish dentists, concluded that in addition to the stressfulness of dental practice and having to deal and manage anxiety, the most prevalent additional stressors included:

- running behind;
- causing pain;
- heavy workload; and
- late-arriving patients.

In a study of general practitioners in England and Wales, Wilson et al.[83] reported similar results, citing that running behind schedule, coping with difficult or uncooperative patients, and lack of patient appreciation as main occupational stressors. In 2005, Yamilik[84] stated that every step of oral care involves a dentist–patient interaction, built on the perceived roles of each of the participants, their characteristics, personalities, and values, which are influenced by economics, culture, fears, and health beliefs, and that all these factors influence stress on both patient and dentist.

In 2008, Hill et al.[85] suggested in their evaluation of perceived dental needs regarding treatment of the anxious patients in the United Kingdom that the majority of practitioners felt current teaching to be less than adequate, and that further training in psychological approaches would be beneficial; in most dental schools today, as a result of these needs, students are receiving the very behavioral and psychological training that past graduates did not receive. In this study, the vast majority of practitioners also stated that they did not have enough time to devote to fearful patients, especially the time that would be required in the use of these advanced psychological modalities.

Still, advances in technology resulting in less discomfort in patients undergoing dental treatment are not mirrored by a visible decline in the fear of dentistry. This may suggest that inherent aversiveness and negative sensitivity toward treatment stimuli may only be part of the explanation of the continued prevalence of dental anxiety in the population. Major factors also include the cognitions, past experiences and expectancies that patients bring to the treatment room, and their appraisal of both the procedures and the dental practitioner. Patients seeking dental care often state that there are a variety of specific dentist and staff behaviors that affect the levels of fear and fear-related behaviors associated with treatment. In 2000, Weiner and Forgione, utilizing a questionnaire developed from an earlier study at the Tufts University School of Dental Medicine,[86] investigated the existence of a variety of these behavior complaints associated with dentists.[87] The questionnaire was structured around five categories of potential fear provoking behaviors (Figure 2.3).

| Most prevalent fear-provoking behaviors by category[87] | |
| --- | --- |
| **Category** | **Behavior** |
| I—The dentist appeared rushed | The dentist did not bother to ask any questions before beginning treatment |
| II—The dentist failed to provide sufficient information regarding treatment | The dentist did not explain the risks and benefits of the treatment |
| III—The patient was concerned whether the anesthetic would be effective | The dentist often begins to work before the anesthetic has taken effect |
| IV—The patient worried about the neatness of the dentist and staff | The patient worries if the instruments have been properly disinfected and sterilized |
| V—The dentist and staff failed to demonstrate concern for the patient's feelings | The dentist did not provide me with a signal to stop treatment if needed |

**Figure 2.3** Results of clinical investigation of top the five most fear-provoking patient observations and associated negative dentist's behavior. Reprinted with permission from *General Dentistry* 48(4):466–471, 2000, copyright Academy of General Dentistry.

The most fear-provoking experiences for the patient were:

- The dentist appeared rushed.
- The dentist failed to provide sufficient information.
- The dentist failed to pay attention to my needs and goals.
- The dentist did not explain the risks and benefits of treatment.

In 2007, Klages et al.[88] suggested that in addition to being able to provide desired and needed treatment information to patients, the dental practitioner who encounters a patient with strong interpersonal concerns should encourage the patient to ask questions and to make a special effort to devote time in listening and answering to whatever concerns are presented.

## Common findings in the literature

Practitioners perceive that increased stress in practice is due to:

- running behind;
- uncooperative and manipulative patients;
- anxious, fearful and uncooperative patients;
- individuals who require extra time with inadequate fees;
- dentists' lack of confidence in knowledge of behavioral science;
- dentists' lack of basic knowledge concerning emotions of fear/anxiety;

- dentist lacks knowledge of various behavior management modalities; and
- a lack of availability of continuing education course in behavior science and its application.

## Chairside clinical implications

- Dental practitioner who are conversant and able to communicate and provide patients with information about their fears, often contributes to reducing their patients' anxiety and in tandem lessens the effects of stress upon themselves.
- Reassuring patients by providing sufficient information, not rushing, and paying attention to a patient's motivations, concern, needs, and goals can greatly aid in reducing treatment anxiety and number of cancelled appointments
- If necessary, the practitioner should do something early that coincides with that which has motivated the individual to seek care and meets the needs and goals of a patient.

For example, a young woman comes into the office seeking treatment for a badly discolored front central incisor. She wishes it to be taken care of initially so she can smiles during family photos at her sister's wedding. The dental practitioner instead feels that two other teeth are in worse shape and require immediate attention, especially since they are presently asymptomatic. If the practitioner follows his professional instinct, and proceeds to care for the two badly diseased teeth, he, in reality, (1) has failed to take into consideration that which has motivated the individual to seek treatment, namely the discolored incisor; and (2) the patient's needs and immediate goal, which is to be able to smile during the wedding pictures. The result is dissatisfaction, anger, and loss of trust with the dentist. These two common behavior patterns that some dentists exhibit[87] may be perceived by patients as a lack of caring and empathy on the part of the practitioner, and may reflect poorly on the practitioner's image.

## Psychological and emotional determinants of dental fear

The difficulty and stress encountered by dental practitioners in treating the subset of the dental population afflicted with various emotional, anxiety, and psychiatric disorders has often left practitioners frustrated and reluctant to treat these individuals. Some patients suffering from these disorders often miss appointment and exhibit disruptive behavior, while others may display misplaced anxieties over planned treatment, leading to mistrust and the belief that the agreed-upon treatment is not working. These negative and aversive behaviors can often interrupt, delay, and misdirect treatment goals. Often, early signs of unrealistic goals and demands are present as subtle signs, but lack of training in the early years in dental school makes it difficult for the inexperienced clinician to detect. Clearly, there is a small proportion of individuals who because of some emotional instability, have difficult completing agreed upon treatment.

*Warning signs:* Patient obstacles to successful treatment.[89] These subtle signs can manifest themselves in many ways such as:

- changing chief complaints;
- repeated questioning after agreed-upon treatment;
- overreaction to mild pain and discomfort;
- dentist shopping;
- attempts at self diagnosis;
- preference for unrealistic treatment.

According to Centore et al.,[89] it is important to assess behavior and psychological factors early in daily practice in order to achieve treatment compliance and optimal outcomes. The authors state that emotional stability can complicate and interfere with dental treatment. They claim, and excellently instruct, that dentists can learn to identify easily emotional problems such as fear, strong dependency needs, alcohol or drug abuse, uncontrolled depression, poor impulse control, or obsessive compulsive, and somatic focus disorders. Proper, accurate history taking can help the practitioner through the use of specific questions that are designed to identify complex hidden emotional disorders and behaviors. Having been fortunate to spend a day with Dr. Centore, watching and learning from her has been one of the most beneficial learning experiences for this clinician, and a plus for those with whom I have been able to share such teachings.

Disorders such as uncontrolled depression may cause patients to have more somatic complaints. Uncontrolled anxiety may increase the likelihood for poor treatment outcome. Impulsive behaviors may surface as exaggerated emotional outbursts. Such behavior can become evident when patients fret over filling out forms or waiting too long in the reception area. Patients may try to impose their own beliefs as to which treatment plan might be best, especially if they have surfed the web and feel they know as much as the dentist.

The dental practitioner also plays a role in inserting barriers to successful and completed treatment, such as:

- Failing to reevaluate working diagnosis when treatment is unsuccessful or does not reach completion.
- Failure to properly recognize signs of fear, anxiety depression somatic or compulsive disorders, and agoraphobic behavior.
- Allowing patient to rush or control pace of treatment.
- Believing he or she can succeed where others have failed.
- Failing to address negative behavior in the early stages of treatment.

Dental fear and anxiety has also been studied in relation to mental health and personality factors. In 2002, Hagglin and Hakeberg[104] studied dental fear and anxiety in relation to other fears, depression, neuroticism, extraversion/introversion, and psychiatric impairment among middle-aged women over a 24-year period. They found that psychiatric impairment was more common in the high-fear group, and that depression and anxiety disorders were more prevalent in women than men. Armfield,[90] in a 2008 study investigating the relationship of dental fear to other specific fears, concluded that dental fear was correlated with a large number of specific fears, which included fears of failure, of heights, of various dental stimuli such as the dental injection, and of loss of perceived control.

In 2009, Carleton et al. suggested that pain-related anxiety is generally comparable across anxiety and depressive disorders and that pain-related anxiety is found to be higher in individuals with anxiety and depressive disorders.[91]

Dental fear is a proliferated determined reaction, often complicated by comorbidity with other anxiety and mood disorders, and simultaneously occurring with numerous other fears. Both coexisting fears, past experiences, and personality traits, help determine an individual's dental fear experience.

## Common findings in the literature

- *Individuals* with high levels of dental fear are more likely to express other specific and general fears.
- *Dental fear* seems to be related to a diverse range of fears relating more to perceived loss of control, personality traits, vicarious learned fears, and various anxiety and depressive disorders.
- *Those fears* that are harbored and remain unrecognized by the dental practitioner may present a variety of complications that will interfere with dental treatment.

## Clinical chairside implications

- Practitioners need to become aware of the likelihood of other psychological fears and develop both efficient screening and appropriate behavioral management modalities to minimize the negative effect on treatment with which these psychological disorders are associated.
- Failure to recognize these patients may result in increased stress during treatment, prolonged treatment time, miscommunication, ill feelings, and, in rare cases, litigation.[89] Possessing the ability to be able to recognize the presence of possible psychological and emotional conditions in their patients may provide an opportunity to confront an individual's fear of the dentist better, which it may be hoped will lead to improvements in oral health and regularity of dental visits.

# ORAL HEALTH, QUALITY OF LIFE, AND THE IMPACT OF DENTAL ANXIETY

High levels of dental anxiety have been shown to be associated with poor clinical oral health: Dentally fearful and anxious patients have been shown to have greater numbers of decayed and missing teeth, less restored teeth, and greater levels of periodontal disease. Dental anxiety affecting on the status of an individual's oral health also may have an impact on the quality of life. Patients with high levels of dental anxiety also frequently report high levels of psychological stress, suffer from negative social consequences, and, in some cases, can be psychologically handicapped.[92]

In 2004, McGrath and Bedi studied the prevalence of dental anxiety in Great Britain and the association between levels of dental anxiety and the overall impact on the oral-health quality of life.[93]They found that those experiencing high levels of dental anxiety were among those with the poorest oral-related quality of life. They suggest the reason that dental anxiety and poor oral health-related quality of life coexist is that they seem to both be associated with psychological, especially neurotic disorders.

Another reason for this coexistence is that dentally anxious people may neglect their oral health to such a degree that the untreated dental disease, may detract from every day living and a positive quality of life. In 2007, Vemaire et al.[94] concluded that the importance of applying effective treatment for dentally anxious patients was not only to help them alleviate their fear of dentistry, but also because ameliorating those fears enhances the individual's quality of life through more frequent utilization of dental service and lessening of oral problems. Impaired quality of oral health and dental fear seem to coexist as determinants of dental fear ,[95] which affect the quality of life in some individuals.

*General life style, gender, socioeconomic status, and occupational status* also play a role in determining dental health behavior. General health behavior and dental service use was found to be worse among men and individuals of lower socioeconomic status.[96,97] Sakki et al., in their 1998 study on the effects of gender, lifestyle and occupational status, concluded that differing beliefs, attitudes, education, and traditions, were more influential in explaining the effects on oral health, than purely economic status. However, a lower occupational status clearly limited the use of dental service. Women demonstrated more frequent dental utilization due to aesthetic concerns and perhaps a greater sensitivity towards illness, pain, and discomfort, and a willingness to seek help. Generally, individuals with positive oral health habits seem to be related to individuals dedicated to a health oriented lifestyle, and effected to a lesser extent by socioeconomic factors.[98,99]

In 2009, Muirhead et al., studied the predictors of dental care in working poor Canadians.[100] They found *male working* individuals less likely to seek dental care than females. In context to length of time working, *male poor persons* worked longer with less flexible hours, limiting access to dental services. *Single poor working* parents at a financial disadvantage, sought less care, probably due to economics and child rearing responsibilities. Age, gender, out-of-pocket dental payments, lack of insurance, self-related oral health determined frequency of dental visits.[100]

*The dental provider* also plays a role in determining the level of dental fear, and is a key figure in both determining the degree of fear/avoidance and importance of regular care, as influenced by his or her efforts in establishing and maintaining a positive inter-personal patient-doctor relationship. Patient satisfaction with the dental provider and its effect on regularity of attendance has mainly been examined as it affects the adult population.[101,102] In 2004, Okullo et al.[103]studied the effect on perceived provider performance among adolescents, especially during their last dental care appointment. Evaluation of the provider was based on factors that included (1) freedom to explain problems with sufficient time allowed, (2) provision of information by provider regarding patient's problem, (3) provision of information regarding tooth decay, gum disease, and preventative measures, and (4) understanding the patient's needs and requirements. The behavior of the providers in this study received a 75%–80% satisfaction score, suggesting that communication with and information from the oral health provider contributed substantially to the explanation of the adolescents overall satisfaction. These findings are similar to those of Weiner and Forgione in their study of practitioner behaviors that added to anxiety.[87] This may support the theory that higher levels of satisfaction are associated regular dental care, increased compliance and reduction in levels of dental fear.

## Common findings in the literature

- *Patients* with dental fear/anxiety suffer considerably from impaired "oral health quality of life" and the degree of this impairment is directly proportional to their degree of dental fear.
- *Provider behaviors*, as perceived by a patient, greatly affect patients' satisfaction with their care in the adolescent years, and has a direct bearing on adult behavior and regularity of dental service use.

## Clinical chairside implications

- *Patient satisfaction* plays a major role in determining a whether or not a patient is satisfied with oral health services rendered.
- *Interpersonal interaction with the dentist* is a key factor in establishing satisfaction, and it involves both a strong effort to create and maintain a positive patient–doctor relationship and the provision of information in a manner that can be fully understand and appreciated by the patient.

- *Sincere and honest communication* between the dentist and adolescent patients in the early years during visits, might serve to increase patient satisfaction while lessening dental anxiety, help correct falsely learned vicarious cognitions, and to promote regular dental care and attendance. This might even carry through the adult years, contributing to the continued enhancement of a person's quality of oral health.

## SUMMARY

Dental fear is a multifaceted phenomenon whose etiology stems from a variety of factors that include pain-related fear, personal experience, vicarious learning habits, behavioral, emotional, and psychological disorders, to name a few. Behavioral assessment and patient management must become a major component of dental practitioners' skills in order to enable them to overcome the negative behavior and stress associated with the emotions of fear in dental practice. Without adequate knowledge of behavioral science, practitioners cannot hope to understand or effectively treat their fearful patients. Unless dentists broaden their diagnostic skills and management abilities, dental fear will remain as prevalent in the future as it has been in the past. All the modern equipment and technical skills are useless, if the practitioner does not know how to get and keep the patient coming for regular care.

## REFERENCES

1. Hakeberg M, Berggren U, and Carlsson S. 1992. Prevalence of dental anxiety in an adult population in a major urban area in Sweden. *Community Dent Oral Epidemiol* 20:97–101.
2. Milgrom P, Fiset L, Melnick S, et al. 1988. The prevalence and practice management consequences of dental fear in a major US city. *J Am Dent Assoc* 116:641–7.
3. Stouthard M and Hoogstraten J. 1990. Prevalence of dental anxiety in the Netherlands. *Community Dent Oral Epidemiol* 18:139–2.
4. Vassend O. 1993. Anxiety, pain and discomfort associated with dental treatment. *Behav Res Ther* 31:659–66.
5. Kleinknecht RA. 1978. The assessment of dental fear. *Behav Ther* 9:626–34.
6. Gatchell R, Ingersoll B, Bowman L, et al. 1982. The prevalence of fear and avoidance: A recent survey study. *J Am Dent Assoc* 107:609-610.
7. Locker D, Poulton R, and Thomson W (2001). Psychological disorders and dental anxiety in a young adult population. *Community Dent Oral Epidemiol* 29:457–63.
8. Cohen S, Fiske J, and Newton J. 2000. The impact of dental anxiety on daily living. *Br Dent J* 189(7):385–90.

9. Lindsey S, Humphris G, and Barnaby G. 1987. Expectations and preferences for routine dentistry in anxious adult patients. *Br Dent J* 163: 120–4.

10. Milgrom P, Weinstein P, Kleinknecht R, et al. 1995. *Treating Fearful Dental Patients: A Patient Management Handbook*, 2nd edn. Seattle: University of Washington.

11. Domoto P, Weinstein P, Melnick S, et al. 1988. Results of a dental fear survey in Japan: Implications for dental public health in Asia. *Community Dent Oral Epidemiol* 16:199.

12. Weiner AA. 1994. *The Difficult Patient: A Guide to Understanding and Managing Dental Anxiety*, 3rd edn. Randolph, MA: Reniew Publishing Co.

13. Miller N and Dollard J. 1950. *Personality and Psychotherapy*, Vol. 1, 1st edn. New York: McGraw-Hill, pp. 76–84, 161.

14. Freeman RE. 1985. Dental anxiety: A multi-factorial etiology. *Br Dent J* 159:406–8.

15. Eli I. 1992. *Oral Psychophysiology: Stress, Pain and Behavior in Dental Care*. Boca Raton, FL: CRC Press.

16. Lindsy S and Jackson C. 1993. Fear of routine dental treatment in adults: Its nature and management. *Psychol Health* 8:135–53.

17. Kent G. 1997. Dental phobia. In: G Davey (ed.), *Phobias: A Handbook of Theory and Research*. London: J. Wiley & Sons.

18. McNeil D and Berryman M. 1989. Components of dental fear in adults. *Behav Res Ther* 27:233–5.

19. Carter L, McNeil D, Vowles K, et al. 2002. Effects of emotions on pain, tolerance, and physiology. *J Pain Res Manag* 7:21–30.

20. Mersky H and Spear F. 1967. *Pain: Psychological and Psychiatric Aspects*. Baltimore: Williams and Wilkins

21. Mersky H and Bogduk N. 1994. *Classification of Chronic Pain*, 2nd ed. Seattle, WA: IASP Press.

22. Dworkin S, Ference T, and Giddon D. 1978. *Behavioral Science and Dental Practice*. St Louis, MO: C.V. Mosby, pp. 242–3.

23. Mowrer O. 1939. A stimulus response analysis of anxiety and its role as a reinforcing agent. *Psychol Rev* 46:553–66.

24. Davey G. 1989. Dental phobias and anxieties: Evidence for conditioning processes in the acquisition and modulation of a learned fear. *Behav Res Ther* 27:51–8.

25. Davey G. 1989. UCS revaluation and conditioning models of acquired fear. *Behav Res Ther* 27:521–8.

26. Reiss S and McNally R. 1985. Expectancy model of fear. In: Reiss S and Bootzin R (eds.), *Theoretical Issues in Behavior Therapy*. San Diego, CA: Academic Press.

27. Mostofsky D, Forgione A, and Giddon, D. 2006. *Behavioral Dentistry*. Oxford, UK: Blackwell Munksgaard, pp. 83–5.

28. Reiss S and McNally R. 1985. Expectancy model of fear. In: Reissand S and Boootzin RR (eds.), *Theoretical Issues in Behavior Therapy*. San Diego: Academic Press, pp. 107–21.

29. Zvolensky M, Eifert G, Lejuez C, et al. 2000. Assessing the perceived predictability of anxiety-related events: A report on the perceived predictability index. *J Behav Ther* 31:201–18.

30. Asmundson GJ. 1999. Anxiety sensitivity and chronic pain: Empirical findings, clinical implications and future directions. In Taylor S (ed.), *Anxiety Sensitivity: Theory Research and Treatment of the Fear of Anxiety*, Marhwah, NJ: Erlbaum, pp. 269–85.

31. Schmidt N, Lerew D, and Jackson R. 1999. Prospective evaluation of anxiety sensitivity in the pathogenesis of panic: Reaction and extension. *J Abnorm Psychol* 108:532–7.

32. Asmundson GJ, Norton P, and Norton G. 1999. Beyond pain: The role of fear and avoidance in chronicity. *Clin Psychol Rev* 19:97–119.

33. McCracken L, Zayfert C, and Gross R. 1992. The Pain Anxiety Scale: Development and validation of a scale to measure pain. *Pain* 50:67–73.

34. Eifert G, Zvolensky M, Sorrell J, et al. 2000. Predictors of self reported anxiety and panic symptoms: An evaluation of anxiety sensitivity, suffocation fear, heart focused anxiety, and breath holding duration. *J Psychopathol Behav Assess* 21:293–305.

35. Zvolensky M, Goodie J, McNeil D, et al. 2001. Anxiety sensitivity in the prediction of pain related fear and anxiety in a heterogeneous chronic pain population. *Behav Res Ther* 39:683–96.

36. Vassend O. 1993. Anxiety, pain and discomfort associated with dental treatment. *Behav Res Ther* 31:659–66.

37. Locker D, Shapiro D, and Liddell A. 1996. Negative dental experiences and their relationship to dental anxiety *Community Dent Health* 13:86–92.

38. Maggirias J and Locker D. 2002. Pyschological factors and perceptions of pain associated with treatment. *Community Dent Oral Epidemiol* 30(2):151–9.

39. Klages U, Kianifard S, Ulusoy O, et al. 2006. Anxiety sensitivity as a predictor of pain in patients undergoing restorative dental procedures. *Community Dent Oral Epidemiol* 34(2):139–45.

40. Dworkin S and Chen A. 1982. Pain in clinical and laboratory context. *J Dent Res* 61:772–4.

41. Gatchel R. 1992. Managing anxiety and pain during dental treatment. *J Am Dent Assoc* 123:37–41.

42. Eli I. 1992. *Oral Psychophysiology. Stress, Pain and Behavior in Dental Care.* Boca Raton, FL: CRC Press.

43. Sullivan M and Neish N. 1999. A psychological intervention for reducing pain during dental hygiene treatment. *Probe* 33:23–30.

44. Feldner M and Hekmat H. 2001. Perceived control over anxiety-related events as a predictor of pain in a cold pressor task. *J Behav Ther Exp Psychiatry* 32:191–202.

45. Law A, Logan H, and Baron R. 1994). Desire for control, felt control and stress inoculation training during dental treatment. *J Pers Soc Psychol* 67(5):926–36.

46. Domoto P, Weinstein P, Kamo Y, et al. 1991. Dental fears of Japanese residents in the United States. *Anesth Prog* 38(3):90–5.

47. Holtzman J, Berg R, Mann J, et al. 1997. The relationship of age and gender to fear and anxiety in response to dental care. *Spec Care Dent* 17(3):82–7.

48. Liddell A, Locker D. 1997. Gender and age differences in attitude to dental pain and dental control. *Community Dent Oral Epidemiol* 25:314–8.

49. Gadbury-Amyot C and Williams K. 2000. Dental hygiene fear: Gender and age differences. *J Contemp Dent Pract* 1:42–59.

50. Setteneri S, Tati F, and Fanara G. 2005. Gender difference in dental anxiety: Is the chair position important? *J Contemp Dent Pract* 6:155–22.

51. Heft M, Meng X, Bradley M, et al. 2007. Gender differences in reported dental fear and fear of dental pain. *Community Dent Oral Epidemiol* 35:421–8.

52. Eli I, Baht R, Kozlovsky A, et al. 2000. Effect of gender on acute pain prediction and memory in periodontal surgery. *Eur J Oral Sci* 108:99–103.

53. Locker D. 2003. Psychosocial consequences of dental fear. *Community Dent Oral Epidemiol* 31:144–51.

54. Locker D and Liddell A. 1991. Correlates of dental anxiety among older adults. *J Dental Res* 70:198–203.

55. Liddell A and Locker D. 1997. Gender and age differences in attitude to dental pain and dental control. *Community Dent Oral Epidemiol* 25:314–8.

56. Street R. 2002. Gender differences in health care provider communication: Are they due to style, stereotypes or accommodation? *Patient Educ Couns* 48:201–6.

57. Moore R, Brodsgaard I, and Rosenberg N. 2004. The contribution of embarrassment to phobic dental anxiety: A qualitative research study. *BMC Psychiatry* 4:10.

58. Brener N, Grunbaum J, Kann L, et al. 2004. Assessing health risks behaviors among adolescents: The effect of question wording and appeals for honesty. *J Adolesc Health* 35:91–100.

59. Fendrich M, Wislar J, and Johnson T. 2003.The utility of debriefing questions in a household survey on drug abuse. *J Drug Issues* 33:267–84.

60. Ost L. 1987. Age of onset of different phobias. *J Abnorm Psychol* 96:223–9.

61. Milgrom P, Fiset L, Melnick S, et al. 1988. The prevalence and practice management consequences of dental fear in a major US city. *J Am Dent Assoc* 116:641–7.

62. Locker D, Liddell L, Dempster L, et al. 1999. Age of onset of dental anxiety. *J Dent Res* 78(3):790–6.

63. Weiner A and Sheehan D. 1990. Etiology of dental anxiety: Psychological trauma or CNS imbalance. *Gen Dent* 22: 39–43.

64.  Rachman S. 1991. Neo-conditioning and the classical theory of fear acquisition. *Clin Psychol Rev* 11:155–73.

65.  Ooternink F, de Jongh A, and Hoogstrate J. 2009. Prevalence of dental fear and phobia relative to other fear and phobia subtypes. *Eur J Oral Sci* 117:135–43.

66.  Poulton R, Waldie K, Locker D, et al. 2001. Determinants of early-vs late onset dental fear in a longitudinal-epidemiological study. *Behav Res Ther* 39:777–85.

67.  Sohn W, Ismail A. 2005. Regular dental visits and dental anxiety in an adult dentate population. *J Am Dent Assoc* 136(1):58–66.

68.  Corah N. 1969. Development of a dental anxiety scale. *J Dent Res* 48:596.

69.  Smoller J, Gardner-Schuster E, and Misiaszek M. 2008. Genetics of anxiety: Would the genome recognize DSM? *Depress Anxiety* 25(4): 368–77.

70.  Chaki S and Okuyama S. 2005. Involvement of melanocortin-4 receptor in anxiety and depression. *Peptides* 26(10):1952–64.

71.  Lui J, Garza J, Truong H, et al. 2007. The melanocortinergic pathway is rapidly recruited by emotional stress and contributes to stress-induced anorexia and anxiety-like behavior. *Endocrinology* 148(11):5531–40.

72.  Raimondi S, Sera F, Gandini S, et al. 2007. MC1R variants, melanoma and red hair color phenotype: A meta-analysis. *Int J Cancer* 122(12): 2753–60.

73.  Liem E, Lin C, and Suleman M. 2004. Anesthetic requirement is increased in redheads. *Anesthesiology* 101(2):278–283.

74.  Liem E, Joiner T, Tsueda K, et al. 2005. Increased sensitivity to thermal pain and reduced subcutaneous lidocaine efficacy in redheads. *Anesthesiology* 102(3):509–14.

75.  Binkley C, Beachham A, Neace W, et al. 2009.Genetic variations associated with red hair color and fear of dental pain, anxiety regarding dental care and avoidance of dental care. *J Am Dent Assoc* 140:896–905.

76.  Corah N, O'Shea R, and Ayer W. 1985. Dentist's management of patient fear and anxiety. *J Am Med Assoc* 110:734–6.

77.  Corah N, O'Shea R, and Skeels D. 1981. Dentists' perceptions of problem behaviors. *J Am Dent Assoc* 104:829–33.

78.  Menola P, O'Shea R, Corah N, et al. 1991. General practitioners'opinions on the treatment of anxious patients. *Gen Dent* 39:444–7.

79.  Moore R and Brodshaard I. 2001. Dentists' perceived stress and its relation to perceptions about anxious patients. *Community Dent Oral Epidemiol* 29(1):73–80.

80.  Weiner A and Weinstein P. 1995. Dentists' knowledge, attitudes, and assessment practices in relation to fearful dental patients: A pilot study. *Gen Dent* 43:164–8.

81.  Tay K, Winn W, Milgrom P, et al. 1993. Effects of instruction on dentist motivation to manage fearful patients. *J Dent Educ* 57:444–8.

82.  Milgrom P, Cullen T, Whitney, C, et al. 1996. Frustrating patient visits. *J Pub Health* 56(1):6–11.

83. Wilson R, Coward P, and Capewell T. 1998. Perceived sources of occupational stress in general dental practitioners. *Br Dent J* 184:499–502.

84. Yamalik N. 2005. Dentist-patient relationship and quality care 5: Modification of behavior. *Int Dent J* 55: 395–7.

85. Hill K, Hainsworth J, Burke F, et al. 2008. Evaluation of dentists' perceived needs regarding treatment of the anxious patient. *Br Dent J* 2048(E13):442–3; discussion.

86. Weiner AA, Forgione AG, Weiner LK, et al. 1998. Survey examines patients' fear of dental treatment. *J Mass Dent Soc* 47:16–21.

87. Weiner A, Forgione A. 2000. Potential fear-provoking patient experiences during treatment. *Gen Dent* 48(4):466–71.

88. Klages U, Sadjadi Z, Lojek L, et al. 2007.Development of a questionnaire measuring treatment concerns in regular dental patients. *Community Dent Oral Epidemiol* 36:219–227.

89. Centore L, Reisner L, Craig A, et al. 2002. Better understanding your patient from a psychological perspective: Early identification of problem behaviors affecting the dental office. *J Calif Dent Assoc* 30(7):512–9.

90. Armfield, J. 2008. A preliminary investigation of the relation-ship of dental fear to other specific fears, general fearfulness, disgust sensitivity and harm sensitivity. *Community Dent Oral Epidemiol* 36:128–36.

91. Carleton R, Abrams M, Asmundson G, et al. 2009. Pain-related anxiety and anxiety sensitivity across anxiety and depressive disorders. *J Anxiety Disord* 23(6):791–8.

92. Abrahammsson K, Berggren U, and Carlsson S. 2000. Psychological aspects of dental and general fears in dental phobic patients. *Acta Odontol Scand* 58(1):37–43.

93. McGrath C and Bedi R. 2004. The association between dental anxiety and oral health-related quality of life in Britain. *Community Dent Oral Epidemiol* 32:67–72.

94. Vamaire, J, deJong A, and Aartman A. 2007. Dental anxiety and quality of life: The effect of treatment. *Community Dent Oral Epidemiol* 36(5):409–16.

95. Mehrstedt M, John M, Tonnies S, et al. 2007. Oral health related quality of life in patients with dental anxiety. *Community Dent Oral Epidemiol* 35(5):357–63.

96. Peterson P and Nortov B. 1989. General and dental health in relation to life-style and social network activity among 67 year-old Danes. *Scand J Prim Health Care* 7:225–30.

97. Steele J, Walls A, Ayatollahi S, et al. 1996. Dental attitudes and behavior among a sample of dentate older adults from three English communities. *Br Dent J* 180:131–6.

98. Sakki T, Kuuuttila M, and Anttila S. 1998. Lifestyle, gender and occupational status as determinants of dental health behavior. *J Clin Periodontol* 25:566–70.

99. Green C, Pope C. 1999. Gender, psychosocial factors and the use of medical services: A longitudinal analysis. *Soc Sci Med* 48:1363–72.

100. Muirhead V, Quinonez C, Figueiredo R, et al. 2009. Predictors of dental care utilization among working poor Canadians. *Community Dent Oral Epidemiol* 37:199–208.

101. Newsome P and Wright G. 1999. A review of patient satisfaction: 1. Concepts of satisfaction. *Br Dent J* 186:161–5.

102. Newsome P and Wright G. 1999. A review of patient satisfaction: 2. Dental patient satisfaction in an appraisal of recent literature. *Br Dent J* 186:166–70.

103. Okullo I, Nordrehaug-Astom A, and Haugejorden O. 2004. Influence of perceived provider performance on satisfaction with oral health care among adolescents. *Community Dent Oral Epidemiol* 32(6):447–55.

104. Hagglin C, Hakeberg M, Hallstrom T, et al. 2001. Dental anxiety in relation to mental health and personality factors. *Eur J Oral Sci* 109:27–33.

# Factors affecting the psychological collection and identification of the fearful dental patient

## Arthur A. Weiner

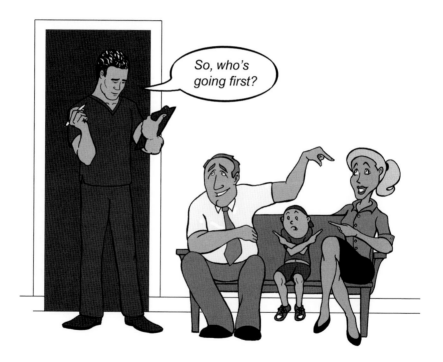

## INTRODUCTION

The assessment and identification of dental fear and anxiety, although it appears deceptively simple, can actually be rather difficult. Although

*The Fearful Dental Patient: A Guide to Understanding and Managing*. Edited by Arthur A. Weiner
© 2011 Blackwell Publishing Ltd.

dentistry is a technically oriented profession, the way a dentist communicates can significantly influence the behavior of his or her patients. The dental situation does not generally favor two-way conversation. The dentist is often seen as an individual carrying on a one-sided conversation with the patient, who is unable to participate.

Communication is a two-way street. The dentist needs not only to have the ability to receive messages from, but also to convey information, to the patient. The ability to receive a patient's verbal and nonverbal messages is of paramount importance in developing rapport and mutual trust. When a practitioner fails at this, it can lead to mistrust, anger-increased fear and anxiety and eventual avoidance. Collection of information concerning a patient's past and present history should ensure that the dental practitioner acquires a complete understanding of the needs and dental problems of his or her patients. But this is not often emphasized or even taught within the dental curriculum.

The identification of this multifaceted emotion we call fear requires the accumulation of complete and accurate information in order to ensure that the desired result is achieved. The essential components are:

- enhanced communication-listening skills;
- a positive dentist-patient interpersonal relationship;
- rapport building and establishing trust;
- good interviewing skills;
- empathy; and
- willingness to cooperate and learn to overcome one's fears.

The most critical and potent component of effective communication is not speaking, but rather *listening*. Listening is far more potent a tool then speaking. Listening not only helps determine what is heard, but more significantly, what is often said after the hearing. When the dental practitioner begins to listen effectively to what the patient is saying, he or she has taken the first steps toward understanding the thoughts, feelings, goals, and needs of that patient. It is the initial building block of a doctor–patient relationship, one built on mutual trust and rapport.

## PREREQUISITE COMPONENTS FOR ENHANCED COMMUNICATION SKILLS

Good active listening skills are largely comprised of "attention skills." These imply a direct interest of the part of the listener practitioner. Attention skills include:[1,2]

*Eye contact*: Eye contact is the principal means of expressing involvement. Establishing and maintaining eye contact throughout a conversation is an essential listening skill. It should be steady, frequent, and focused on the face and eyes of the speaker. However, one should also avoid prolonged eye contact, which can be intimidating, especially in some cultures. Eye contact and facial expressions are fairly reliable indicators of how good the speaker–listener contact is, and may indicate the quality of the information being communicated. If eye contact is lessened by the patient, it may be difficult for the dentist to acquire adequate information without these nonverbal cues.[3]

*Body orientation*: This pertains to the degree to which one's shoulders and legs are turned in the direction of the speaker. Bodily facing the speaker is the correct position.

*Posture*: The listener's body posture conveys important messages concerning interest and attention. A listener should maintain a slight forward lean. To do so communicates a positive attitude and interest, while leaning back often implies a negative attitude and disinterest on the part of the listener.

*Silence:* Silence is an extremely effective listening tool. Silence on the part of a dentist during a conversation, especially during the initial consult and interview, often gives patients the time to formulate their thoughts and facilitates continued communication. A listener should avoid interruptions.

*Following cues*: "Cues" are verbal and nonverbal behaviors that occur in response to a patient's statements and can reinforce the patient's desire to continue communicating. For example, the listener could make such statements like "That's interesting," or I'd like to hear more about that." Vocal interjections such as "really?" and the use of facial expressions that denote interest serve to convey interest and empathy. Nodding the head occasionally indicates that the listener is interested in what the patient is saying. A timely smile can indicate a genuine feeling, implying "I'm looking forward to working with you," or "it's a privilege to have met with you."

*Establishing appropriate distance*: A distance of 3–4 ft (36–48") is considered to be an appropriate distance for interpersonal communication. Closer distances make evoke feelings of intrusion, while a greater distance may imply a lack of interest and involvement.

*Eliminating distracting behaviors*: Many practitioners have personal habits that can be distracting and annoying to a patient. Pencil tapping, continuous shifting of positions, nervous movement of the hands and feet, playing with objects, or glancing at watches should all be avoided. These may indicate to the patient that the consultation is taking up too much valuable time. Conduct the interviews and consults in a setting where telephone calls will not be a distraction.

*The physical environment*: The environment or room for the consult or interview should make it easy for both the patient and dentist to give their undivided attention to one another. It should provide sufficient privacy so that a patient's conversation cannot be overheard. It should be well lit, pleasant, and comfortable.

*Attending to content*, not the delivery. Most patients are not good speakers, and often they are anxious and frightened. Some may have an unpleasant voice, while others may have speech defects. Ensuring positive and successful communication requires a deliberate attempt to attend to what the patient is saying, despite the manner in which it is said.

*Listening to feelings*: While factual knowledge is essential for proper diagnosis and treatment, it is also important that a dentist listen for affective and attitudinal messages. Very often feelings, concerns, and attitudes are expressed in offhand remarks, asides, and by-the-ways. A patient may often insert casual comments to his or her messages to see how the dentist will respond. A lack of response to these messages may be interpreted by the patient as a lack of interest on the part of the practitioner. Practitioners must constantly be alert for such cues.

*Attending to nonverbal forms of communication.* Patients communicate through nonverbal channels, as well as verbal ones. Nonverbal behavior is influenced by many factors, including personality, culture, and time context, to name a few. Most of what a patient feels and thinks are communicated through gestures, tone of voice, and body actions. Positive and effective listening necessitates that a listener pay as much attention to nonverbal forms of communication as to the spoken words of the patient.

Nonverbal behaviors are potent cues in the communication process because they lend context to the patient's words, thoughts, and feelings. They also reveal the distress and discomfort patients may be experiencing during treatment. The value for the dentist of attending to these non verbal messages has been shown to including the following;

- Yields a more accurate understanding of what the patient feels and needs.
- Helps provide a determination of the emotional flavor behind the patient's words or feelings. Did you hear an angry "no" or a questioning "no"?
- Helps to provide feedback to the patient demonstrates that the dentist is an interested and attentive listener/observer.
- Demonstrates to the patient that a non verbal communication links exists, which can be reassuring to the patient, and helps reveal that the dentist is concerned.
- Helps regulate the flow of speech, conveys emotional feeling and thoughts, and most importantly, helps build and maintain a positive relationship.

When the dentist uses positive nonverbal communication (smiles, nods, gestures, facial expressions), he or she demonstrates a capacity to understand, listen, and identify with the feelings and concerns of their patient.

- Avoid questions or words that might cause emotional arousal such as "drill," "scrape," "needle," and "grind."
- Develop calming statements such as "Try not to let it upset you" or "Try to relax, it is not as bad as you think it is." Some individuals prefer to be called by their full first name rather than by a shortened version or nickname (William instead of Bill). Some individuals become antagonized by the shortened use of their name. Try to avoid the overuse of technical jargon. Such language can intimidate patients and cause them to withdraw and avoid giving needed information.

*Reflective listening and response*: In any given point in a conversation in reflective listening, the dentist combines both verbal and nonverbal information captured and feeds back to the patient in his or her own words the patient's expressed or implied feelings, in an effort to reiterate correctly what the patient perceives the message to be. The goal is to provide the patient with specific feedback about the dentist's understanding of the needs, goals, and concerns of the patient. It allows the patient the opportunity to correct any misinterpretations and avoid any misunderstandings. It can also be utilized when a treatment plan is presented to a patient, allowing patients to present their interpretation of the suggested treatment plan in their own words, and correct any misunderstandings that may have risen during the practitioner's explanation.

With this technique, you can reinforce the patient's emotional state, clarify vague statements, and help the patient assess and take ownership of his or her feelings. Remember, feelings can often color content. The art of listening is essential to establishing a positive working relationship between patient and dentist. Affective responses such as "You seem anxious," "You seem concerned and uncomfortable," or "I can understand why you would feel anxious and upset" can elicit responses providing valuable information that may help complete the picture and explain a patient's negative and emotional behavior, fear, and cognitions more fully.

*Provide positive feedback*: Refrain from using language that discourages rather than encourage solutions to an ongoing problem. Avoid responding to the patient solely when the individual's response illustrates a past negative response or behavior. Provide positive feedback to counteract the patient's negative outlook; it helps to motivate and promote a brighter outlook. For example, during a new patient consultation, the patient stated that "all her previous dentists were only interested if she had insurance, did not provide her with sufficient information or answer her questions fully, never explained the risks and benefits of what was to be done, and were always in a rush to get started." Try using the *I* statement technique to communicate a positive attitude and counteract the patient's negative experiences. For example, "*I* am very sorry you have experienced these past difficulties. *I* do not practice like that. Each of my patients is adequately informed each visit. Before I start, *I* give each of my patients the opportunity to ask any and all questions they may have. *I* believe we all forget sometimes, information previously given, and many times, *I* myself am guilty of momentary lapses. Please be assured if *I* at any time seem to be rushing or you have any question, *I* want you to feel free to interrupt me; in fact my staff and *I* insist upon it." The idea is to communicate to the patient that you are a different type of person, more caring and responsive to the needs and feelings of your patients. It allows them to feel they will be a part of the overall treatment.

## Clinical chairside implication

- The reflective listening/response technique can help insure treatment compliance in that it permits (1) a checking the accuracy of information and (2) the elimination of misunderstandings through the giving and receiving of feedback by all parties involved. It can be a potent factor in assuring treatment compliance and building trust.

I know that many times during this text, I can be accused of repetition, but I always remember one of my first dental school professors saying:

*Repetition is the mother of learning.*

I feel so strongly about many of the ideas and concepts this text advocates that I feel no quilt in constantly restating them.

# ESTABLISHING A POSITIVE PATIENT–DENTIST RELATIONSHIP[2]

Key elements in creating a positive patient–dentist interpersonal relationship are:

- Establishing rapport and trust;
- utilizing two-way communication—verbal and nonverbal;
- understanding a patient's perception of control, relative to past dental experiences and effects on fear levels; and
- accommodating initial patient-dentist priority differences.

## Creating rapport

Rapport is a relationship that must be established early in the cycle of dental treatment. Most individuals, especially fearful and mistrustful ones, form their impressions of a practitioner within the first few minutes of their encounter. Therefore, early communication should consist of listening to the concerns and needs of the patient.

A patient's perception of a practitioner as warm, caring, and empathetic helps build trust and rapport. Patients should be made to feel comfortable, and encouraged to ask questions and interrupt at any time should they become confused and not understand what the practitioner is trying to communicate. Avoid embarrassing or belittling the patient over lack of care or poor oral hygiene. Do not appear to rush, and be alert to nonverbal cues. Sometimes an individual's verbal message may convey conviction while their gestures, facial expressions and tone of voice may indicate a sense of doubt.

During the initial consultation, get to know to the patient. Try to establish a mutual connection. For example, ask "How long you have lived in the area?" The dentist can respond, "Well, I have also lived here for some time." Ask "What high school did you go to? Great, I went there also." "When did you graduate?" "Who was your dentist when you were growing up? Really? He was mine also." Try to make a connection, through your children, college, soccer, Little League, anything that can equal a shared similarity, or common background. It helps create a friendly beginning to what may potentially be a long association.

## Clinical chairside implication

- Communication and rapport are essential for understanding and trust.
- Listen; listening builds trust, the foundation of all successful relationships. The more you listen, the more people will trust you and feel that you are genuinely interested in their well being. The greater the trust and rapport, the greater the likelihood a patient will agree to a recommended treatment plan.

Past studies cited below, which were concerned with communication between patient and dentists and the many interpersonal variables that can be found in the patient–dentist encounter, demonstrate an increased attention by the profession to this particular interaction.[4–8]

In the establishment of a positive dentist–patient relationship, the dental practitioner must possess certain interpersonal skills, including active listening and the ability to capture both verbal and nonverbal cues, such as displayed and repressed emotions. Patients use these two forms of expression to display their feelings and concerns and inner emotions. It is a way in which a patient expresses their problems, and often reveal any hidden fears. The dentist must be able to recognize these cues and be responsive to them. They may appear as nervousness, fear, shame, and distrust. Some of these emotional cues may be in the form of body language: sitting at the edge of the chair, for example, or nervous rubbing of hands, or crying at the thought of having to discuss treatment. Patients may manifest shame, not wishing the dentist to look in their mouth and see the condition of their teeth.

To establish and maintain this relationship between patient and doctor, the dentist is required to be sensitive to the patient's communication or lack of it, and to be skillful in recognizing these emotional expressions, verbal or nonverbal, that the patient is sending during conversation. The dentist must also play the role of a sympathetic human being, displaying empathy, respect, and an air of understanding. If the dentist fails at this, he or she could fail to gain a complete understanding of the patient's overall dental problems. There are some patients who are distrustful of dentists or dentistry in general and who want to control the entire consultation in order to learn more about who the practitioner is. Some may constantly blame a previous clinician for their poor oral health, while others may hide their fears during the initial consultation, either because they do not want or are unable to express or verbalize their fears and anxieties to the dentist. Also, some individuals repress expressing their anxieties as a strategy for coping with their discomfort, while others joke and minimize their fears as a way to hide their shame and embarrassment.

In 2000, Karoly and Kulich,[9] in their study of the dentist–patient consultation in a clinic specializing in dental phobic patients, suggested, regarding to the dentist's interpersonal skills and as role as a clinician, that the healthcare provider must listen intently to the patient's concerns, learn from the patient, teach the patient, and be open and nonjudgmental in order to understand the patient's complaints and dental problems. They also concluded that the practitioner's overall interpersonal skills must consist of demonstrating empathy and paying attention to both what patients say and also what they are often unable to express verbally but convey through nonverbal forms of communication. The dentist must continuously offer encouragement and understanding.[10–12]

# TWO-WAY COMMUNICATION[2,13–16]

The dental practitioner is often characterized as an individual who usually carries on a one-way conversation, either asking questions, then interrupting before the speaker has completed a response, or making conversation with a patient whose mouth is filled with a variety of equipment and accessories, preventing a reply. Two-way communication between patient and dentist is essential because the patient needs to know that he or she can exercise some degree of control over situations perceived to be threatening. Patients should be informed, each time they present for either a consultation or treatment, that it is perfectly acceptable to interrupt if they feel any unpleasant discomfort during treatment or have any questions needed for clarification during a consult. In the treatment phase, always:

- Inform patient what you wish to do.
- Explain the reason for doing it.
- Ask if any questions or concerns exist before starting.
- If the patient requests, inform how much time is involved.

When patients are well informed and knowledgeable, there is less chance for anticipatory anxiety on their part and less likelihood of surprise during treatment.

## Perceptions of control—effect on levels of fear

There are patients who never avoid dental care and whose attitude towards their dentist and the dental profession is always very positive. This may be due to early childhood treatment that was relatively painless, caring attitude by the dentist, and parental support while receiving care. There are individuals who have endured negative experiences, but with the aid of the dental practitioner, have been able to attain a measure of control, thereby lessening their anxiety. The perception of control can be enhanced by the practitioner suggesting a signal to indicate that the patient needs a break. When a patient experiences pain and is able to gain some measure of control over it, fear is lessened. However, it takes cooperation between patient and dentist, working in harmony to help lessen the level of fear. People have always associated pain and fear with dental treatment, and this has led to avoidance and negative behavior. I firmly believe that fearful dental patients can be successfully treated, and that negative and aversive behavior can be greatly reduced and in many individuals ameliorated. It is my hope that this text will play a role in helping dental practitioners experience less fearful, less stressful, and more satisfied patients.

# ACCOMMODATING PATIENT–DENTIST PRIORITY DIFFERENCES

Dentists are trained to treat dental problems usually in the order of priority pain first, followed by treatment of existing periodontal disease and needed restorations of existing dentition. Cosmetic procedures almost always occupy a lower position on the scale of treatment priorities. In order to build trust and rapport, the dental practitioner must take care to remember that whatever has motivated the patient to seek treatment must take precedence over whatever the practitioner might think has priority. The reason might be as mundane as having a simple but embarrassing badly discolored anterior tooth restored first, regardless how much in need of care several other teeth are. When the practitioner's priorities differ from those of the patient, the dentist must respect the motives of the patient even though each has a different preference. It is the practitioner's responsibility to inform the patient of the difference in priorities and the risks, if any, associated with the two positions. However, the practitioner must respect and accept the patient's wishes and restore the anterior teeth, since it is what motivated the patient to seek care. By doing, this the practitioner has accomplished two things; first, as an agent of change, and second, by allowing the patient to be involved in the decision making and the decision to proceed with treatment. This provides the patient with the perception of having some degree of control over his or her care. This action on the part of the dentist serves as the first stepping stone in the formation of mutual trust and rapport. Over time, the patient should become more open to the practitioner's recommendations.

## Clinical new patient chairside considerations

- Do something that both shows early and fulfills the patient's primary reason for seeking treatment.
- This avoids anger and mistrust that would most probably lead to loss of the patient from the practice.
- It shows a respect for the wishes of the individual over those of the dentist
- Permits the beginning of trust and rapport, essential ingredients for a positive dentist–patient relationship.

# THE INITIAL PATIENT–DENTIST CONSULTATION

## Considerations in developing one's own personal interview model

There are certain basic goals that the dental practitioner should attempt to accomplish. The primary goal is to gain a perception and understanding of what the patient's perceives needs and objectives. To that end, the practitioner will wish to do the following:

- Demonstrate concern and listen attentively.
- Establish trust.
- Always obtain the patient's viewpoint.
- Provide for sufficient two-way communication.
- Avoid carrying on a one-way communication.
- Determine the patient's motivations and goals.
- Determine the patient's attitudes and expectations.
- Do not rush.
- Attempt to learn how the patient copes with stress, and how he or she has handled past difficult dental care.

Some individuals have their own ways to cope with negative experiences, while others do not, and so they avoid them. This last observation will help inform the practitioner how the patient deals with difficult situations, and determine what type of behavior modification to use.

In addition, the dentist should provide information in a positive manner, so as to dispel the fear of receiving "bad news." Statements such as "things are not as bad as they seem, I have patients far worse off than you" often help a patient put things in perspective and lessen the fear of the situation. Patient should understand that they will be consulted concerning any treatment preferences, and will be provided with suitable treatment options which they are free to accept or reject.

Again, the primary goal is to gain an understanding of what the patient perceives his or her needs to be. Hence, the dentist should always allow sufficient time to obtain the patients' views, understand their goals and needs, and demonstrate a continuous concern for what the patients have to say. The dentist must recognize the patient's negative behaviors or emotions, and let the patient know that it is okay to express them. Often by doing this, the practitioner helps to lessen their effect. The dentist must also decipher, from the patient's attitude and points of view, whether or not expectations are unrealistic and possibly influenced by the presence of a psychological or emotional disorder. To assist in the patient's self-disclosure, the practitioner must be supportive while at the same time avoiding an evaluation or grading of the patient's responses, such as "It has been that long since you have seen a dentist? How come?" Such a response could be perceived as judgmental and cause the patient to become angry and defensive, interfering with the development of rapport.

## First visit

(1) *The patient should be greeted* by both the staff and practitioner with a smile, and a welcoming gesture or some other gesture of support. It is up to the dentist to initiate the consultation and make the patient feel comfortable. The consultation should be conducted in a nondental setting and all vocabulary should be kept at a level that the patient can comprehend. Early in the interview, the dentist should impress upon patients that he or she takes their concerns seriously and realizes that they are legitimate. It is important from the beginning that the dentist demonstrates sincere empathy and the ability to understand the individuals' needs and concerns. If patients believe that the practitioner is sensitive to their feelings and emotions, it is a major step in building trust and a positive interpersonal relationship.

(2) *The interview should be designed* to initiate the flow of information, establish trust and help the patient to organize his or her thoughts about precipitating circumstances, sequence of events, and past experiences, in order gradually to form a picture of the entire problem. The discussion must make sense to both the patient and practitioner. The dentist's understanding of the patient's needs and concerns should be consistent with the patient's understanding of the overall problem as he or she perceives it.

(3) *Use open-ended questions* during this initial consultation and history gathering process. Begin with a what, where, when, how, why word,

for example, "What brings you in today?" "What caused you to become fearful?" or "What seemed to make the pain worse?" Open-ended questions are an invitation for the patient to provide a fuller and more detailed response, rather than a simple one- or two-word answer. This mode of questioning demonstrates that the practitioner has a concern and respect for the patient's observations. It promotes patient input and a more active participation, resulting in the acquisition of more pertinent information. Avoid using the "why" question. Such questions are frequently perceived as threatening, because people sometimes do not have a clear reason behind their actions, and therefore are unwilling to disclose what motivated them.[13] Additionally, such questions may appear as evaluations rather than an open minded request for information. Utilize such questions as "What is the reason for today's visit?" Allow patients time to answer and describe their particular problem. Asking another question before the patient has completed their answer may result in the loss of needed information by the dentist and cause the patient to perceives the dentist as distant and uninterested.

(4)    Repeating a patient's main concern and chief reason for seeking treatment, at the end of the consultation, demonstrates to the patient that the dentist was listening and sincerely cared. It also gives the practitioner the opportunity to inquire if there are any other concerns the patient would like to address, before ending the interview.

(5)    As the consultation proceeds, look to see if *tension and stress* have been reduced and the flow of information has increased. Observe whether or not interest has been stimulated and if significant relaxed changes in posture, position, and expression have occurred. If little change in the patient's negative behavior is evident, the practitioner must assume that other factors are present and influencing the event, such as general anxiety, or an emotional/psychological disorder. Early failure to recognize these behaviors or attach any importance to them may result in increased stress during treatment, as well as prolonged treatment time, miscommunication, and potential ability to complete treatment.

(6)    *Use simple language.* When you use too many technical words, you imply a difference in status or intelligence, which may evoke patients' passivity. The dental setting can be intimidating to some, either due to their fears or because they do not want to hear the solutions to their dental problems. When you add technical phrases and words, they can be quickly overwhelmed and back away, complaining that "the explanation is beyond me, too complicated and difficult to understand." Patients can also become angry when they hear multiple complex phrases, which may cause the patient to think that the practitioner is showing off and trying to impress with his or her knowledge. Still, there are times when dental or medical language is appropriate: It may be a rapid way of finding out if a patient is dentally educated and has the ability to understand a treatment plan. The

dentist should be guided by the level of the patient's understanding of dental terminology to determine the manner in which a treatment plan or any other discussion should proceed between them.

## Clinical chairside implication

- The initial contact is extremely important. It is the foundation from which the practitioner begins the patient–doctor relationship. It must be based on genuine empathy and understanding, combined with respect and a feeling of warmth and friendliness. These characteristics serve to reduce existing fears and anxieties and act as the cornerstone for building mutual trust, rapport, confidence. and respect.
- Providing clear and understandable answers that speak to the patient's concerns and needs demonstrates caring and interest on the part of the practitioner. It can affect a patient's decision to remain a patient and accept a proposed treatment plan. It demonstrates empathy and good listening skills on the part of the practitioner.
- "Why" questions should be avoided. They may tend to impede cooperation or even significantly damage the dentist–patient relationship, since the patient may view them as threatening rather than informational.

## Ending the interview

Up to this point, the prime concern of the practitioner has been to listen and gain an understanding of the patient's problem and the reason for the visit. Once the patient has provided all the appropriate information, the the practitioner should use the skill associated with reflective listening, along with notes taken during the consult, to summarize in his or her own words what he or she understands the patient has verbally and non-verbally communicated. This demonstrates that the practitioner was an interested, concerned, and empathetic listener, and gives the patient the opportunity to correct any misinterpretations that may have occurred. The patient should be allowed to restate his or her goals and needs and the practitioner to inquire if there are any other concerns or questions that the patient needs to ask. Be sure to set realistic expectations, defining what is actually meant by successful treatment and what is meant by the practitioner's efforts to reduce anxiety and fear to tolerable levels that will enable the patient to keep appointments.

## Clinical chairside considerations

- Remember that the goal of the interview is not only to acquire information, but to reduce fear and anxiety and establish mutual trust and rapport.

- The patient must leave feeling that the practitioner has his or her best interest in mind.
- The best way to accomplish this is to address the patient's needs as if you needed them yourself.
- Promote a positive feeling of trust, assurance and knowledge that successful management of the patient's concerns will ensue.
- End the consultation with both verbal and nonverbal gestures tailored to this end.

## PRACTITIONER'S VERBAL INQUIRY AND COLLECTION OF PAST AND PRESENT HISTORY

The assessment of dental anxiety by the dental practitioner is important for two main reasons: first, to aid the dentist in the management of the anxious patient, and second, to provide evidence-based clinical research for construction of those psychological factors that may predict avoidance behavior. Humphris in 2006 concluded that the use of a short dental anxiety questionnaire by adult patients immediately before seeing their general dental practitioner does not raise fear or anxiety levels. Completion of a brief modified dental anxiety scale has a nonsignificant effect on state anxiety.[17,18]

I believe all dentists should use dental anxiety and fear questionnaires as part of their general patient assessment. In my practice, we routinely utilized these questionnaires, never taking for granted that a silent patient was a nonfearful patient.

There are a multitude of questions that need to be asked during the collection of information at the initial visit in order to collect the total amount of information required to formulate the best possible treatment plan suited to the specific needs of a patient. The information collected is gathered both through verbal communication and the use of multiple specially designed questionnaires for specific situations as they arise from information as it is collected. These questionnaires are carefully structured from items contained within a number of validated clinical studies and from my personal chairside experiences.

I believe that any time a patient poses a question to me, that question has to be considered as a valid one, regardless of whether or not it has appeared as part of a controlled study. When I hear it repeated several times by different individuals, I consider it to be a common concern, most likely to have been heard chairside by many practitioners and therefore one needing to be included in my own study questionnaires in order to determine its general level of concern. We decided, early in our practice, that the information we required in our efforts to manage the fearful dental patient would be best gathered by questionnaires sent and responded to in the privacy of the new patients' homes. As mentioned earlier, many of the questionnaires we send are derived from variations of selected items from prior published clinical studies carried out at various dental schools and clinical research facilities, combined with those frequently asked by patients themselves both in my practice and within the undergraduate clinic of Tufts School of Dental Medicine (TUSDM).[19-40]

## Collection of information: past and present medical–dental history

The quality and quantity of information that the practitioner is able to collect and evaluate will be directly proportional to the dentist's expertise in history taking. All practices have difficult and fearful patients with histories full of complaints, anxieties, personal and psychological issues, as well as individuals with complicated medical histories. In gathering information, we try to subdivide patients into two categories from information gathered in the initial telephone contact.

One category is composed of individuals who profess little to no fear of dental treatment and/or are trustful because of a friendly referral, or who may state they do not relish dental care but go because it is necessary for good oral health. This patient can be initially seen by the hygienist, who can collect past medical and dental history, including medications, allergies, and family history, as well as take the required radiographic surveys. Such a patient can usually be interviewed within the dental operatory setting, as the sight of instruments and equipment are not a source for arousal or initiation of anxiety. Treatment plans and an overall discussion of the patient's needs and goals, as well as time and cost involved, can be comfortably discussed in this environment by the practitioner. The visit should also include a prophylaxis, since we have found that some patients feel that in addition to discussing their concerns and formulating a treatment plan, a dental visit should include some form of treatment. You need to have the patient leave with a feeling of positive accomplishment, especially in those cases where the patient expresses anxiety. Nothing being done can create the feeling "Is talking all we were going to do? I thought we could begin treatment, especially since I worked up courage to come to this appointment."

The second category consist of individuals who by their responses to the receptionist, indicate past negative experiences, prolonged absence of treatment, complaints like "The Novocain never works," or simply "I'm afraid all my teeth need to come out," or "I hate going to the dentist." Practitioner-specific complaints may include "The dentist always rushes to get started," "He never answers my questions to my satisfaction," "He treats me as if I do not know anything." This type patient needs to be seen by the practitioner in a private, comfortable area of the office, not in the dental operatory. Since patients form their initial impressions of the practitioner in the very first few moments of the consultation, holding the consultation in an area where past dental images and experiences can surface is ill advised.

## Clinical chairside consideration

- Utilizing pretreatment anxiety and psychological profile assessment questionnaires does not have any short-term measurable effect on a patient's state of anxiety, nor does their use initiate or exacerbate any existing pretreatment anxiety.
- Fearful patients find it difficult to respond correctly and completely to questionnaires within the reception area, due to nervousness, varying degrees of anticipatory anxiety, and the sights, noises, and smells associated with the dental environment.
- Experience has taught us that this preconsultation technique—an offsite questionnaire responses with return envelope—provides an opportunity to better recognize and develop management skills that will enable the practitioner to construct individual management programs to fit the specific needs of the patient.
- Questionnaires are sent to the patients at their homes seeking information concerning past medical, dental experiences. These questionnaires are designed to reveal any and ideally all concerns, negative and positive, related to past care and present desired care. Questions are also constructed that elicit any indication of a hidden psychological or emotional disorder. Those questions that are not answered are covered in the following initial consultation utilizing follow-up questions designed to reveal similar information. Examples of the cover letter as well as the questionnaires are listed in Figures 3.1–3.5.

Cover letter:

**Dear New Dental Patient:**

It is our goal to make your dental care and treatment as professional, efficient and caring as possible. To help us achieve this goal, we ask you to take a few moments of your time, in the quiet and privacy of your home to respond to this multiple page questionnaire. **All responses are strictly confidential. Please answer all of the questions to the best of your ability.**

   This initial questionnaire is designed to help us assess any past or present medical, dental and patient management concerns that may or may not affect your overall dental care. It also allows you the patient to express your feelings, concerns, needs and goals and provide whatever additional information you feel necessary to ensure successful treatment. It is our goal to provide excellent and optimal care to each and every individual we care for.

Thank You

**Figure 3.1**   Cover letter for new patient personal questionnaire inventory.

Name…………………………………………………..

Age…    gender. M  F      Language spoken….. Translator
required ….. Yes  No

## PART  A

Medical History: Past- Present- The medical portion of the initial
questionnaire seeks responses to the following:

| | | |
|---|---|---|
| Changes in health past three years?…………………….. | Yes | No |
| Date of last complete physical exam_____ | | |
| Any hospitalization in past five years? | Yes | No |
| List all medications both prescription and over the counter medicines. Include all Vitamins, herbal supplements, contraceptives | | |
| Do you take any **MAOI inhibitors** like NARDIL | Yes | No |
| Do you now take or have taken: (Please circle) Amitriptyline- Paxil, Zoloft, Celexa, Prozac, Effexor XR) Valium, Xanax, Lithium, Migraine medications, Opiods, any others not listed. | | |
| Do you use now or in the past any recreational Drugs, tobacco, alcohol and how much? _____ | Yes | No |
| Are you Pregnant, if so in what month? Yes No | Yes | No |
| Do you now or have you ever had any of the following: | | |
| Heart disease, irregular heart beats or pacemaker | Yes | No |
| Difficulty with breathing | Yes | No |
| Chest pain or history of Angina Pectoris, heart attack? | Yes | No |
| Rheumatic heart disease, heart murmurs, mitral valve prolapse? | Yes | No |
| Stroke, numbness , tingling sensations or severe headaches? | Yes | No |
| High blood pressure. | Yes | No |
| Fainting spells, convulsions or epileptic seizures? | Yes | No |
| Lung disease? Asthma- emphysema- breathing problems? | Yes | No |
| Emotional problems including general anxiety, depression or or other psychological problems/. Any associated hospitalizations? | Yes | No |
| Liver disease, cirrhosis, jaundice or alcohol drinking disorders? | Yes | No |

**Figure 3.2**  Patient past and present medical history profile.

| | | | |
|---|---|---|---|
| Do you suffer from any autoimmune disorders, HIV, Scleroderma, Lupus, Rheumatoid arthritis  Reynaud's Syndrome? | Yes | No |
| Arthritis, rheumatism, painful joints, joint replacements? | Yes | No |
| Diabetes? | Yes | No |
| Blood disorders? | Yes | No |
| Thyroid disease? | Yes | No |
| Cancer? | Yes | No |
| Eye disorders, glaucoma? | Yes | No |
| Hay fever, skin rashes, hives, food sensitivities? | Yes | No |
| Allergies to any of the following?<br><br>Novocain<br>Penicillin or any antibiotics<br>Aspirin, codeine, barbiturates or pain medications | Yes | No |
| Medications not listed and if so please list.... | Yes | No |
| Have you ever smoked cigarettes .... Cigars... Pipe...? | Yes | No |
| Do you take Disulfiram (Antabuse) for excessive alcohol intake? | Yes | No |
| Do you take or have you taken methadone? If yes, how long?.... | Yes | No |
| Have you undergone counseling for alcohol or substance abuse? | Yes | No |
| Are you fearful about medical care? | Yes | No |
| Do you take medications for anxiety or depression.  If so, please list them........................................................ | Yes | No |
| Do you diet frequently? | Yes | No |
| Have you undergone or contemplated cosmetic surgery? | Yes | No |

If you have answered **yes** to any of the above questions, please explain in the space provided below. Your completeness will greatly help us help you.
Thank you.

Use this space for additional information

NOTE: The health and medical portion of our questionnaire (long form) follows that recommended by the ADA and is most likely used by all practitioners.

**Figure 3.2** *Continued*

Name:                    Age:                 Gender:    M    F

Below is a list of experiences, situations, feelings and thoughts that are sometimes associated with dental treatment and that often cause individuals to become more or less fearful. Please circle to what degree each of the following situations or experiences causes you to feel fearful regarding treatment. This questionnaire is designed to help us help you. Your responses are very important to us and are strictly confidential.

**Please do not skip any items.**

**1=No Effect    2=Very Relaxed   3=Somewhat Relaxed   4=Somewhat Fearful   5= Very Fearful**

**I FEEL:**
1.  By the thought of the dental appointment before the actual visit.................1 2 3 4 5
2.  By the thought of past dental experiences.............................................1 2 3 4 5
3.  While waiting in the reception area......................................................1 2 3 4 5
4.  Having the same bad experience a parent had.......................................1 2 3 4 5
5.  When the dentist does not do as they say they will................................1 2 3 4 5
6.  With regard to the dental appointment and treatment in genera.................1 2 3 4 5
7.  When the dentist and staff always make me feel comfortable....................1 2 3 4 5
8.  When the dentist pokes fun at my fears................................................1 2 3 4 5
9.  At the sight of the dental instruments.................................................1 2 3 4 5
10  By the lack of attention given me before, during and after treatment...........1 2 3 4 5
11. At being alone anytime in the dental chair............................................1 2 3 4 5
12. When the dentist seems rushed and I feel he is rushing my care...............1 2 3 4 5
13. When the dentist always asks me questions if I have any concerns............1 2 3 4 5
14. When the dentist answers my questions to my satisfaction.......................1 2 3 4 5
15. When I hear the sound of the drill.......................................................1 2 3 4 5
16. When the dentist appears rushed and insensitive...................................1 2 3 4 5
17. When having my teeth drilled and worrying if the Novocain will work..........1 2 3 4 5
18. When the dentist fails to provide me with a signal to stop.........................1 2 3 4 5
19. When trapped in the dental chair........................................................1 2 3 4 5
20. When the dentist or hygienist make me feel guilty about my teeth..............1 2 3 4 5
21  When the dentist and staff praise my being a cooperative patient..............1 2 3 4 5
22. When the dentist fails to explain the risks and benefits of the treatment.......1 2 3 4 5
23. When the dentist fails to pay attention to my needs and goals...................1 2 3 4 5
24. Knowing the dentist treats individuals with infectious diseases.................1 2 3 4 5
25. Having to avoid certain places, things or activities because of fear.............1 2 3 4 5
26. When the dentist minimizes my need for additional Novocain....................1 2 3 4 5
27. When not informed by the dentist what is to be done this visit...................1 2 3 4 5
28. When the dentist makes me feel uncomfortable about asking questions......1 2 3 4 5
29. When I see the dental injection coming towards me...............................1 2 3 4 5
30. When all the dentist wants to know is how much dental insurance
    have or do nothave......................................................................l 1 2 3 4 5

**Figure 3.3**  Past and present dental history survey (long-form).[38]

Note: Portions of the above questionnaire are reprinted from Weiner, Zemnick, and Ganda K.[38] © Journal of the Massachusetts Dental Society. Reprinted with permission. All rights reserved.

Below is a list of symptoms and complaints that individuals sometimes have when frightened or anxious during dental treatment. Please circle one of the numbers to the right that best describes how much you are bothered or distressed when frightened or anxious during the past and up until today, either when contemplating the dental visit or during it. The information provided by this self report of feelings and experiences, will help us help you in your special areas of concern. Our goal is to provide you with the very best dental care available. Please take your time and respond to all the questions.

**RATINGS:0 = not at all  1 = a little  2 = Moderately  3 = Markedly**
**4 = Severely**

**How much are you bothered by the following complaints:**

1. Fluttery stomach..................................................................................0 1 2 3 4
2. Sweaty palms ....................................................................................0 1 2 3 4
3. Warm all over feeling..........................................................................0 1 2 3 4
4. Skipping or racing of your heart...........................................................0 1 2 3 4
5. Fine tremors of the hands....................................................................0 1 2 3 4
6. Mouth drier than usual........................................................................0 1 2 3 4
7. Shaky inside and out...........................................................................0 1 2 3 4
8. Lightheadedness, faintness or dizzy spells..........................................0 1 2 3 4
9. Chest pain or pressure........................................................................0 1 2 3 4
10. Choking or smothering sensations......................................................0 1 2 3 4
11. Tingling or numbness in parts of the body..........................................0 1 2 3 4
12. Shortness or difficulty in breathing....................................................0 1 2 3 4
13. Bouts of excessive sweating..............................................................0 1 2 3 4
14. Sensation of rubbery or jelly legs.......................................................0 1 2 3 4
15. Episodes of diarrhea.........................................................................0 1 2 3 4
16. Severe anxiety or panic attacks.........................................................0 1 2 3 4

**Figure 3.4**  Associated fear discomfort bodily feelings survey.[33]
Source: Weiner and Sheehan.[33] Reprinted with permission from Elsevier Publishing. All rights reserved.

A severe **anxiety** or **panic attack** is an intolerable situation or occurrence leading to some action such as flight or running away. It may come at any time without warning or visible cause, or it may occur only in certain situations. It is usually accompanied by some or all of the above symptoms or complaints. Please answer the following questions by circling the appropriate number that best describes how much you are bothered, if at all, by these complaints in the past and up until now, whether they occurred in the dental office or not.

**1**. Severe attacks of fear or anxiety only in certain situations
and the cause is readily identifiable to you................................................0 1 2 3 4

**2**. Sudden unexpected attacks of fear or anxiety with symptoms like those listed above, that occur without warning or identifiable cause and that occur any time
spontaneously.......................................................................................0 1 2 3 4

**3**. If you have circled a number from 1-4 in Question # 2, please answer if you feel these unexplained sudden spells of fear or anxiety in your daily activities have played a role in avoiding dental treatment.......................................................................YES.....NO

**Figure 3.5**  Panic attacks occurrence survey.[33,36,46,47]
Source: Weiner and Sheehan.[33] Reprinted with permission from Elsevier Publishing. All rights reserved.

I tend to look for anything in the medical history that would give me a hint of how patients deal with their primary car physician. Do they follow that doctor's directions, fill their required prescriptions, seek routine check-ups, have required vaccinations, ingest more than the recommended dose of prescribed medications? Knowing this sort of information helps me to decide if such new patients are capable of building a trustful relationship. If they do not follow their physician's advice, why should I think they would follow mine? The medical history often helps in revealing a variety of emotional problems, seen in the medications patients are taking, that individuals do not readily provide or discuss with a dentist, such as general anxieties, alcohol, physical and substance abuse.

Due to the nature of my private practice, teaching, and clinical research interests, I found that I required more extensive knowledge of the past and present dental history of my patients as well. We try to establish the best possible psychological profile of each patient, which we hope will aid us in designing an appropriate and optimal treatment plan suitable to the specific needs and goals of each patient. Knowing the past dental history of an individual gives us an insight into what may have caused this person to become fearful of dentistry and the dentist. Remember, no one is born fearful; we become fearful of situations and objects, and either become more fearful or less as time passes. Since our private practice consisted almost entirely of individuals who were extremely fearful of dental care, and whose fears were complicated by other psychological, mental, and emotional disorders, our dental questionnaires were constructed to focus on behavioral feelings, attitudes and conduct in the overall dental environment.

The ability to properly assess the medical and psychological conditions of our patients, and their impact on dental treatment, rests solely on the accuracy and completeness of the information obtained during the history taking. The questionnaires as they are presented in this text are essentially the same that we used in practice, although they were subdivided into separate parts as shown (Figures 3.2–3.5). Sections of them are utilized at the Tufts University Dental School as needed, and are given to new patients during the initial screening appointment, to be responded to at home and returned on the next visit. There are some individuals who, by the nature of their personalities, are always in a hurry, too impulsive and can never find time to be bothered responding to forms and questionnaires. They usually inform the receptionist of this dislike of forms during the initial phone contact in some manner. For those individuals, we utilize a shorter "yes–no" type of questionnaire to collect information and utilize the con-sultation session to fill in information not collected in the written question-naire (Figure 3.6).

All patients in my private practice were required to respond to a preconsultation/questionnaire, or they were not accepted as new patients. There are some individuals who because of embarrassment, type of personality, or some other explained reasons, tend to hide information,

## Past and Present Dental History Survey: PART A
### SHORT FORM

Name:............................ Age          Gender:  M  F

**Have you ever experienced now or in the past any of the following dental experiences listed below?**

**Please circle the appropriate answer**

| | | |
|---|---|---|
| Periodontal treatment including gum surgery? | Yes | No |
| Difficulty or pain on opening and closing your jaw? | Yes | No |
| Any clicking noise on chewing? | Yes | No |
| Dental anesthesia that does not always take effect? | Yes | No |
| Pain in the face, lips, tongue or soft tissue area within the oral cavity? | Yes | No |
| Pain and sensitivity in the teeth? | Yes | No |
| Difficulty with eating or chewing food? | Yes | No |
| Are you fearful of losing your teeth? | Yes | No |
| Do your gums bleed when brushed? | Yes | No |
| Do you suffer from bad breath? | Yes | No |
| Have you ever had orthodontic treatment? | Yes | No |
| Do you experience fear of dental treatment? | Yes | No |
| How do you rate your fear if any? (choose one) Mild… Moderate…. Severe… Avoid completely…. | | |
| Do you wear any dentures?  Complete—Partial | Yes | No |
| Have you ever been dissatisfied with your care? | Yes | No |
| Have you ever been mistreated by a dentist? Hygienist? | Yes | No |
| Trouble with fillings falling out or always breaking? | Yes | No |
| The dental drill cutting your tongue or cheek? | Yes | No |
| Do you find yourself clenching your teeth often? | Yes | No |
| Do you diet often? | Yes | No |
| Do you drink large amounts of soda daily? | Yes | No |
| Do you trust the dentist to treat you as you wish? | Yes | No |
| Have you ever been physically or verbally abused in a dental office? | Yes | No |

**Please use the following space for any additional information you wish to convey.**

**Figure 3.6** Short-form history questionnaires. (a) Past dental history and treatment evaluations. (b) Past and Present Dental Experiences. These forms are used for highly anxious, impulsive patients for whom responding to questions increases anxiety. Portions of the above questionnaire are reprinted from Weiner AA, Forgione A, Weiner LK, et al. 2000. Potential fear-provoking patient experiences during treatment. *Gen Dent* 48(4): 466–71. © Academy of General Dentistry. Reprinted with permission.

**PART B, Short Form: Past and Present Dental Experiences**

Below is a list of situations and experiences that individuals may or may not have encountered in the past when contemplating or undergoing dental treatment. They have been shown in certain occasions to lessen or increase fear and avoidance of dental treatment. If you have experienced any of the situations listed below, please circle the "**YES or NO**" answer that is appropriate for you. The information provided below will help us help you in your special areas of concern. It is our sincere desire to provide you with the very best dental care available. **Please take your time and respond to all the questions.**

| The dentist appeared rushed | Yes No |
|---|---|
| The dentist was impatient and rushed to begin treatment | Yes No |
| The dentist dose not take time to answer my questions | Yes No |
| The dentist does not provide me with clear answers | Yes No |
| The dentist and staff greeted me with a smile and handshake | Yes No |
| The dentist always tells me they have a busy schedule | Yes No |
| The dentist tells me they are running late | Yes No |
| The dentist manners and conversation are usually abrupt | Yes No |
| The dentist always begins without asking me any questions | Yes No |
| The dentist and staff make me feel time outs are an annoyance | Yes No |
| The dentist is always caring and ask me questions before beginning treatment | Yes No |
| The dentist fails to provide me sufficient information | Yes No |
| The dentist fails to explain the reasons for the particular planned treatment to my satisfaction | Yes No |
| The dentist buses terms and language I do not understand | Yes No |
| The dentist does not answer my questions to my satisfaction | Yes No |
| The dentist never takes my questions seriously | Yes No |
| The dentist always answers my questions satisfactorily | Yes No |
| The dentist never tells me what to expect | Yes No |
| The dentist often begins before the Novocain is working | Yes No |
| The dentist always minimizes my need for additional Novocain | Yes No |
| The dentist always uses topical anesthetic before injecting | Yes No |

**Figure 3.6** *Continued*

| The dentist treats me with respect and listens to my concerns | Yes<br>No |
| --- | --- |
| The dentist fails to pay attention to my needs and goals | Yes<br>No |
| The dentist pokes fun at and minimizes my fears | Yes<br>No |
| The office staff is rude and not helpful | Yes<br>No |
| The dentist always provides me with a signal to stop. | Yes<br>No |
| The dentist and staff always worry if I have dental insurance or not | Yes<br>No |
| The dentist is not sufficiently empathetic and does not understand what it feels like to have to be the patient | Yes<br>No |
| The dentist is not interested in my opinion or past experiences | Yes<br>No |

**Figure 3.6**  *Continued*

which can lead to disagreements in treatment plans, interruptions, mistrust, and failure. I try not to allow for midtreatment surprises by a patient commenting "I forgot to mention that I cannot deal with removable appliances in my mouth. I wanted fixed bridgework," or "I wanted tooth-colored restorations, not silver ones," or "I hope this set of dentures will fit better that the last three I had made." Fully knowing your patient is the best guarantee against unneeded stress and treatment failure.

Once we receive the completed questionnaire back and they are evaluated, an appointment is set up for the initial interview, during which we try to get the patient to reveal as much as possible of the reasoning behind the answers he or she has given to on the questionnaire. It has been my experience that patients who genuinely wish to overcome their fear of dentistry and restore their dentition never complain about filling out any of the questionnaires or about the number and type of questions asked during the initial consultation. All of the responses are addressed during this interview because self-reports are not always completely accurate, and some people tend to overdramatize their feelings regarding pain and discomfort levels.

To complete our discussion concerning the data collection and identification of the fearful patient, we must acknowledge that there is a subgroup of patients that present for treatment who are under treatment for various emotional, psychological, psychiatric, and somatoform disorders. The difficulty and stress encountered by dentists in treating this subset of the patient population has often left some reluctant to treat these individuals because they often miss appointments and exhibit disruptive behaviors. These individuals do not always respond positively to written questionnaires. Their identification in the practice will be recognized by the medications they are taking and in the behavior and attitude they present, such as:[41–47,48]

- frequent attempts at self diagnosis;
- changing chief complaints;
- clear preference for nonspecific treatment;
- overdescription of physical symptoms;
- impulsive and demanding behavior;
- impatience with time frame;
- poor tolerance for mild pain;
- inability to commit to a definite treatment plan;
- refusal to permit practitioner to speak with the patient's physician; or
- demonstration of obsessive behaviors.

Some of these individuals may develop displaced anxieties over planned treatment, leading to the belief that agreed-upon treatment is not working and causing mistrust. When taking the patient's history, practitioners often note the presence of psychotherapeutic agents such as selective serotonin reuptake inhibitors (SSRIs), as well as other medications.[49,50]

Frequently, because of lack of training or a prior difficult experience, practitioners harbor some fears of potentially negative and aversive behavior. But with experience, practitioners can learn to recognize and manage these warning signs and gain skills in managing behaviors that left unattended, almost always lead to failed treatment. How we interpret and assess these responses and decide which simple behavioral modality will help facilitate treatment compliance will be discussed in the next chapter.

## SUMMARY

In this chapter, we have discussed some ramifications of the assessment, collection, and identification of the various factors that can affect whether or not a patient decides to receive care and remain with a particular practitioner. There are many factors and variables that need to be considered, and also many individuals involved in the identification, recognition, and collection of a patient's concerns, feelings, and behaviors that eventually determine whether or not optimal dental care will ensue. The task of the practitioner and staff is to carefully examine and prioritize the management of those concerns that have led to the development of fear and avoidance. The information from the patient should also act as a guide to determine whether or not the dentist has the skills to manage such individuals, and feels comfortable in doing so, or not. The use of pretreatment questionnaires, beginning with the initial phone contact, followed by a home mailing, a return of the completed forms, and preconsultation review, may appear unwarranted measures to some of my readers, but they are exceptional tools that according to the positive results of many studies, have been shown to help sharpen diagnostic skills and enable the dental practitioner to plan positive strategies that lead to successful treatment. The knowledge that each patient has conveyed from these questionnaires has proven to be the single most helpful behavioral management tool I have had available in lessening and in some cases ameliorating the fear in some individuals. They should be the first and most important instrument in a practitioner's armamentarium of behavior management instruments.

# REFERENCES

1. Pruett H. 2007. Listening to patients. *J Calif Dent Assoc* 35:183–5.
2. Weiner, A. 1994. *The Difficult Patient: A Guide to Understanding and Managing Dental Anxiety*, 3rd edn. Randolph, MA: Reniew Publishing Co.
3. Buck, R. 1984. *The Communication of Emotion*. New York: Guilford Press.
4. Sondell K and Soderfeldt B. 1997. Dentist-patient communication: A review of relevant models. *Acta Odontol Scand* 5:116–26.
5. Weiner A and Weinstein P. 1995. Dentists' knowledge, attitudes and assessment practices in relation to fearful dental patients: A pilot study. *Gen Dent* 43:164–8.
6. Ong LM, DeHaes J, Hoos A, et al. 1995. Doctor patient communication: A review of the literature. *Soc Sci Med* 40:903–18.
7. Yamalik N. 2005. Dentist-patient relationship and quality care: Modification of behavior. *Int Dent J* 55:395–7.
8. Mauksch L, Dugdale D, Dodson S, et al. 2008. Relationship, communication, and efficiency in the medical encounter. *Arch Intern Med* 168:1387–94.
9. Karoly K, Berggrfen U, and Hallberg L. 2000. Model of the dentist-patient consultation in a clinic specializing in the treatment of dental phobic patients: A qualitative study. *Acta Odontol Scand* 58:63–71.
10. Harris M and Rosenthal R. 1986. Nonverbal aspects of empathy and rapport in the physician-patient interaction. In: Harris M and Rosenthal R (eds.), *Nonverbal communication in the clinical context*. University Park and London: Pennsylvania State University Press.
11. Riggio R. 1992. Social interaction skills and nonverbal behavior. In: Feldman R (ed.), *Application of Nonverbal Behavioral Theories and Research*. Hillsdale, New Jersey: Erlbaum.
12. Luallin M and Sullivan K. 1998. The patient's advocate: A six part strategy for building market share. *Group Pract J* 47(July–August):13–6.
13. Bernstein L and Bernstein R. 1980. *Interviewing: A Guide for Health Professionals*, 3rd edn. New York: Appleton-Century-Crofts.

14. Geboy M. 1984. *Communication and Behavior Management in Dentistry*. Philadelphia, PA: B.C. Decker, Inc.
15. Desmond J and Copeland L. 2000. *Communicating with Today's Patients: Essentials to Save Time, Decrease Risk, and Increase Patient Compliance*. San Francisco: Jossey-Bass.
16. Dworkin S, Ferrence T, and Giddon D. 1978. *Behavioral Science and Dental Practice*. St. Louis, MO: C.V. Mosby.
17. Dailey Y, Humphris G, and Lennon M. 2001. Dental anxiety: The use of dental anxiety questionnaires: A survey of a group of UK dental practitioners. *Br Dent J* 190:450–3.
18. Humphris G, Clarke H, and Freeman R. 2006. Does completing a dental anxiety questionnaire increase anxiety? A randomized controlled trial with adults in general practice. *Br Dent J* 201:33–5.
19. Corah N. 1969. Development of a dental anxiety scale. *J Dent Res* 48: 596.
20. Scott D and Hirshman R. 1982. Psychological aspects of dental anxiety in adults. *J Am Dent Assoc* 104:27–31.
21. Scott D, Hirschman R, and Schroder K. 1984. Historical antecedents of dental anxiety. *Journal of the American Dental Association* 108:42–5.
22. Kleinknecht R, McGlynn F, Thorndike R, et al. 1984. Factor analysis of the Dental Fear Survey with cross validation. *J Am Dent Assoc* 108:59–61.
23. Kress C. 1988. Patient satisfaction with dental care. *Dent Clin North Am* 32(4):791–802.
24. Gatchel J. 1989. The prevalence of dental fear and avoidance: Expanded adult and recent adolescent surveys. *J Am Dent Assoc* 118:591–3.
25. Ayer W and Corah N. 1984. Behavioral factors influencing dental treatment. In: Cohen L and Bryant P (eds.), *Social Sciences and Dentistry: A Critical Bibliography*, Vol. II. Kingston-upon-Thames: England Quintessence Publishing Co., pp. 267–322.
26. Corah N, Zielenzny M, O'Shea R, et al. 1986. Development of an interval scale of anxiety response. *Anesth Prog* 33:220–4.
27. Corah N, O'Shea R, and Bissell G. 1986.The dentist-patient relationship: Mutual perceptions and behaviors. *J Am Dent Assoc* 113:253–5.
28. Corah N, O'Shea R, Bissell G, et al. 1988. The dentist–patient relationship: Perceived dentist behaviors that reduce patient anxiety and increase satisfaction. *J Am Dent Assoc* 116:73–6.
29. Milgrom P, Weinstein P, Kleinknecht R, et al. 1995. *Treating Fearful Dental Patients: A Patient Management Handbook*, 2nd edn. Seattle: University of Washington.
30. Milgrom P, Cullen T, Whitney C, et al. 1996. Frustrating patient visits. *J Public Health Dent* 56(1):6–11.
31. Weiner A, Forgione A, and Weiner L. 1998. Survey: Incidence of fear of treatment in new patients in a dental school clinic. *J Mass Dent Soc* 47(1):16–21.
32. Weiner A, Sheehan D, and Jones J. 1986. Dental anxiety: The development of a measurement model. *Acta Psychiatr Scand* 73:559–65.

33. Weiner A and Sheehan D. 1988. Differentiating anxiety-panic disorders from psychologic dental anxiety. *Dent Clin North Am* 32(4):823–40.

34. Weiner A and Weinstein P. 1995. Dentist's knowledge, attitudes and assessment practices in relation to the fearful dental patient: A pilot study. *Gen Dent* 43:164–8.

35. Baron R, Logan H, and Kao C. 1990. Some variables affecting dentists' assessment of patients' distress. *Health Psychol* 9:143–53.

36. Hendrix W. 1986. Dental stress model and assessment questionnaire. *Dent Clin North Am* 33(Suppl):S1–10.

37. Weiner A, Forgione A, Hwangh J, et al. 2000. Potential fear-provoking patient experiences during treatment. *Gen Dent* 48(4):466–7.

38. Weiner A, Zemnick C, and Ganda K. 2002. Comparison of anxiety responses in HIV positive patients to non HIV individuals. *J Mass Dent Soc* 51(3):12–6.

39. Brosky M, Keefer O, Hodges J, et al. 2003. Patient perceptions of professionalism in dentistry. *J Dent Educ* 67(8):909–15.

40. Kages U, Sadjadi Z, Lojek L, et al. 2007. Development of a questionnaire measuring treatment concerns in regular dental patients. *Community Dent Oral Epidemiol* 36:219–227.

41. Bare L and Dundes L. 2004. Strategies for combatting dental anxiety. *J Dent Educ* 68:1172–7.

42. Corah N, O'Shea R, and Skeels D. 1982. Dentists' perceptions of problem behaviors in patients. *J Am Dent Assoc* 104(6):829–33.

43. Smith T, Weinstein P, Milgrom P, et al. 1984. An evaluation of an institution-based dental fears clinic. *J Dent Res* 63:272–5.

44. Rouse R and Hamilton M. 1990. Dentist's technical competence communication and personality as predictors of dental patient anxiety. *J Behav Med* 13(3):307–19.

45. Clark J and Morton J. 1980. Behavioral assessment: An appraisal of beliefs and behaviors relating to treatment. *Oral Health* 70(1):71–7.

46. Centore L, Reisner L, and Pettengill C. 2002. Better understanding your patient from a psychological perspective: Early identification of problem behaviors affecting the dental office. *Canadian Dental Journal* 30(7):512–9.

47. American Psychiatric Association. 1987. *Diagnostic Criteria from DSM III.* Washington DC: American Psychiatric Association.

48. Psychiatric Association. 2004. *Diagnostic and Statistical Manual of Mental Disorders: DSM–IV Guide Book*, 4th edn., text rev. Washington, DC: American Psychiatric Association, pp. 231–4.

49. Weiner A and Stark P. 2008. Patient-perceived anxiety levels associated with use of selective serotonin and serotonin norepinephrine reuptake inhibitors. *J Mass Dent Soc* 57(1):22–6.

50. Ashok R and Sheehan D. 1999. The use of selective serotonin reuptake inhibitors in panic disorder. *Home Health Care Consult* 6(4):15–19.

# Chairside management of the fearful dental patient: behavioral modalities and methods

Arthur A. Weiner

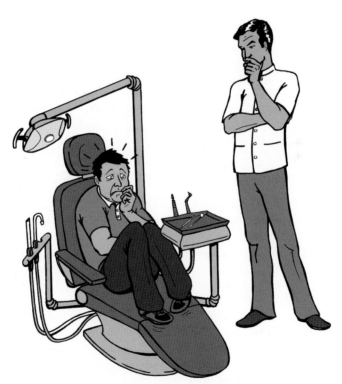

*"Let's see... Do I try distraction, positive attribution, relaxation... or bribery???"*

*The Fearful Dental Patient: A Guide to Understanding and Managing.* Edited by Arthur A. Weiner
© 2011 Blackwell Publishing Ltd.

# INTRODUCTION

In the preceding chapters, we have discussed the basic concepts associated with phobias and emotions of anxiety and fear. We have also mentioned the various common determinants associated with creating fearful dental patients and their chairside implications as determined by the findings of numerous dental and nondental clinical studies. The previous chapters discussed numerous factors that affect the assessment, collection of information, and identification of the dentally fearful individual, as well as chairside implications and considerations that can affect the success or failure of treatment.

In this chapter, I would like to present both a model that brings together findings from past studies and personal experiences, and a cohesive chairside program that follows from that model, for the behavior management and lessening of fear of dental treatment before, during and after the office visit. Using this model and clinical program, dental practitioners should be able easily to formulate and adapt a similar successful chairside model program suitable to their unique needs and practice styles. By utilizing this information and combining it with their own personal experiences, they can construct, as I have done, a successful chairside approach that lessens, and makes manageable, dental fears found in the clinical practices of dentistry.

# THE CONCEPT OF THE DENTAL PRACTITIONER AS A "FACILITATOR OF CHANGE"

One of the first changes I recognized that had to take place before I would see any successful modification of a patient's behavior was that I would first need change my own behavior and approach to both the anxious, fearful person as well as the nonfearful ones. As dental practitioners, we do make changes automatically to accommodate every patient problem, and every patient complaint, whether confronted with it in our office, or when we try to convince patients to improve their home care. We become empathetic, bending in our verbal and nonverbal behavior to make them comfortable and at ease. We modify a technique to make it appear less fearful. Most of the time, we make these changes quite naturally, fitting our responses to meet the demands of the situation better, and sometimes we do this without even realizing that we have, in fact, changed a portion of our routine.

Conversely, patients often do the same to us when they attempt to:

- control their treatment;
- lessen a fee;
- insist upon a certain type of restoration; or
- change an appointment date.

Dworkin[1-3] mentions that one of the basic clichés of any change in behavior or attitude involving an interpersonal relationship between two or more individuals is that when the behavior of one individual within a relationship changes, that change compels others in that relationship to change too. If dental practitioners wish to change the behavior of patients to more positive and well-meaning goals, then it is self-evident that clinicians must first consider examining and modifying their own behavior, and do the same when required. When dental practitioners change their behavior to meet the needs of others in the dentist–patient interpersonal relationship, they demonstrate an understanding that such behavior change is a reciprocal process. When this reciprocal process works well, each individual has changed to behaviors that are both personally and interpersonally acceptable and positive. It is important to remember that when individuals seek dental care, they are in reality seeking a change, a change in their oral health and their well being. The rewards for making these behavioral changes include having a more compliant, appreciative and long-lasting patient relationship, as well as a much easier work environment. The patient becomes more enjoyable, and the dental practitioner feels not only more relaxed, but more satisfied as a healing health professional.

This change on the part of the patient may involve a wish for a different treatment plan or a change in treatment behaviors and attitudes from a past practitioner. There are a number of factors that the dental practitioner can focus upon that influence a patient's behavior, such as:

- physical and psychosocial environment;
- individual patient /dentist's perceptions;
- vicarious patient learning habits; and
- past negative and positive patient experiences.

Thus, the concept of change needs to be understood as it relates to:

- change that concerns the dentist as an agent of change;
- change that concerns the dental patient.

## Change associated with the dental practitioner

It cannot be stressed enough that in order for the dental practitioner to be able to cause a patient to understand, be motivated, accept, appreciate, and continue treatment without negative and disruptive behavior, the practitioner must be able to create changes that favor a positive patient relationship. The interaction and relationship that exist between patient and dentist is a mix of psychological/emotional variables including:

- fear;
- self-esteem;
- variations in personalities,
- environment, and
- parental and cultural influences.

These patient factors are also found to some extent within the practitioner, who inevitably has self-esteem needs, as well as personality traits that were either learned or perhaps inborn. Ideally, these practitioner characteristics are largely positive and can be used to good advantage by the dentist as a change agent. But in any case, the practitioner as a person is an equal contributor to that complex interaction we call "the dentist–patient relationship." When these factors collide with each other and the relationship that ensues is not positively shaped, such a relationship can shift from friendship to anger and frustration. Behaviors that negatively affect and shape the patient–dentist relationship need to be minimized by effecting a change that creates a positive flavor to the dentist–patient interaction.

## Chairside clinical implications of change

The occurrence of positive changes in the dentist–patient interaction permits the practitioner to maximize his or her ability:

- to efficiently gather and provide information;
- to determine and discuss reasons for past inappropriate dental behavior, and develop a positive change strategy for specific individuals; and
- to develop trust and rapport more easily, leading to treatment compliance and patient satisfaction.

The dental practitioner must deal on a daily basis with a variety of inappropriate behaviors and conflicts—having typically received little to no education in how to understand or manage them. Too often, these psychological, emotional, cultural, and economic concerns result in behaviors that lead to uncompleted treatment. That these aversive behaviors present frequent difficulties, which interfere with treatment, is reason enough for dental practitioners to want to take suitable actions to create an environment that permits only positive behavior while minimizing the negative ones. The practitioner must develop an increased willingness to listen, along with an increased sensitivity that causes them to become totally aware of what the patient perceives his or her needs and goals to be. This must include an increased effort and determination to gain an understanding and perception of the cause of a patient's negative actions, along with conduct on the part of the dentist that demonstrates the practitioner perceives these behaviors as problematic and is willing to help the patient cope with them. Practitioners must constantly engage their patients and learn to use a variety of behavioral strategies that minimize conditions the patient perceives to be negative and maximize those the patient perceives to be positive.

## A facilitator of change

The dental practitioner must act as a "facilitator of change" and implement change whenever the dentist–patient interaction is perceived to be either becoming uncomfortable or interfering in the optimal provision of care. In this situation, it is the dentist who must be the first in the relationship to institute change, permitting the patient's behavior change to be the result of the practitioner's new behavior.

For me, the way to attain these goals successfully, and to be able to change when circumstances within the ongoing interaction demand, has been through the use of:

- pretreatment, as well as mid-and posttreatment questionnaires;
- a well-developed set of listening and communication skills;
- a clear set of behavioral change or behavior modification strategies; and
- a readiness to change *my* routine behavior to behavior that meets the needs and goals of the patient without sacrificing any of my own objective and subjective needs and goals.

The information collected from a compilation of items studied on prior on questionnaires[4-20] and presented to patients in the form of self-report questionnaires, provides me with the information necessary, to gain an insight into needs, goals, and make-up of the individuals seeking care. It permits me to be pre-prepared to change from my professionally trained method of providing care to an approach that initially will not appear threatening and in conflict with the needs and care the patient perceives he or she requires.

For example, this is a situation I am sure many practitioners have encountered, the patient who does not wish to have local anesthesia. Dentists, however, routinely works with such anesthesia for the comfort of the patient and the ease of providing pain-free dentistry to their patients. I often used the following example to my students when discussing the need for the practitioner to institute a change in behavior in order to accomplish a desired end result, in this case, the restoration of a large carious lesion.

A young man had presented to our office for the restoration of several large carious lesions. The information collected from our pretreatment questionnaires and initial office consultation provided little information concerning any fear of dental treatment, either past or present. There was no apparent fear of needles, no past negative experience with previous care, and a medical and dental history that was essentially uneventful. The patient stated that after his discharge from active duty and a lengthy period of unemployment, his oral care had slipped.

After completing the required periodontal prophylaxis, we suggested to him that we begin by treating the largest of the decayed teeth first. The patient informed me that he was a former Green Beret and that he could withstand a great deal of pain, and that he preferred no regional anesthetic. He stated he had endured far worse discomfort on the battlefield than that caused by drilling a tooth. I agreed to begin without a local anesthetic even though I doubted he could endure the discomfort that was to follow.

By proceeding in this manner, that is, agreeing to accept the patient's self-perceived lack of need of anesthesia, I have immediately demonstrated:

- That by offering to change my normal operating behavior, I am permitting the patient to realize that his current need for no anesthesia, has been recognized by me and that it supersedes my need to use Novocain routinely.
- That *I am an individual who is sensitive to his motivations and perceptual needs*, and is willing to proceed initially in a manner less threatening to his well-being.

In doing so, I am confirming a willingness to adapt to his needs immediately rather than trying to figure out what other motives are behind his refusal to want anesthesia. However, although I am willing to change my behavior, I expect that the patient will have a mutual and reciprocal willingness to modify his behavior, should circumstances arise that interfere with my ability to provide excellent dentistry. If my change of behavior is to act as a vehicle and initiate a reciprocal positive change in his behavior, when required, a mutual understanding has to be reached: that should during the preparation of the tooth the drill causes undue discomfort and result in frequent interfering movements, the patient must be willing to change and permit me:

- to demonstrate that I can provide a relatively pain-free injection; and
- to complete the dental treatment in a comfortable and pain-free manner thanks to the use of anesthesia.

## Chairside clinical consideration

To be able to facilitate a change in a patient's behavior, the dentist must consistently:

- Recognize when the patient or the practitioner perceives that a problem exists.
- Discuss the existence of the problem, and validate the patient's perception that a problem exists.
- Implement an appropriate strategy to alleviate the immediate difficulty.

If in this case, the patient still refuses to receive anesthesia, and I believe that without it an inability exists on my part to restore the tooth properly, I do not immediately institute treatment without attempting to learn the reasons for the patient's refusal. Highly anxious patients often report more pain during dental injections.[21–29] I find it imperative to know exactly why the patient refuses the dental injection by posing the following questions on a scale of Likert scale 1–5.

This series of questions is posed during the initial consult with the patient, and as the responses are elicited, I discuss each one, attempting to find out what if any past experiences or vicariously learned negative cognitions are influencing the responses. We also attempt to inform patients about newer techniques now available, if I determine that their present thoughts are influenced by past out-of-date experiences and knowledge. If necessary, I will devote additional time to demonstrating my technique using topical anesthetic, and if that is insufficient, I will add the nitrous oxide-oxygen conscious-analgesia concept, the objective being to demonstrate that dental anesthesia administration can be pain free and permit discomfort-free dentistry to occur. I also like to remind the patient that drilling can excessively overstimulate the nerve tissue fibers and that local anesthesia not only prevents pain now, but also keeps the tooth healthier and pain free in the future.

This questionnaire is hand held by the patient as we address and discuss each item on the sheet.

---

**Situations Associated with My Fear of the Dental Injection**

**1.** not at all, **2.** very slightly **3.** Moderately fearful, **4.** severely fearful **5.** Avoid completely

**I am bothered**

1.  Thought of the pain on the needle piercing my gums. 1  2  3  4  5
2.  Thought of the pain before I receive the injection.  1  2  3  4  5
3.  The needle will break requiring surgery to remove. 1  2  3  4  5
4.  I hate the sight of the needle. It terrifies me       1  2  3  4  5
5.  I get very anxious the moment of the injection      1  2  3  4  5
6.  The needle might damage a nerve or blood vessel 1  2  3  4  5
7.  I am very hard to get numb and need extra
    Novocain                                             1  2  3  4  5
8.  I am afraid I might be allergic to the Novocain     1  2  3  4  5
9.  The feeling of numbness might not go away          1  2  3  4  5
10. I fear my throat will be numb and I will not be     1  2  3  4  5
    able to swallow and might choke.
11. I might move and cause the dentist to injure me    1  2  3  4  5
12. Feeling the needle poke through my gums is
    the worst                                            1  2  3  4  5
13. The needle might not be clean                       1  2  3  4  5

---

If after going over the entire questionnaire I cannot change the patient's behavior, I then suggest that a referral might be needed to seek any hidden emotional or psychological disorders influencing the patient's decision in this matter.

## Change associated with the dental patient

The process of helping the patient change begins, obviously, with the practitioner ascertaining what the patient's perception of the problem is, and then providing assurance that the problem is one which is valid—and valid simply because the patient perceives it to be so. It is not necessary most of the time for the practitioner to know the exact and true cause of the fear. The real objective of the dentist in facilitating a change is to identify and manipulate whatever factors exist in the psychosocial–physiological environment that are presently fearful to the patient, so as to be able to deliver the desired optimal dental care today and understand what will be required tomorrow.

## Three chairside clinical objectives

- Determine the needs, goals and motivations of patient.
- Assess the existing relationship between the dentist and patient, i.e., the degree of trust and rapport that exist, in an effort to determine the best behavioral modality to utilize so as to achieve the best behavioral results.
- Relate to the patient in terms and wordings that are designed to minimize circumstances the patient perceives as negative and threatening, and to maximize those conditions the patient perceives to be positive and not threatening or fear provoking.*

In my practice, to accomplish the first of these three objectives—determining needs, goals and relevant past experience—we utilized questionnaires such as those found on Chapter 2.

First, and most important, is the determination of needs and goals of the individual. These factors directly influence the patient's behavior, with a resulting impact on the practitioner's ability to affect change. For the dental practitioner it is necessary to:

(1) *Understand* the patients' needs, the *whys* and where they arise from.
(2) *Acknowledge* those needs and communicate to the patient our understanding of them and our desire to help them achieve and fulfill those needs and goals.
(3) *Convey* the message as dentists, both verbally and nonverbally, of our intentions and objectives in a manner that is persuasive but not overbearing so as to influence and change their behavior to positive and acceptable modes.

In the preceding chapters, we have emphasized the many emotional, anxious/fearful factors, and feelings associated with past dental care or

---

*Portions of this section are reprinted from Dworkin S. 1978. *Behavioral Science and Dental Practice*. St. Louis, MO: CV Mosby, with the permission of the author, Dr. Samuel Dworkin.

avoidance of care. These following factors are also equally important considerations in the second objective in producing change: assessing the dentist–patient relationship and the ability for the practitioner to facilitate change. The practitioner should ascertain

- What is this patient's overall attitude toward dentistry in general?
- Why, if a new patient, has the individual chosen you as his or her new dentist?
- What, if any, are the patient's negative past experiences, and how have they shaped his or her present fears, attitudes, and emotions?
- What are the patient's individual personality traits, age, education level, occupation, and past dental history?
- What degree of positive influence, if any, already exists over this patient? Those referred to you by a former patient may already have a certain level of trust in you, facilitating a greater willingness on the part of the patient to accept help offered by the practitioner in coping with such patients perceive to be their problem.
- What are your behavior management and treatment objectives regarding this patient, and how do you intend to achieve them? What are your long term goals?
- What strategy will best suit this individual? How and when will you present this change strategy? Can you reason with this individual? Does the patient have the ability to understand the need and importance of the intended treatment?

The third objective affecting the patient's change is determining what behavioral strategy a practitioner decides to implement. The dental practitioner, in making this decision, must understand and deal with all of the factors that play a role in the patient's behavior. The practitioner, in attempting to change a patient's behavior, must be confident that his or her messages are heard, understood, and accepted as truth by the patient. The message, whether it be a strategy to overcome fear and anxiety or the presentation of a treatment plan, should be presented in an orderly and logical sequence in a manner that will positively influence the behavior of a specific patient.

To construct and influence strategies that will have positive effects on a patient, one must constantly assess a patient's physical and psychological state of well-being. A periodic review and update of a patient's history, as well as the degree of positive progress an implemented strategy has provided, will allow the practitioner to identify potential sources of influence clearly as they develop. Constant monitoring of behavioral progress using mid treatment questionnaires also helps eliminate any minor existing negative influences still being perceived by the patient as a problem. I realize that all these tasks must seem monumental and requiring time that may not immediately appear to be rewarding financially. But I can emphatically state that if you are looking to reduce stress, lessen negative behavior, increase patient satisfaction, lessen cancelled and broken appointments, add this modality of "behavior change" to your treatment armamentarium and watch treatment compliance increase.

This concept that I advocate is not a difficult one; in reality, it is quite simple. The issue from where I see it is not that it is difficult to get patients to change away from their negative, aversive and fearful behavior, because it is not; the difficulty is trying to get the dental practitioner to change from only paying attention to the things needed to fix the patient's dentition. Two elements must change if a practitioner wishes to improve his management skills in treating the fearful patient, and they are the patient and the dentist. I try to attach a change in behavior to a patient's importance and value they may place on treatment previously rendered or presently needed.

For example:

- For the patient who has recently completed extensive periodontal treatment, I would suggest:

   The reason you undertook such intensive and expensive treatment was to improve your oral health, lessen your embarrassing bad breath, and improve your smile and well being. In the past, the cause for your periodontal disease was your lack of brushing, flossing and regular check-ups. Studies have shown that patients who maintain regular dental visits, and exhibit good home care habits, demonstrate fewer reoccurrences of previous periodontal disease and loss of teeth. I believe, that after all you have gone through, this has to motivate you to change your past neglectful behavior. You would not want to go through all that time and expense again, would you?

- A similar approach can be used to motivate the patient who has extensive caries involvement in their dentition, due to neglect and avoidance. To motivate this type of patient, I often search the past dental history, looking for some factor or occurrence that the patient has emphasized as hoping never to experience. A good example is the patient whose history demonstrates parents who wear dentures and who constantly has to listens to them complain about their difficulty with eating or speaking, or with dentures falling out when the wearer is talking. To such patients' complaining how they hate to always see that or worrying that the same fate could befall him or her, I express empathy and attempt to initiate a change in behavior by trying to use their dislike of their parents' situation, and to encourage these patients that by restoring their own badly decayed teeth, they prevent a similar repetition of their parents' problems happening to them.

*Remember that it is the dentist who must change first, because it is the dentist who is the vehicle of change for the patient's change. It is the key to behavioral management success.*

However, the dentist as a change agent does not seek to change the patient, per se, but only to change some of the patient's behaviors and negative emotions, like anxiety, when they arise in the dental office.

# STEP-BY-STEP CHAIRSIDE MODEL FOR FEAR AMELIORATION IN THE FRIGHTENED DENTAL PATIENT

## Part 1: The office model

The first management technique begins with the first contact the patient has with our office, and that is with the receptionist. Our receptionist has been trained to ask a specific set of questions when a new patient calls for an initial appointment and to listen intently, paying attention to tone and content of the conversation. The receptionist must at all times be dignified, calm, empathetic, and understanding. After securing the patient's name and phone number in case a disconnection occurs, the receptionist is instructed to ask specific questions regarding the following topics:

- Reason for appointment: The reason for the appointment—emergency or regular check-up. This allows us to determine the exact reason for the appointment.
- Any special concerns, fear, anxieties over treatment, past and present?: This question ideally will inform us of any fears or concerns about specific treatment, dentist's attitudes, past experiences, or negative thoughts and cognitions. The tone of the patient's expressions are noted, angry, calm, demanding, full of questions, or only statements of fear and concern about changing dentists. (Answers are noted.)
- Who referred you to this office?: It is important to know this for a couple of reasons: First is so as to be able to thank the individual responsible both for the referral and for having the sort of confidence in our ability to refer another person; second, to determine if individual was a prior frightened individual whom we successfully treated and lessened their fears. If so, it makes the referral even more meaningful. It indicates a past success. (Answers are listed.)
- Specific reason for changing dentist: What specific reasons are influencing changing dentist? This gives us the opportunity to learn past negative feelings or experiences a prior practitioner may have visited on the individual, which we prefer not to duplicate. We are also interested in any positive experiences the patient wishes to relate.
- How long ago was last dental visit?: How long has it been since the patient's last regular visit to a dentist? It permits us to learn what issues have influenced the avoidance of care, what, if any, negative cognitions in the patient's psychosocial sphere played a role in influencing the lack of care. (Answers are listed.)

- Specific physical needs, if any: Any special physical needs that the patient requires to ensure their comfort? This permits us to become aware if any special accommodations are required due to a physical handicap or medical disorder.
- The most convenient time for appointments: It is important to inquire whether a patient prefers a morning or afternoon appointment. Some individuals seem to function better during different times of the day, including coping better with fear or anxiety. Handicapped individuals and those with other medical conditions also have their own time of day that they function optimally.

During the initial phone contact, the receptionist can also begin the process of fear/anxiety reduction by informing the frightened patient that this dentist has a special interest in working with individuals who are apprehensive of dental treatment. Whatever the tone or reasons for requesting an appointment, the receptionist should always find a way to comment, "Well, you have come to the right office; Dr. Weiner is known for being very successful in treating fearful and anxious individuals. We have many, many wonderful patients who would gladly attest to that." Remember, the first contact and the first opportunity to make a favorable impression starts with your receptionist and the initial phone call.

After I have consulted with my receptionist and reviewed both the patient's responses to the questions and the receptionist's impressions, notes are entered into the patient's record concerning the overall impression of the initial contact. This extra time we take helps me to understand the patient's needs and goals better, and serves as an opportunity to begin to establish trust and rapport. From this point, the patients are mailed a set of questionnaires as determined from their tone, content of information given and overall impression of the initial contact. These are described in Chapter 3, Figures 3.1–3.6. A stamped return envelope is included in the mailing. Usually, the initial appointment will be set up in a well-lit, comfortable area devoid off any equipment or relationship to dental care, and scheduled to permit adequate time for a complete and informative discussion.

## Reception room phase of program

The behavior in the reception area can serve to provide and early indication of the emotional state of the patient, whether or not he or she is anxious, calm, etc. The individual best suited to monitor this behavior is the receptionist. We utilize a patient observation form that permits the receptionist to note the patient's behavior; the receptionist is instructed, if uncomfortable or anxious behavior is noted, to meet and engage the patient in person (see Figure 4.1).

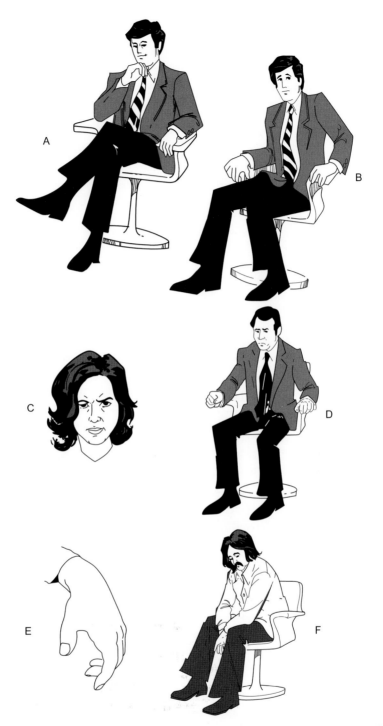

**Figure 4.1** Reception room monitoring. (A) relaxed, (B) sitting with white-knuckle grip, demonstrating possible anxiety or tendency to leave, (C and D) anger—frustration, (E and F) depression, feeling of hopelessness, "why me?"
Source: Dworkin S. 1978. *Behavioral Science and Dental Practice*. St. Louis. MO: CV Mosby. Used with permission.

---

**Receptionist Patient Observation Assessment**

**0 – None at all, 1 – a little, 2 – Moderately, 3 – Severely**

Fidgeting with hands or object                                           _____

Sitting on edge of chair or leaning forward            _____

Pacing                                                                                _____

Frequent changes in sitting position                        _____

Repetitious hand or leg movements                          _____

Frequent visits to rest room                                       _____

Arrive on time?   Yes___ No___ Never on time     _____

---

The dental practitioner can utilize the information relayed by the receptionist from his or her phone observations, and combine it with the information collected from the return of the previously mailed questionnaires to construct a specific plan for the approaching initial consult. The practitioner upon reviewing all the collected data can determine which areas need to be attended to and which areas in the sphere of dental care the patient does not perceive as presenting major concerns. All the bits of information received from the initial phone call and the returned questionnaires serve as pieces of the puzzle that when put together with the additional information gained during the consultation, guide us in determining what direction we need to proceed to lessen the individual's fear. The questionnaires and consultation represent a compilation, a log book of the patient's past fears, experiences, likes and dislikes, needs and goals. It is an up-to-date diary of their life's experiences with dentistry.

## Assessing the patient's individual questionnaire responses

The most common fears that we note seem to be the same encountered by the average practitioner, only to a much greater degree of severity because they have been allowed to grow in intensity and overtake the individual's ability to cope. When this occurs, most individuals will invoke their built in defensive mechanisms, which is to avoid subjecting themselves to such threatening experiences.

When I review the material sent back by the patient, which contains both past and present medical and dental history, I first focus in on the responses found on the dental part of the questionnaire and the responses describing the bodily physical effects of their fear and anxieties. The reason for this is simple: the patient is seeking help in overcoming what they perceive to be problems related to dentistry, not medicine. True, their medical history will play an important role in determining the use of certain techniques, pharmacological agents, and length of treatment, but for the patient, it is not the prime reason for them sitting in my office. Let us take a sample dental questionnaire from a patient and follow it as I would in the consultation.

**Past and Present Dental History Survey**

**Example**

**Name:**          **Age:**          **Gender:  M  F**

Below is a list of experiences, situations, feelings and thoughts that are sometimes associated with dental treatment and that often cause individuals to become more or less fearful. Please circle to what degree each of the following situations or experiences causes you to feel fearful regarding treatment. This questionnaire is designed to help us help you. Your responses are very important to us and are strictly confidential. **Please do not skip any items**.

**1 = No Effect, 2 = Very Relaxed, 3 = Somewhat Relaxed, 4 = Moderately Fearful, 5 = Very Fearful**

**I FEEL:**

| | | | | | | |
|---|---|---|---|---|---|---|
| 1. | By the thought of the dental appointment before the actual visit............1 | 2 | 3 | X | 5 |
| 2. | By the thought of past dental experiences..................................................1 | 2 | 3 | X | 5 |
| 3. | While waiting in the reception area................................................................1 | 2 | 3 | 4 | X |
| 4. | Having the same bad experience a parent had............................................1 | 2 | X | 4 | 5 |
| 5. | When the dentist does not do as they say they will................................1 | 2 | 3 | X | 5 |
| 6. | With regard to the dental appointment and treatment in general...........1 | 2 | 3 | X | 5 |
| 7. | When the dentist and staff always make me feel comfortable................1 | X | 3 | 4 | 5 |
| 8. | When the dentist pokes fun at my fears............................................. | 1 | 2 | 3 | X | 5 |
| 9. | At the sight of the dental instruments..........................................................1 | 2 | X | 4 | 5 |
| 10. | By the lack of attention given me before, during and after Treatment.......1 | 2 | 3 | 4 | X |
| 11. | At being alone anytime in the dental chair.................................................1 | X | 3 | 4 | 5 |
| 12. | When the dentist seems rushed and I feel he is rushing my care................1 | 2 | 3 | X | 5 |
| 13. | When the dentist always asks me questions if I have any concerns..........1 | X | 3 | 4 | 5 |
| 14. | When the dentist answers my questions to my satisfaction....................1 | X | 3 | 4 | 5 |
| 15. | When I hear the sound of the drill.................................................................1 | 2 | X | 4 | 5 |
| 16. | When the dentist appears rushed and insensitive.....................................1 | 2 | 3 | 4 | X |
| 17. | When having my teeth drilled and worrying if the Novocain will work.................................................................................................1 | 2 | 3 | 4 | X |
| 18. | When the dentist fails to provide me with a signal to stop....................1 | 2 | 3 | 4 | X |
| 19. | When trapped in the dental chair.................................................................. 1 | 2 | X | 4 | 5 |
| 20. | When the dentist or hygienist make me feel guilty about my teeth........1 | 2 | X | 4 | 5 |
| 21. | When the dentist and staff praise my being a cooperative patient...........1 | X | 3 | 4 | 5 |
| 22. | When the dentist fails to explain the risks and benefits of the treatment.....1 | 2 | 3 | X | 5 |
| 23. | When the dentist fails to pay attention to my needs and goals..............1 | 2 | 3 | 4 | X |
| 24. | Knowing the dentist treats individuals with infectious diseases................X | 2 | 3 | 4 | 5 |
| 25. | Having to avoid certain places, things, activities because of fear.................X | 2 | 3 | 4 | 5 |
| 26. | When the dentist minimizes my need for additional Novocain.................1 | 2 | 3 | X | 5 |
| 27. | When not informed by the dentist what is to be done this visit.................1 | 2 | 3 | 4 | X |
| 28. | When the dentist makes me feel uncomfortable about asking Questions...............................................................................................1 | 2 | 3 | X | 5 |
| 29. | When I see the dental injection coming towards me.................................1 | 2 | 3 | X | 5 |
| 30. | When all the dentist wants to know is how much dental insurance I have or do not have.................................................................1 | 2 | 3 | 4 | X |

We initiate the consultation by going over each of the items on the questionnaire, allowing the patient sufficient time to explain how and why that particular item is a determinant of fear in his or her special case. This exercise allows patients to feel some degree of control over the interview while they inform me of what they perceive their problems to be and what caused them. If I am to succeed, patients must be able to tell me their likes, dislikes, and what they perceive has caused them to be fearful of care. During the consult, I constantly take notes of what the patient is saying. The purpose of this is at the end of the interview, I want to be able to repeat back in my own words, what I believe the patient has tried to tell me. In doing this, I accomplish two important tasks: (1) I demonstrate to the patient that I have been an interested listener and a willing and active participant in the conversation. (2) By relaying my interpretation of the consultation, I give the patient the chance to clear up any misinterpretations that may have occurred on my part. This avoids any chance of error and confusion that could later lead to anger and mistrust.

Once I have gone over the questionnaire, I also like to include a set of four questions suggested to me by Peter Milgrom of the University of Washington School of Dentistry back in the 1980s when I first asked for some help in initiating a fear amelioration program at Tufts Dental School. They are:

- What has caused you to seek treatment today?
- Has fear of dental treatment ever caused you to cancel or not appear for an appointment?
- Have you experienced any anxiety last night or today before the visit?
- What can I do as your dentist that would help you maintain your treatment and regular appointments? And conversely, what would I do that would make it more difficult and fearful for you, causing you to cancel and avoid treatment?

Once again, we take notes and allow the patient adequate time to respond, making sure we understand the response to the questions, and that the patient has been made to perceive that we do by our verbal and nonverbal responses. We also take notes at times during the conversation, and after going over all of the questionnaire, ask ourselves:

- If the patient appears more or less relaxed,
- Whether still frustrated over his or her dilemma.
- Did the patient more easily provide feedback to my inquiries at the end of the interview than in the beginning?
- Is the emotional flavor and tone of the patient's conversation more positive than it was earlier, and more open to new ideas?
- Does the patient's musculature and facial expressions appear more relaxed than at the beginning?

All this can be noted by the practitioner, by both listening to the verbal communication and observing the various nonverbal behavior cues being exhibited by the patient (Figure 4.2).

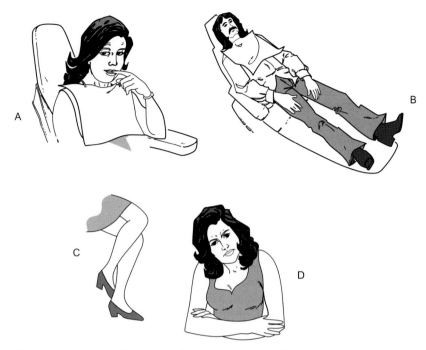

**Figure 4.2**   Noting the nonverbal cues being exhibited by the patient. Is the patient (A) deliberating or not sure, (B) relaxed, (C) with legs crossed, displaying anxiety and discomfort, or (D) anger—frustration?
Source: Dworkin S. 1978. *Behavioral Science and Dental Practice*. St. Louis. MO: CV Mosby. Used with permission.

During the entire length of the conversation, we are continuously cognizant of the three most fear-provoking situations individuals claimed during repeated investigations at Tufts School of Dental Medicine[8,15] (Figure 4.3, contains three most provoking fears as responded in two clinic studies.)

It is during the initial consultation that I attempt to discuss those responses noted in the preconsultation questionnaire mailed to the patient and returned prior to the interview. I feel that whatever extra time I spend, and whatever information I can gather by allowing the patient to express their fears and concerns freely, will greatly aid me in constructing a clear and specific program to help this patient. I also utilize this time to try to pose additional questions relating to those items responded to as major factors responsible for elevated levels of fear and avoidance, for example, fear of the dental injection. Dentist must be constantly aware of the fact that dental patients who have suffered negative experiences, especially regarding dental injection, may feel and exhibit elevated levels of pain, which most probably will lead to negative expectations for pending treatment.[10,11] Highly anxious dental patients usually feel more pain than do relatively less fearful individuals.[21–27] And fear of the dental injection is almost always a major cause of avoidance. If a patient expresses or has responded to this specific fear, I like to pose the following questions

Top 3 Questions Eliciting Fear

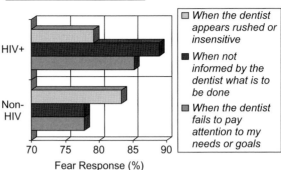

**Figure 4.3** Three most common fear-provoking situations. Reprinted from Weiner A, Zemnick C, and Ganda K. 2002. Comparison of anxiety responses in HIV positive patients to non HIV individuals. *J Mass Dent Soc* 51(3):12–6. © Journal of the Massachusetts Dental Society. Reprinted with permission. All rights reserved.

directly during the consultation, so as both to listen and to observe the verbal and nonverbal cues accompanying the responses. I keep various preprinted sets of questionnaires pertaining to a variety of known fear-causing stimuli for presentation during the consultation. I present them with the specific questionnaire and together we go over the responses.

---

### Needle Phobia Follow-Up Questionnaire

I ask the patient to respond to the following questions on a Likert scale of 1–5: 1 = not at all, 2 = somewhat fearful, 3 = moderately fearful, 4 = severely fearful, and 5 = avoid completely.

I become more or less fearful:

1. When I see the dental needle.
2. When I think of the needle penetrating my gums.
3. When I worry that the needle might break and require surgery to remove.
4. That the needle may damage a nerve or blood vessel.
5. Realizing I am hard to get numb, and the dentist might not believe me.
6. When the Novocain numbs my throat and I think I cannot swallow.
7. When I think the needle might not be clean.
8. That the dentist might slip and injure me.
9. When I worry if I might be allergic to the Novocain.
10. That the numbness will not go away and wondering whether or not the dentist will poke fun at my fears.

I listen to each response, paying attention to the tone of the response, the individual's interpretation of the cause of the fear of the injection, and always repeat back what he or she perceives caused the fear. I try to counter the negative perception of each item with a positive response; for example, I will explain the use of topical anesthetic to eliminate the feeling of penetrating the gums. For those who hate the prolonged feeling of numbness, I provide information about short-acting anesthetics. I explain the fine quivers and palpitations that some experience by explaining the effects of epinephrine and the reason for its incorporation into some local anesthetics, and, if necessary, how we can use anesthetic without it. For those that feel it will not wear off, we invite them to remain in the reception area as long as they wish, knowing well how long the anesthetic will last. We explain our methods on sterilization for those concerned about infection, and provide information regarding the flexibility and virtual non-breakable characteristics of the newer metals as well as the thinness to minimize discomfort. There is much the practitioner can do to overcome fear of injections once they learn the individual's specific thought and concerns.

Another fear-causing factor is the noise of the drill. Many patients state, "I can't stand the feeling and noise of the drill cutting through my teeth. It gives me a terrible feeling and fright. What if the dentist slips and, drills away more than is required?" There are numerous ways patients discuss their sensations and experiences. To help ease the terror and false cognition of grinding associated with this experience I try to associate the noise of the drill with the following explanation.

I ask the individual whether when they are out for a Sunday drive, they have ever passed by an old grist mill or seen a water wheel attached to a building and being powered by the stream of water. I explain to them that in olden days, the wheel powered by the water turned a stone within the house that milled the grains for flour. I then show them a small turbine saved from inside my dental hand piece. It looks similar to the paddles on the water wheel, except that this turbine is operated by forced air from a compressor within the dental office.

I explain that in order to keep the drill bit turning, the air travels to the small hole at the end of the dental drill by decreasing the diameter of the piping to maintain a certain air pressure. I allow them to feel the forced air exiting the hand-piece and demonstrate that I can regulate the pressure, sound, and speed of the drill via the foot pedal. The next step is to ask them to try and whistle without puckering their lips. They can do this but produce no sound. I then instruct them to whistle with lips puckered and in doing so, they are able to produce a whistling sound. I explain to them that the noise of the drill is produced in the same way the whistling was, by increasing the pressure of air as it passes through a very small passageway. The noise is not produced by the drill bit cutting tooth structure, but by forced air exiting through a tiny hole. It is sort of the *"drill whistling while it works."* It may sound like kid stuff, but to the frightened, dentally uneducated person, it is a fear-lessening story. Try it some time; you may be pleasantly surprised.

I could fill the pages with many similar explanations we utilize to explain a patient's past negative experiences, false cognitions and concerns of repetitions of past negative experiences.

Many patients worry about gagging when they have to have impressions or x-rays taken. We try to reassure them that I have two ways to prevent their gag reflex:

(1)   the use of nitrous oxide-oxygen analgesia; and
(2)   neurosensory distraction.

First, I utilize light levels of nitrous oxide-oxygen conscious sedation to do away with the gag reflex. This is a technique that I can readily demonstrate to a concerned patient without actually doing any dental treatment. I utilize the technique advanced by Harry Langa,[28] which involves an explanation and careful introduction to the patient of this conscious sedation technique. It is well known that nitrous oxide at low level (10%–15% $N_2O$ and 30% $O_2$) will eliminate the gag reflex. When the patient has reached a very light level of sedation and is alert and capable to understand and visualize the technique, I place a impression tray in the mouth, rub the soft palate with a tongue blade, and may even place an instrument down on the rear of the tongue to demonstrate that none of these actions cause gagging. It is a simple systematic way of illustrating a positive result to a previously negative and dreaded dental technique. It may also be utilized to expose a long forgotten and hidden past severe traumatic event that unconsciously may be influencing the present negative and aversive behaviors.

I would like to present a related technique that I have used quite successfully that utilizes the concept of nitrous oxide-oxygen inhalation conscious sedation. It concerns the insertion, at appropriate levels of sedation, of a post–hypnotic suggestion geared to elicit a hidden fear.[29]

I would like to add that in using this technique, one must be aware that many fearful patients are also fearful of the nasal mask and the sensation of losing control, so we thoroughly question patients concerning their feelings regarding these aspects associated with this technique. For this reason, the dental practitioner must proceed very slowly, introducing the patient to each of the steps that lead up to positive inhalation–sedation. That means properly teaching the patient correct breathing methods, as well as giving him or her the time to experience, slowly and gradually, the body and emotional changes that individuals experience with this technique, to become familiar with the nasal mask in place, allowing for adequate instruction and time for the patient to become receptive to this therapeutic regimen.

## Nitrous oxide-oxygen analgesia and the posthypnotic effect

This gaseous mixture produces an altered state of consciousness, enhancing right brain hemispheric activity. It permits the patient to be more concerned with inner thoughts and less concerned with what is happening in the operatory. Nitrous oxide-oxygen analgesia depresses the limbic centers, enabling patients to be more in touch with their feelings. During this time of increased right brain activity, patients can be guided toward introspection. Here, the practitioner can attempt to elicit the cause of the patient's extreme fear that has not been explained during the initial consultation.

After thorough and careful explanation of the techniques, making sure the patient's medical history permits the use of nitrous oxide-oxygen, and that there is willingness on the part of the patient, the practitioner slowly introduces the patient to the gaseous mixture. The level of nitrous oxide is raised until the mixture reaches 40%–55% of nitrous oxide. One must be sufficiently experienced so as not to allow the patient to approach the second stage of anesthetic excitement. When the patient is relaxed, I present the following suggestion: "Because you are very relaxed and completely at ease with your fear now gone, whatever is hidden in your subconscious, whatever you are unable to remember that has caused you to fear dentists and dental treatment, will now be remembered. It is perfectly safe for you to remember the traumatic event; no harm will come to you. When I remove the nasal mask, you will remember what has kept you from receiving dental care, it will come to the surface and you will no longer be fearful". I keep repeating this suggestion as the nitrous oxide is gradually reduced to 0%, and after 2 minutes of oxygenation, the mask is removed. In almost all of these cases, the response is usually spontaneous and informative, eliciting a variety of hidden fears that when fully discussed with the patient, markedly reduce the previous existing fear. It is a great technique but should only be used by the most experienced of clinicians.

*Neurosensory distraction*: For the practitioner who does not have this modality in their office, I recommend trying the following technique. It involves the principle of reciprocal inhibition, somewhat similar to the theory that a person cannot be relaxed and anxious at the same time. That is, if one can initiate a relaxation response strong enough, it will block out the anxiety response. Using this principle, we have found that if we can initiate a strong stimulation of the chorda tympani branch of the facial nerve, which supplies the dorsal anterior portion of the tongue, it will block out the activity of the glossopharyngeal nerve and its complex somatic sensory innervations of the base of the tongue, mucous membranes of the pharynx, fauces and palatine tonsil, and the nerve of taste to the posterior part of the tongue.

We place a small bolus of ordinary table salt on the tip of the tongue just prior to inserting the impression tray. I instruct the patient to touch the roof of his or her mouth twice with the salt, but not to swallow any of it. At this point, we have overexcited the sensory innervation of the chorda tympanic nerve, and have distracted the sensory stimulation of the glossopharyngeal complex. The impression tray is inserted, and it is very rare that we encounter the gag reflex utilizing this technique. Of course, this technique has limitations that are associated with diet and certain medical conditions.

Many times, patients are not fearful of the usual stimuli associated with heightened levels of anxiety, but rather, their concerns and anxieties are directed to whether or not the extensive restorative procedures they are about to undertake will be successful. These concerns are often detected in the initial phone call, and, if so, an additional questionnaire is enclosed in the preconsultation package (Figure 4.4).

The returned responses afford us the time to detect the major anxieties the patient is concerned about that might interfere with the sought-after treatment. It also gives us the time to construct positive responses to these concerns, the goal being to create a supportive environment that will help alleviate the patient's anxieties and ensure treatment compliance.

For the practitioner who is willing to spend the extra few moments, the initial consultation affords the opportunity to explain how he or she can help overcome each of the items the patient has noted as causing heightened levels of fear and avoidance. The average general dental practitioner instinctively uses a variety of behavioral techniques as a comprehensive part of everyday practice. Some are successful, while others fall short, the result being treatment failure and loss of the patient. The lack of self-awareness of how practitioners change to help fearful patients change too often results in the practitioner viewing the patient as a "problem patient"; this only decreases the chance that treatment will be successful, while it increases the chance that not only will the practitioner feel more stressed when working with a problem patient, but the patient will pick up on those cues and leave the dentist for someone else.

## Chairside clinical considerations for consultation success

To ensure positive and complete collection of the information needed to completely evaluate the patient and be able to construct a specific behavioral strategy that will meet the needs and goals of both the patient and the practitioner, the following steps should be considered:

- The use of pretreatment questionnaires mailed to the new patient's home, with a stamped return envelope enclosed.
- A preconsult evaluation of the returned forms followed by an initial consultation in a well lighted and comfortable room devoid of all things associated with dentistry.

## PATIENT ESTHETIC ANXIETY AND CONCERN QUESTIONNAIRE

Below is a list of situations, experiences, thoughts and feelings that some individuals may or may not have experienced in the past before today's office visit. The items mentioned below have been shown in certain cases to cause fear and avoidance of needed and recommended cosmetic dental treatment. Please circle the number to the right of each question that best describes the amount of anxiety and/or avoidance the following situations and concerns NOW cause you. Circle only one number of each question and do not skip any items. This questionnaire is designed to help us help you in your pursuit of that beautiful smile and healthy set of teeth.

**0 = Not at All Anxious      1 = A Little Anxious      2 = Moderately Anxious
3 = Markedly Anxious      4 = Severely Anxious      5 = Avoid Completely**

Do you fear dental treatment?      ☐ Yes      ☐ No

I become anxious and concerned.........

1.  When I think about visiting my dentist..............................................0 1 2 3 4 5
2.  About past negative experiences....................................................0 1 2 3 4 5
3.  Whether or not I will be happy with the outcome..............................0 1 2 3 4 5
4.  The dentist might not listen to my concerns and goals......................0 1 2 3 4 5
5.  That the cosmetic dentistry cost will be more than I can afford...........0 1 2 3 4 5
6.  That the outcome may look false and unnatural...............................0 1 2 3 4 5
7.  That the dentist might promise more than can be accomplished.........0 1 2 3 4 5
8.  That the dentist might object to my opinion and concerns.................0 1 2 3 4 5
9.  That the outcome might not be as I had hoped...............................0 1 2 3 4 5
10. That the dentist might not redo it if I am not satisfied with the          0 1 2 3 4 5
    outcome........................................................................................
11. Thinking about the degree of discomfort associated with these          0 1 2 3 4 5
    procedures.....................................................................................
12. When I compare other peoples' great smiles with mine....................0 1 2 3 4 5
13. That the resulting shape and shade will not be flattering...................0 1 2 3 4 5
14. That the dentist will not fully explain the associated risks and          0 1 2 3 4 5
    benefits.........................................................................................
15. That TV commercials only present the positive while leaving out        0 1 2 3 4 5
    negative results..............................................................................
16. That the dentist might rush and not confer with me..........................0 1 2 3 4 5
17. That my concept of beauty may differ from the dentist......................0 1 2 3 4 5
18. That the dentist will not compromise if we differ on color, shape and   0 1 2 3 4 5
    size..............................................................................................
19. That I may not be happy with my new smile...................................0 1 2 3 4 5
20. That my family and friends might not like my new smile....................0 1 2 3 4 5
21. That the long appointments will interfere with my employment............0 1 2 3 4 5
22. That the TV advertisements and cosmetic dentistry commercials        0 1 2 3 4 5
    might be misleading........................................................................
23. That my dentist might not have pictures or models of some prior        0 1 2 3 4 5
    cases...........................................................................................
24. That my teeth might need more than the available material can         0 1 2 3 4 5
    deliver...........................................................................................
25. That my dentist will not give me a suitable guarantee of success.........0 1 2 3 4 5

**Figure 4.4** Fear/anxiety questionnaire prior to anticipated esthetic restorative dentistry.
Source: Weiner A and Stark P. Fears and concerns of individuals contemplating esthetic restorative. In *Compendium of Continuing Education in Dentistry*, 31(6):446–454, July/August 2010.

- A careful item-by-item review of each of the major items marked as the cause of severe fright and avoidance, permitting the patient adequate time both to explain and to receive answers to these problems.
- Practitioner patience, both in not rushing the consultation and not neglecting and to ask and answer fully all the patient's questions and concerns.
- Constant demonstrations of concern and empathy for the patient. The dentist's actions and attitude must be such as to permit the patient to recognize and perceive that the practitioner is an attentive listener and a willing participant in the consultation. This is greatly facilitated by the practitioner repeating back to the patient what he or she perceives the patient's problems, needs, and goals to be thereby eliminating the chance for any misinterpretations.
- Be constantly alert aware for favorable and positive nonverbal cues of behavior, noting whether or not they demonstrate a decrease in tension and stress, or if the flow of information and interest has increased, and anger, fear, and frustration still remain or have decreased.
- Lastly, the practitioner's understanding of the patient's needs and concerns must correspond to the patient's understanding and perception of them.

Fearful individuals who receive a systematic approach aimed at making them calm and relaxed in a comfortable environment, supported by the dentist's positive and relaxed behavior, attitude and attentive, and supportive listening skills, experience a greater reduction in dental fear and anxiety than do individuals who have a standard interview in the dental chair.

## Presence of psychological and emotional disorders

The use of pretreatment questionnaires not only provides valuable information that might not be fully collected during a consult, but also allows the practitioner the advance opportunity and knowledge to construct a positive format for the interview. It enables the practitioner to structure the interview so as to meet the needs and goals of all the participants. It affords the practitioner advance knowledge about when to institute changes in behavior and attitudes of the patient by informing the practitioners as to when they themselves need to change their routine approach to one that permits their patients to realize that the dentist understands and is a eager partner, ready to help them overcome their problems of fear and anxiety.

Once the dental portion of the initial consultation is completed, we review the medical history, seeking any contraindications to treatment, allergies, or presence of any medications that might indicate the presence of an emotional or psychiatric disorders such as noted by Centore et al.[33] such as:

- tricylics for depression;
- selective serotonin reuptake inhibitors (SSRIs) eating disorders, obsessive-compulsive disorders, anxiety disorders;
- benzodiazepines for anxieties
- lithium for bipolar disorders; and
- opioids for chronic pain.

The medical history is the source that allows the practitioner to become aware of these problems, and its success depends on the practitioner's acumen in history taking. It invites an open and frank discussion concerning the reasons for these medications. It may help expose cases of depression, misplaced ideas concerning a particular obsession, some specific misdirected somatic anxiety, or potential problems with a particular phase of treatment. Outburst of anger and disruptive behavior during the consultation might be indicative of an impulsive behavior, for example, early assessment allows the practitioner a further opportunity to assess the patient's behavioral and dental concerns. It also allows practitioners to become aware of their own attitudes, and to determine whether they wish to treat this subsection of the dental population or not.

All practices contain difficult, frightened, highly anxious, and emotional patients. The medical history of some of these patients indicate treatment for various emotional psychological, psychiatric, and somatoform disorders with various psychopharmacological agents, such as SSRI and serotonin/norepinephrin reuptake inhibitor (SNRI) agents like Effexor XR, Paxil, Zoloft, Cymbalta (duloextine), and Prozac. Many practitioners are sometimes reluctant to treat such patients due perhaps to the belief that these patients will be difficult to deal with and may at times be disruptive. Many practitioners believe that the presence of these agents is a predictor of missed appointments, lack of trust, poor treatment response, and prolonged treatment time.

However, patients taking these above-mentioned psychopharmacological agents recently responded to a questionnaire, graded on a Likert scale of 1–5, with 5 being severely anxious, in a clinical study completed at Tufts Dental School.[30–32] It was noted that all the individuals in the study who were being treated with SSRIs seemed to recollect experiencing greater varying levels of fear and anxiety to a variety of previously experienced dental situations before being treated with their individual-specific drug regimens, as noted by their responses to the study questionnaire.

They did not present any of the negative behavior patterns that one would have expected, and, to date, have not presented any of the anticipated negative behaviors thought to occur. Further clinical studies in the future are required to validate this phenomenon, because the results rely on the patient's recollections of their attitudes and past behaviors prior to initiating drug therapy. It should be noted that it is not possible to assess the accuracy of patient's responses regarding past fears and emotions, as the effects of the current medications may cloud these recollections. It is important to note, though, that such a phenomenon was detected.

Once I summarize all that we have discussed during the consultation and allow the patient to correct any misinterpretations by me, I try to decide on a mutually agreeable plan to proceed, beginning with radiographs.

# CHAIRSIDE MANAGEMENT RESULTING FROM PATIENT'S CONSULTATION AND DETERMINANTS OF FEARS ELICITED

Having both agreed upon an initial plan at the end of the consultation, we begin by paying attention to the patient's self-reported primary reason for seeking care. The patient often is focused primarily on treating the cavities, restoring his or her smile and oral health. However, the real primary problem is often fear. That is why it is essential to have this initial interview to clarify the existence of these problems, the reasons for them, and the need to attend to their understanding and management, if within the realm of dentistry, before embarking on treatment. Regardless of the particular management therapy chosen, an agreement with the patient that the first objective is lessening fear first helps keep the patient's attention on that goal. This is important because patients tend to be eager for rapid dental care, which, if occurring too fast, can be counterproductive and undo any gains accomplished in emotional and behavioral changes. Attempts to change behavior must proceed first. Most patients claim on their question-naires that the dentist:

- rushes;
- does not ask questions or answer questions satisfactorily;
- does not explain the risks and benefits of the recommended treatment; and
- expect the patient to do whatever is needed without questioning why.

Patient responses like these do not need any specific behavioral technique, they just need the practitioner to be nice, polite, and mindful that the patient is not a dentist and has the right to know what is going on. All this demands is simple respect and courtesy, yet you would be astounded if you knew the extent of this type of criticism that exists in the patient pool.

If the patient self-identifies as a *gagger* during the interview and x-rays are needed, our first effort to create a change in the patient's behavior would be to introduce the nitrous oxide-oxygen technique I discussed earlier with the patient. I firmly believe, as Berggren claims,[34,35,42] that to achieve the amelioration of fear in patients, the dental practitioner must at times use cross-disciplinary methods that involve behavioral, pharma-cological, and psychological efforts. Being well trained in the use of the

$N_2O-O_2$ technique, I use it in combination with a modified version of the behavior modification techniques known as "systematic desensitization." Earlier, I mentioned that many times practitioners intuitively use this technique without realizing it. When a patient says "I hate/fear the needle," the practitioner explains the use of a topical to hide the discomfort of the initial penetration and picks an easy site like the tissue above a premolar to demonstrate how pain free the injection can be. If necessary, the practitioner may repeat this demonstration without depositing any anesthetic solution. He or she does the very same thing for the patient who fears that the Novocain will not work by restoring the smallest of cavities first, despite the need to do others. Here, the practitioner has instinctively changed his or her routine behavior in order to effect a positive change in the patient's behavior and attitude toward the fear of the drill, the failure of the Novocain, and anticipated associated pain. I do the same with each of the major fear provoking stimuli that the patient expresses on their pre-treatment questionnaires.

The program that I have followed, and hope I have improved over the years, has led to much success simply because it involves nothing more than using questionnaires to gather information, and using that information to change both my behavior and my routine to meet the fears, needs, and goals of the patient when the situation demanded it. I always work with the patient, and listen carefully, no matter how long it takes, the goal always being to ameliorate the existing fear and to strengthen the patient's feelings of self-efficacy. There are times I use techniques such as systematic desensitization and reciprocal inhibition in combination with progressive relaxation[36,37] when heightened levels of fear demand more specialized management. However, these cases turn out be few and far between, and are usually referred to a psychologist, because I have found that sometimes utilizing simple cognitive behavioral approaches in combination with a technique like nitrous oxide-oxygen analgesia or conscious sedation utilizing IV Valium is necessary to ensure initial success and build trust. My ultimate goal is always to end this type of joint behavior therapy with conventional treatment, without the need for any supplemental forms other than behavior management. Sometimes, you need to use both psychological and medicinal modalities to make it possible for the patient to acquire new and positive experiences that can lead to a lasting ability to cope and reduce their fears and anxieties. To utilize adjunctive techniques continuously, however, means that one has failed in behaviorally helping this individual lessen his or her fears. Patients do not unlearn past negative cognitions or feelings with continued use of psychopharmacological agents.

I know that many readers will feel all this takes too much time, for which we will not be financially compensated. Nothing can be farther from the truth. Keep in mind that many fearful patients have avoided dental care for pronged times. Their dentition requires extensive and often expensive rehabilitation. When they are able to meet a caring practitioner who will take the time to help them overcome their fear and anxieties, they make the best patients, never break or cancel appointments, and become an excellent source of new patient referrals. Try taking that extra few moments: It will be a priceless experience. Remember, one of the main objectives of the dental practitioner is to make every fearful patient a patient for life, and every emergency patient a permanent patient. By taking the few extra trivial minutes in the beginning, you are assuring the current and long-term objectives associated with building a positive and stable practice. My greatest feeling of achievement comes when a patient says to me, "Nobody ever took this amount of time to explain all of this to me or bother to find out why I was so terrified of dentists." When I hear this, I know I have a patient for life, one who will refer many others to my office.

## Determining the effectiveness of a given management program

The introduction of any type of behavioral management program needs to proceed on the basis of careful assessment of each patient's level of dental anxiety. To ensure whether or not an individual program is successful, the practitioner must evaluate its efficacy. The last step in managing dental fear and anxiety is to assess the performance of the particular management program utilized. To accomplish this, all one has to do is to utilize the same pretreatment questionnaires, permit the patient to respond to these questionnaires midway during the cycle of treatment and at the completion and compare the responses. This affords the patient the opportunity to witness the improvement in behavior and decreases in anxiety that has occurred over the span of visits. It illustrates the success of everybody's efforts. The use of this information collected at various times demonstrate the ultimate integration of identification and management of dental fear and anxiety.

# DOCTOR–PATIENT RELATIONSHIP AND ITS ROLE IN REDUCING ANXIETY AND GAINING TREATMENT ACCEPTANCE
*This section by Samuel Shames*

Anxious patients, in addition to fearing invasion of a very intimate portion of their body, often dread the cost of treatment. It seems appropriate to include a section concerning this everyday occurrence, which often burdens the practitioner and effects treatment. If a dentist can be successful in creating a positive trusting first impression with a patient, develop rapport and trust, many obstacles, including cost, will cease to be a factor in the patient's decision to proceed with treatment.

## Fear of cost

When fear of cost is a major motivator not to initiate treatment, the practitioner might wish to inform and remind patients of the and benefit of committing to treatment now, as opposed to the risks of escalating cost by deferring treatment to a later date, which usually translates to more and costlier treatment.

## The psychology of spending

This concept is a variable every dental practitioner should contemplate. A patient who earns $50,000 a year will somehow try harder to find a way to purchase a $3000 flat-screen TV than to find the same financial resources to save a posterior tooth. Yet conversely, that same patient will forgo that TV to save an anterior tooth. Why? Because patients place a greater degree of importance on anterior teeth, psychologically and emotionally, for a number of reasons, for example:

- personal appearance;
- ego;
- overall health of the oral cavity;
- embarrassment;
- public speaking; and
- ability to present positive smile.

Anterior dentition with missing teeth, or in a state of poor condition, engulfed with caries or chipped, has the possibility of creating a negative impression of that individual to the people he or she meets. Patients must be educated to perceive that a costly treatment plan is really an inexpensive plan if it will maintain the health of the teeth and surrounding structures for many years and provide a feeling of well-being and a pleasant appearance.

Patients must be reminded that teeth are something they use almost 24 hours a day, to eat and to maintain physical, oral, and even mental health. The practitioner must gain a grasp of each of the patient's motivations and, as frequently as possible during the presentation of the treatment plan, remind the patient of the positive goals and objectives they both wish to pursue. The strongest motivations are always the *emotional* ones, such as:

- avoiding pain;
- looking more attractive; and
- avoiding embarrassment.

*Logical* motivators include:

- eating better;
- speaking better; and

- ability to perhaps advance one's career owing to an attractive and cosmetically appealing smile that exudes confidence and indicates "I care enough to look to look well."

All these can be used as patient motivators to help insure implementation of needed dental treatment. It is sometimes difficult to translate to a patient the need for asymptomatic dental treatment when the individual has no physical or cosmetic concerns at the moment. However, determined and successful practitioners find a way to present needed treatment plans to patients without giving them a course in dentistry. The patient should always be adequately informed so as to gain at least a basic understanding of his or her diagnosis, treatment options, possible complications, and cost. Practitioners should remember to de-jargonize their presentations, using words that patients can understand, so that the patient will be able to perceive not only the need for treatment, but understand the value and positive effect it will bring to the patient's overall health and welfare. The suggested treatment must be made to appeal to the patient's inner need for personal betterment.

No matter what type of dentistry is being explained to the patient, people are sensitive and influenced by the practitioner's enthusiasm and body language. If a clinician appears disinterested, not proactive or presses too much to obtain a patient's compliance, the patient will recognize this behavior and most probably be turned off.

## Summary

All practices have difficult and fearful patients that many times cause treatment delays and bring needless stress to the office. To combat this, practitioners must find creative ways to work with these individuals. Practitioners must not only serve as agents of change, permitting their positive behavioral changes to cause a patient's negative behaviors to change to more acceptable and positive ones. Dentists must also be aware of the negative attitudes they often present. These include:

- failure to exude empathy;
- failure to identify a patient's priorities; and
- failure to observe and respond to non verbal cues that patients exhibit during periods of discussion and communication that are often the cause of unwanted behavior and stress.

The use of efficient information gathering questionnaires will greatly aid the clinician's knowledge of the determinants of fear for a given individual. Successful behavior modification results when the practitioner utilizes motivational and behavioral strategies for each of the responses a patient deems a major obstacle to treatment, and when, as treatment progresses, there occurs a lessening of resistance and stress and an increased willingness for treatment compliance on the part of the patient. Although a combination of behavioral and psychopharmacological techniques may be initially required to begin the amelioration of fear anxiety, reliance on pharmacological approaches too exclusively leaves the patient no better off with regard to being a vessel for dental fear and anxiety, even though the dentition may be better off. The long-term benefit to the patient of acquiring simple fear-reducing strategies that can, in some cases, be temporarily facilitated with drugs as adjuncts fosters long-term dental patient relationships that are rewarding for both the dentist and the patient.

# ALTERNATIVE BEHAVIOR MODIFICATION AND TREATMENT MODALITIES[11,48]

I would like, for the sake of completeness, to mention briefly other modalities available to the dental practitioner to modify a patients negative and aversive behaviors. They are:

- systematic desensitization and reciprocal inhibition;
- progressive relaxation;
- modeling positive association and reinforcement;
- imagery flooding;
- hypnosis;
- learning by attribution and appraisal;
- minimizing fear-provoking cues;
- biofeedback.

I would like to discuss the two most widely used and simple methods of behavior modification. They are systematic desensitization and reciprocal inhibition involving the use of progressive relaxation. These two initial modalities assume that negative or erroneous behavior has been learned, and that these behaviors interfere with the provision of optimal dental care.

Systematic desensitization is a highly structured program whereby an individual is gradually desensitized to a particular fear or event causing stimulus. It requires that the patient correctly identify the fear and become proficient in relaxation, and that the practitioner work with the patient to help him or her construct a hierarchy of the specific fear or fears ordered from the least to the most fear eliciting. It may consist of 10 or 12 steps from the least fear provoking exposure to the greatest. Both the patient and the dentist first must correctly identify the specific feared object, action or situation that currently hinders the patient from receiving dental care. Once the individual's fear has been correctly identified, such as the "simple calling and making" of a dental appointment, the next step in the process of desensitization involves the teaching of proper breathing and muscle relaxation. In order for these techniques to be successful, the dentist must be assured that the patient understands and agrees that they wish to attain the specific end point—that is, the overcoming of the specific fear that both have correctly identified as the major obstacle to treatment.

*Reciprocal inhibition*, as described by Wolpe,[36] proposes that a person cannot be relaxed and anxious at the same time. If a patient can engage in a relaxation response to a strong degree, the relaxation created will then inhibit the anxiety response. Generally, inhibition is effective only if a person can experience the feared thought or situation one segment at a time. This is because contemplation of the experience in its entirety is impossible to control.

*Progressive relaxation* was first introduced by Jacobson in 1938, and followed by Benson in 1975.[37,38] It is also called self-relaxation and auto-relaxation. It includes the patient self-inducing as much muscular relation as possible in combination with proper breathing exercises. The patient is taught to tense individual groups of muscle for 10–15s, then relax and exhale completely. The idea is that to feel muscle relaxation, a person must experience the muscles in a state of tension. After this is mastered, a specially constructed hierarchy of fears is developed, and with the aid of a therapist, is taught to master their fears.[6,10,39–42]

The third step in this process is the establishment of the hierarchy, the slow step-by-step method the patient will follow to lessen and overcome the correctly identified fear. The protocol for this segment requires developing with the patient a series of steps (actions) that are ordered along a dimension of increasing degrees of anxiety from the least noxious to the most noxious, and form the basis for the hierarchy. The first scene or step is structured for the patient to visualize or imagine the least amount or degree of the feared anxiety-arousing obstacle associated with the previously identified fear. The imagery is maintained until the individual begins to experience anxiety interfering with the muscular relaxation. When this occurs, the scene is abandoned, and muscular relaxation is again induced.

This step is continued once relaxation is again achieved, and repeated until all anxiety associated with that particular scene is extinguished and the patient can visualize the scene while experiencing total muscular relaxation. Once anxiety related to that scene has been eliminated, the next step (scene) in the hierarchy is introduced and so forth until the point is reached, where it may be hoped the individual does not experience any anxiety or fear about the particular feared dental situation.

When developing a specific hierarchy, it is of prime importance that increases from one scene to the next are minimal. This procedure can produce superior results only when the patient first become desensitized in imagination before tackling the real-life situation.

## Example: Dental hierarchy

(1) Making an appointment to go to the dentist six months in advance.
(2) Thinking about going to the dentist a month before you go.
(3) Thinking about going to the dentist the day before you go.
(4) Going to the dentist.
(5) Waking up and realizing this is the day to go to the dentist.
(6) Driving to the dentist's office.
(7) Standing in front of the building where the dentist's office is.
(8) Walking into the dentist office.
(9) Sitting in the dentist's reception area.
(10) Sitting in the dental chair waiting to have your teeth drilled.
(11) Sitting in the dental chair having your teeth drilled.

The goal of the hierarchy must be formulated to deal with the specific fear stimulus the patient has correctly identified.

## Modeling

Also called positive association and reinforcement, this method is aimed at building and reinforcing new and more positive associations with dental care. These methods are designed to help patients unlearn old associations. Positive reinforcement provides the patient with pleasant rewards for performance of a requested behavioral pattern. The reward for positive behavior can be in the form of praise or small material gifts that orthodontists or general dental practitioners usually hand out for good brushing habits to their young patients. These gifts act as reinforcers of good behavior, and can be extremely effective.

Two other methods of unlearning can also be extremely effective: *familiarization* (as in "tell–show–do" using video-taped or other educational tools) and *modeling*, behavioral procedure utilized to increase cooperative behavior especially in children. Most often children learn behaviors through observation and imitation. Therefore it is easy to understand how a child who has never visited a dentist or experienced the dental situation may acquire apprehension and fear-related responses from just hearing the experiences of others. Since children learn much from watching, the technique of modeling can be applied to reduce fear-related behaviors Studies by Melamed, Weinstein,[43-47] and others demonstrated that a child's behavior could be affected by viewing a video-taped model who demonstrated appropriate cooperative behavior. Children exposed to those films were found to have a higher degree of cooperation and a greater reduction in dental anxiety and disruptive behavior. Care must be taken that the model is known to be one who is cooperative and relatively anxiety free. Modeling accomplishes two feats: First, it provides a vicarious experience of rewards, whereby the prospective patient observes the patient receiving positive reinforcement for appropriate behavior; and second, it demonstrates relevant information concerning upcoming treatment. For modeling to be successful, both these components must be present.

## Imagery flooding

This psychological technique is based on the concept that phobic individuals can experience reductions in anxiety levels when repeatedly imagining feared stressful situations. This technique involves:

- patient confidence;
- muscular relaxation; and
- flooding phase of fear stimulus.

The patient must be made to feel that it is perfectly safe to re-experience an imagined fearful event and to let out those emotions that have been held in. It is of prime importance to remember that for these techniques to be successful, the practitioner must be assured that the correct feared stimulus has been identified and the proper degree of anxiety recognized.

## Hypnosis

While a much more complex technique, hypnosis is currently experiencing reawakening of great interest, based on scientific brain research showing where and how it is effective. The efficacy of hypnosis for pain control is now an evidence-based treatment possibility and will be discussed in its entirety in a subsequent chapter.

## Learning by attribution and appraisal

This group of behavioral modalities focuses less on learning by association and more on learning by attribution and appraisal of objects and situations. These methods are designed to provide information to patients that encourages nonanxiety-provoking attributions and more positive appraisals of the dental experience, and include explaining what kind of procedure the patient will undergo, the effects, what to expect and feel, and the benefits that will achieved as a result of this procedure. While such information is being provided, alternative attributions can be offered to the patient. An example would be to explain to the patient that the fine tremors or shaky feeling some experience with the dental injection is normal. Some individuals experience palpitations and rapid heartbeats and fear they may be allergic or having a heart attack. Explain to patients that such feelings are in reality normal and are felt by most. The adrenaline contained within the anesthetic is a natural-occurring substance within our bodies utilized to permit the anesthesia to last longer. Since it occurs naturally, one would not become allergic to its presence. This allows the patient to perceive that he or she is not alone in experiencing these sensations, and since almost everyone feels them, they are quite normal. This explanation serves to reduce fear and anxiety in almost all patients. Another example of providing positive information to object that usually invokes fear, the sound of the drill, we have explained in a previous section.

## Minimizing cues

This group of techniques concentrate on minimizing those cues that elicit dental fear and anxiety. They are modalities that attempt to break the learned association between fear and dental treatment. Such techniques can occur at the biological level, such as use of topical anesthetic before the dental injection to reduce the pain often associated with it as a cause of anxiety. Another method advises patients against the ingestion of excessive stimulants such as caffeine to reduce arousal, which is often a cue to anxiety. The minimization of cues can also occur at the sociological level. For example, the dental office can be structured to reduce or prevent anxiety by "hiding the hardware," that is, by eliminating the sight of instruments patients are exposed to. Second, the reception area can be a breeding ground for anxiety due to the large amount of time some individuals spend waiting their turn. They can be subjected to ongoing noises of the drill, certain smells, and various types of literature, all of which can elicit anxiety. The removal of posters often supplied by makers of toothpaste that picture comic cartoon-like characters swarming all over the teeth with drills and chisels is enough to frighten the most hardened individual. Certain types of pamphlets and literature can promote feelings of guilt; for example, a parent who takes time to read information of concerning orthodontic treatment and its benefits can develop arousal and guilt over not being able to afford such treatment for their children. It is better to limit reading material in the reception area to popular magazines and no dental literature.

## Biofeedback[49–52]

In recent years, a great deal of attention has been given to this technique. This procedure requires the use of very sensitive and sophisticated electronic instruments that are designed to measure minute changes in muscular activities of the autonomic nervous system. The theory involved is that a person should be able to develop improved relaxation responses by being informed via the feedback signal, as small decreases in tension occur. The sensitivity of the biofeedback monitoring technique permits a more direct and precise appraisal of the patient's state of relaxation.

One of the most significant aspects of biofeedback is that it shifts the control center of the individual from external to internal dependence. The patient, after appropriate training, no longer depends on a therapist, drugs, or any other external variables. The control of the individual's physiological functioning can and does come from within. The technique leads not only to control over involuntary functions, but also to transitional states of awareness and heightening of mental perspective.

Electromyographic biofeedback is used in teaching patients with TMJ pain to relax masseter, internal pterygoid and temporal muscles, which are the principle muscles used in closing the jaw and in the regulation of the position of the mandible in space, as well as in the treatment of tension headaches.

# REFERENCES

1.  Dworkin S. 1978. *Behavioral Science and Dental Practice*, St. Louis, MO: CV Mosby.
2.  Dworkin S. 1973. A rationale for obtaining change in attitudes and behavior of dental patients. *J Tenn Dent Assoc* 53:147–52.
3.  Dworkin S. 1977. Psychiatry and dentistry. In: Wollman B (ed.), *International Encyclopedia of Neurology, Psychiatry, Psychoanalysis and Psychology*, Vol. 4, New York: D.Van Norstrand Co.
4.  Eifert G, Zvolensky M, Sorrell J, et al. 2000.Predictors of self reported anxiety and panic symptoms: An evaluation of Anxiety sensitivity, suffocation fear, heart focused anxiety, and breath holding duration. *J Psychopathol Behav Assess* 21(4): 293–305.
5.  Maggirias J and Locker D. 2002. Pyschological factors and Perceptions of pain associated with treatment. *Community Dent Oral Epidemiol* 30(2): 151–9.
6.  Gatchel R. 1992. Managing anxiety and pain during dental treatment. *J Am Dent Assoc* 123:37–41.
7.  Feldner M and Hekmat H. 2001. Perceived control over anxiety–related events as a predictor of pain in a cold pressor task. *J Behav Ther Exp Psychiatry* 32:191–202.
8.  Weiner A and Forgione A. 2000. Potential fear-provoking patient experiences during treatment. *Gen Dent* 48(4):466–71.
9.  Weiner A and Weinstein P. 1995. Dentists' Knowledge, attitudes, and assessment practices in relation to fearful dental patients: A pilot study. *Gen Dent* 43:164–8.
10. Milgrom P, Weinstein P, Kleinknects R, et al. 1995. *Treating Fearful Dental Patients: A patient Management Handbook*, 2nd edn. Seattle: University of Washington.
11. Weiner A. 1994. *The Difficult Patient. A Guide to Understanding and Management*, 3rd edn. Randolph, MA: Reniew Publishing Co.
12. Corah N, O'Shea R, Bissell G, et al. 1988. The dentist-patient relationship: Perceived dentist behaviors that reduce patient anxiety and increase satisfaction. *J Am Dent Assoc* 116:73–6.
13. Milgrom P, Cullen T, Whitney C, et al. 1996.Frustrating patient visits. *J Public Health Dent* 56(1):6–11.

14.  Weiner A and Sheehan D. 1988. Differentiating anxiety-panic disorders from psychologic dental anxiety. *Dent Clin North Am.* 32(4):823–40.
15.  Weiner A, Zemnick C, and Ganda K. 2002, Comparison of anxiety response levels in patients who are HIV-positive and patients who are not. *J Mass Dent Soc* 51(3):12–6.
16.  Baron R, Logan H, and Kao C. 1990.Some variables affecting Dentists' assessment of patients' distress. *Health Psychol* 9:143–53.
17.  Malamed B. 1979. Behavioral approaches to fear in dental settings. In: Hersen M, Eisler R, and Liller P. (eds.), *Progress in Behavior Modification*, New York: Academic Press.
18.  Kulich K, Berggren U and Hallberg L. 2000.Model of the dentist-patient consultation in a clinic specializing in the treatment of dental phobic patients: A qualitative study. *Acta Odontol Scand* 58:63–71.
19.  Berggren U and Meynert G. 1984. Dental fear and avoidance: Causes, symptoms and consequences. *J Am Dent Assoc* 109:247–51.
20.  Berggren U. 1993. Psychosocial effects associated with dental fear in adult dental patients with avoidance behaviors. *Psychol Health* 8:185–96.
21.  Weisenberg M, Aviram O, and Raphaeli N. 1984. Relevent and irrelevant anxiety in the reaction to pain. *Pain* 20:371–83.
22.  Milgrom P, Coldwell S, Getz T, Weinstein P, et al. 199. Four dimensions of fear of dental injections. *J Am Dent Assoc* 128:756–66.
23.  Rhudy J and Meagher M. 2000. Fear and anxiety: Divergent effects on human pain thresholds. *Pain* 84:65–75.
24.  Klages U, Ulusoy O, and Wehrbein H. 2004. Dental trait anxiety and pain sensitivity as predictors of expected and and experienced pain in stressful dental procedures. *Eur J Oral Sci* 112:477–83.
25.  van Wijk A and Makkes P. 2008. Highly anxious dental patients report more pain during dental injections. *Br Dent J* 205:583, 1–5.
26.  Mehta N, Maloney, G, Bana D, et al. 2009. *Head Face and Neck Pain: Science, Evaluation and Management*. Hoboken, NJ: John Wiley and Sons Inc.
27.  Van Wijk A and Hoogstraten J. 2005.Experience with dental pain and fear of dental pain. *J Dent Res* 84:947–50.
28.  Langa H. 1968. *Relative Analgesia in Dental Practice*. Philadelphia: W.B. Saunders Co., pp. 116–35.
29.  Weiner A. 1987. Nitrous oxide-oxygen analgesia and the post-hypnotic effect: Eliciting the hidden fear. *J Am Dent Assoc* 114:589–90.
30.  Weiner A and Stark P. 2008. Patient perceived anxiety associated with use of selective serotonin and selective serotonin nor-epinephrine reuptake inhibitors. *J Mass Dent Soc* 57(1):22–6.
31.  Sheehan D and Sheehan K. 1996. The role of SSRI's I panic disorder. *J Clin Psychiatry* 57(10 Suppl):51–8.
32.  Askor R and Sheehan D. 1999.The use of selective serotonin reuptake inhibitors in panic disorder. *Home Health Care Consult* 6(4):15–9.
33.  Centore L, Reisner L, and Pettengill C. 2002. Better understanding your patient from a psychological perspective: Effective identification of

problem behaviors affecting the dental office. *J Can Dent Assoc* 30(7): 512–9.

34. Bergrren U and Linde A. 1984. Dental fear and avoidance: A comparison of two modes of treatment. *J Dent Res* 63:1223–27.

35. Bergrren. 2001. Long term management of the fearful adult patient using behavior modification and other modalities. *J Dent Educ* 65(12):1357–68.

36. Wolpe J. 1958. *Psychotherapy for Reciprocal Inhibition*. Stamford, CA: Stamford University Press.

37. Jacobson E. 1938. *Progressive Relaxation*. Chicago: University of Chicago Press.

38. Benson H. 1975. *The Relaxation Response*. New York: Avon.

39. Klepac R. 1982. Characteristics of clients seeking therapy for the reduction of dental avoidance: reaction to pain. *J Behav Ther Exp Psychiatry* 13(4):293–300.

40. Berggren U. 1986. Long tern effects of two different treatment for dental fear and avoidance. *J Dent Res* 65:874–6.

41. Harrison J, Carlsson S, and Berggren U. 1985. Research in clinical process and outcome methodology: Psycho-physiology, systematic desensitization and dental fear. *J Behav Ther Exp Psychiatry* 16:201.

42. Berggren U and Hakeberg M. 2000.Relaxation vs.cognitively oriented therapies for dental fear. *J Dent Res* 79(9):1645–51.

43. Malamed B, Weinstein D, Hawes R, et al. 1975. Reduction of fear related dental management problems with use of filmed modeling. *J Am Dent Assoc* 90:822–6.

44. Weinstein P. 2006. Provider versus patient-centered approaches to health promotion with parents of young children: What works/does not work. *Pediatr Dent* 28(2):192–8.

45. Weinstein P, Harrison R, and Benton T. 2006. Motivating mothers to prevent caries: Confirming the beneficial effects of counseling. *J Am Dent Assoc* 136(6):789–93.

46. Weinstein P. 2008. Child-Centered child management in a changing world. *Eur Arch Paediatr Dent* 9(Suppl) 1:6–10.

47. Weinstein P, Raadal M, Naidu S, et al. 2003. A videotaped intervention to enhance child control and reduce anxiety of dental injections. *Eur J Paediatr Dent* 4(4):181–5.

48. Weiner A, Moore P, and Sheehan D. 1982. Current Behavioral modes of reducing dental anxiety. *Quintessence Intern Dent Digest* 9:981–5.

49. Schwartz M and Andrasik F. (eds.). 1995. *Biofeedback: A Practitioner's Guide*, New York: Guilford Press.

50. Kasman G, Crom J, and Wolf D. 1997. *Clinical Applications in Surface Electromyography*, Gaithersburg, MD: Aspen Publications.

51. Motofsky D, Forgione A, and Giddon D. 2006. *Behavioral Dentistry*, Ames, Iowa: Blackwell Publishing Co.

52. Mehat N, Maloney G, Bana D, et al. 2009. *Head, Face, Neck Pain: Science, Evaluation and Management*. Hoboken, NJ: John Wiley and Sons.

# The pharmacological basis of pain and anxiety control

## Morton Rosenberg and Michael Thompson

## INTRODUCTION

Despite their ability to reduce fear, anxiety, and apprehension, behavioral techniques may be inadequate for some patients, and pharmacological interventions may be necessary in addition to and/or in combination with behavioral strategies. The use of sedation and even general anesthesia may be necessary to access dental care for some severely phobic patients. Local anesthesia continues to be the foundation of clinical dentistry, and, unfortunately, is related to many of the dental phobic's fears. This chapter is intended to present an overview of the use of sedation in dentistry and not intended as one directed at teaching technique.

Studies continue to affirm a significant percentage of the population is very anxious or even terrified of the dental environment.[1] Despite the advances in understanding of these issues, the incidence of dental anxiety has remained basically unchanged for the last 50 years.[2,3]

Many of the causative factors surrounding the development of dental phobia and avoidance of care center upon pain. These factors include if the patient has had painful dental experiences in the past, or if the patient believes that painful treatment is inevitable.[4-6] Fear of dental pain and avoidance of care has even been linked with genetic variations associated with red hair color. Subjects with red hair color caused by variants of the MC1R gene are less sensitive to subcutaneous local anesthetics,[7] and report more anxiety and fear of dental pain than participants lacking the MC1R gene variations.[8]

---

*The Fearful Dental Patient: A Guide to Understanding and Managing.* Edited by Arthur A. Weiner
© 2011 Blackwell Publishing Ltd.

## LOCAL ANESTHESIA

The administration of local anesthesia is one of the most stressful and difficult procedures for the dental phobic. Many of the psychogenic medical emergencies encountered in dentistry occur in the period prior, during, or immediately after the injection.[9] Unfortunately, intraoral injections are administered into a region of the body that is richly innervated, in addition to having deep psychological implications. For many dental patients, it is the local anesthetic injection procedure that often represents the most fear-provoking portion of the dental experience. When patients are asked to judge their dentists, the most important criteria is "a dentist who gives a painless injection."[10]

Nondrug techniques such as behavior modification, hypnosis, distraction, and other methods of reducing the anxiety and fear surrounding the dental injection can be useful. The attention to the patient's fears and apprehension by a concerned dentist makes the greatest difference in the injection period, which many feel is the most stressful part of the dental appointment. For example, the use of a topical anesthetic prior to injection will provide a degree of anesthesia to nonkeratanized tissues to a depth of 2–3 mm, which reduces the pain of needle insertion and has become a patient expectation. Benzocaine 20% and lidocaine 5% are the most popular topical anestheteics and gels, ointments, and sprays for this purpose are available. Additionally, eutectic mixtures of local anesthetics (prilocaine and lidocaine) are available in a vehicle (Oraqix®, Dentsply International, Philadelphia, PA) that is expressed as a liquid and becomes an adherent gel at body temperature when deposited in the periodontal space. Using this technique, full quadrant periodontal curettage can be accomplished without the use of multiple local anesthetic injections.[11] The compound can also be used as pre-injection topical anesthetic.[12] More recently, it has been reported that using a refrigerant (1,1,1,3,3-pentafluoropropane/1,1,1,2-tetrafluoroethane) as a preinjection anesthetic was more effective than a topical anesthetic gel of 20% benzocaine in reducing the pain of posterior palatal injection.[13]

Alternative anesthetic techniques and equipment have also been introduced to make the administration of local anesthesia less stressful, more dependable and easier for many patients.

The attempt to modify the medical technique of transcutaneous electrical nerve stimulation (TENS) to dentistry with the use of intraoral electrodes was termed electronic dental anesthesia (EDA). Although initially thought to have great promise, its lack of consistency in providing reliable pulpal anesthesia and equipment issues has decreased its popularity and utility in dentistry.[14]

Techniques or devices that create pressure or vibration have been shown to inhibit painful sensations prior to or at the same time as a painful stimuli is applied. A battery-powered attachment to the regular dental syringe, Vibraject® (VibraJect LLC, Irvine, CA), produces a series of fine vibrations that has been reported to reduce pain during needle insertion.[15]

Computer-controlled local anesthetic delivery systems (CCLDS), beginning with the Wand™, enable the dentist to accurately control needle placement with fingertip accuracy. The system replaces the classical dental syringe with a lightweight handpiece, and the dentist delivers the local anesthetic by a foot activated control.[16] Flow rate of the local anesthetic solution is computerized and thus very consistent. Randomized clinical studies confirm a significant reduction in pain perception with the use of CCLDS as opposed to the use of standard equipment.[17]

The ability to anesthetize a single tooth rather than an entire quadrant is very important for some phobic patients. In addition to simple infiltration techniques, the periodontal ligament injection (PDL) or intraligamentary injection (ILI) and intraosseus anesthesia, provide pulpal anesthesia to a single tooth with only localized soft tissue anesthesia surrounding that tooth developing. The success rate for the PDL injection is high although it can be painful.[18] The introduction of a new iteration of the CCLAD, Single Tooth Anesthesia (STA™, Milestone Scientific, Piscataway, NJ) incorporates dynamic pressuring sensing technology that continually measures the exit pressure of the local anesthetic solution during a PDL injection. By strictly regulating pressure of the local anesthetic being infused into the periodontal ligament space, most patients experience less discomfort than with traditional syringes.[19]

Intraosseous anesthesia is the technique of injecting local anesthesia directly into the cancellous bone spaces adjacent to the target tooth and results in rapid onset of local anesthesia. It allows for profound single tooth anesthesia and has a high degree of success in teeth unable to be anesthetized by standard injection techniques.[20,21]

There are patients who do fear the prolonged lingering soft tissue numbness following routine dental local anesthesia. While pulpal anesthesia from local anesthetics containing vasconstrictors may last approximately 45–60 min, the soft tissue anesthesia and associated functional deficits may last 3–5 h. Phentolamine mesylate (OraVerse™) is FDA approved to reduce the time necessary to return of normal nerve function following the administration of local anesthesia. OraVerse™ acts by dilating the blood vessels constricted by the vasoconstrictor in the local anesthetic, increasing the blood flow to carry away the local anesthetic, and is thus not a true reversal agent or antagonist to the local anesthetic itself. It does the decrease the duration of mandibular inferior alveolar block anesthesia 121% faster than control and maxillary infiltration 166% faster than control.[22,23]

## Sedation

Despite the advances in local anesthesia administration and the application of behavioral technique, there are many phobic patients who will need sedation and anesthesia to access dental care. The need of sedative services has been documented, but unfortunately there are not enough qualified dentists to provide sedative services for the population especially for patients requiring more than minimal sedation. Need and demand studies indicate 23 million more Americans would access dental care on a routine basis if sedation services were available.[24] Among dentists using sedation on their patients, a majority use minimal sedation (82.3%), with fewer utilizing moderate sedation via the enteral route (28.3%), moderate sedation via the parenteral route (12.4%), and less than one in 10 are trained to competency in deep sedation.[25] The perceived invasiveness or stress of the dental procedure dramatically increases the need for sedation/anesthesia with patient preference rising from 2% for a dental cleaning to 47% for an extraction, to 55% for an endodontic procedure to 68% for periodontal surgery.[2]

Dentistry and medicine sedative/anesthesia providers have come to consensus and are unified as to the fact that sedation/anesthesia is a continuum and therefore it is not always possible to predict how an individual will respond to a central nervous system depressant. It is imperative to practice with one's educational qualifiers and state permitting. The most important concept of this continuum is that ability to rescue (diagnose and manage) patients who enter a deeper level of sedation (e.g., from moderate to deep sedation) than initially intended. For all levels of sedation, the practitioner must have the training, skills, and equipment to identify and manage such an occurrence until either assistance arrives (emergency medical service) or the patient returns to the intended level of sedation without airway or cardiovascular complication.

The American Dental Association has always recognized the right of and privilege of educationally qualified dentists to deliver sedation/anesthesia to their dental patients (Box 5.1).

The levels of the continuum are:

(1) *Minimal sedation*—a minimally depressed level of consciousness, produced by a pharmacological method, that retains the patient's ability to independently and continuously maintain an airway and respond *normally* to tactile stimulation and verbal command. Although cognitive function and coordination may be modestly impaired, ventilatory and cardiovascular functions are unaffected.

(2) *Moderate sedation*—a drug-induced depression of consciousness during which patients respond purposefully to verbal commands, either alone or accompanied by light tactile stimulation. No interventions are required to maintain a patent airway, and spontaneous ventilation is adequate. Cardiovascular function is usually maintained.

(3) *Deep sedation*—a drug-induced depression of consciousness during which patients cannot be easily aroused but respond purposefully following repeated or painful stimulation. The ability to independently maintain ventilatory function may be impaired. Patients may require assistance in maintaining a patent airway, and spontaneous ventilation may be inadequate. Cardiovascular function is usually maintained.

---

**Box 5.1**

AMERICAN DENTAL ASSOCIATION POLICY STATEMENT: THE USE OF
SEDATION AND GENERAL ANESTHESIA BY DENTISTS
As adopted by the October 2007 ADA House of Delegates

Introduction

The administration of sedation and general anesthesia has been an integral part
of dental practice since the 1840s. Dentists have a legacy and a continuing
interest and expertise in providing anesthetic and sedative care to their patients.
It was the introduction of nitrous oxide by Horace Wells, a Hartford, Connecticut
dentist, and the demonstration of anesthetic properties of ether by William
Morton, Wells' student, that gave the gift of anesthesia to medicine and dentistry.
Dentistry has continued to build upon this foundation and has been instrumental
in developing safe and effective sedative and anesthetic techniques that have
enabled millions of people to access dental care. Without these modalities, many
patient populations such as young children, physically and mentally challenged
individuals and many other dental patients could not access the comprehensive
care that relieves pain and restores form and function. The use of sedation and
anesthesia by appropriately trained dentists in the dental office continues to have
a remarkable record of safety. It is very important to understand that anxiety,
cooperation and pain can be addressed by both psychological and pharmacological techniques and local anesthetics, which are the foundation of pain control
in dentistry. Sedation may diminish fear and anxiety, but do not obliterate the
pain response and therefore, expertise and in-depth knowledge of local anesthetic techniques and pharmacology is necessary. General anesthesia, by definition, produces an unconscious state totally obtunding the pain response.

Anxiety and pain can be modified by both psychological and pharmacological techniques. In some instances, psychological approaches are sufficient.
However, in many instances, pharmacological approaches are required.

---

Due to risks inherent in general anesthesia and/or deep sedation, only
dentists with the most advanced training, oral and maxillofacial surgeons,
have the ability to provide deep sedation and/or general anesthesia and
thus the majority of general dentists and other specialists utilize minimal
and moderate sedative techniques. This discussion will be limited to
minimal and moderate sedation.

The Guidelines for the Use of Sedation and General Anesthesia by
Dentists and The Guidelines for Teaching Pain Control and Sedation to
Dentists and Dental Students adopted by the American Dental Association
in 2007 provide the framework for the safe and effective use of sedation
and anesthesia in dentistry. For each level in the sedation/anesthesia continuum, these documents describe in detail the educational qualifiers for
dentists and their staff, equipment, facility and personnel requirements,
patient preoperative evaluation, monitoring and documentation, recovery
and discharge, and emergency management. Moderate and deep sedation

and general anesthesia are regulated in all states, and permitting processes have been established to ensure educational qualifiers, office and staff requirements, and reporting criteria.

There are many possible routes of administration for the introduction of sedative drugs (e.g. topical, sublingual, intranasal, rectal, transdermal, subcutaneous, intramuscular), but the majority of general dentist practicing minimal or moderate sedation rely on the inhalational route for nitrous oxide-oxygen, the oral (enteral) or intravenous route.

## Nitrous oxide-oxygen sedation

Nitrous oxide-oxygen sedation is the most commonly used sedative agent in dentistry, and is used by dentists, and, in some states, by dental hygienists, as a safe and effective minimal sedative agent. With minimal cardiovascular and respiratory effects in the healthy patient, combined with its advantageous pharmacokinetic property of being very insoluble, thus making induction, maintenance, and recovery very rapid, nitrous oxide sedation has a long history and excellent safety record in dentistry.[26] Its ease of administration and the demand by some patients as the only way they have been treated in the past, and its lack of significant complications, make nitrous oxide useful for phobic dental patient for many procedures. The ability to titrate easily to a level where the patient will become relaxed, comfortable, less anxious, and may experience a tingling sensation in the fingers, toes, cheeks, lips and tongue, heaviness in the extremities, and perhaps a lighter, floating feeling without a prolonged recovery explains the popularity of the nitrous oxide-sedation technique.[27] The amnesic properties of nitrous oxide and its ability for the patient to feel that time is compressed are other positive attributes of the drug.[28] The combination of nitrous oxide and local anesthetic make oral surgical procedures more tolerable and provide superior pain relief.[29]

Early childhood negative experiences can be reduced with the administration of nitrous oxide sedation along with lowering anxiety on sequential visits and facilitating positive behavior.[30] Patients with dental fear that were given nitrous for dentistry to reduce anxiety have been reported to show positive effects lasting for years.[31]

Nitrous oxide has been reported to be very useful when combined with behavioral and psychological techniques. The importance of psychological preparation of the patient prior to administration has a marked increase in the effect of nitrous sedation.[32] Nitrous oxide sedation is enhanced by the calming words and actions of the dentist, addition of music and "white noise,"[33,34] hypnosis,[35] and electronic dental anesthesia.[36]

## Minimal and moderate oral and intravenous sedation

Oral (enteral) sedation has become increasing more popular in minimal and moderate sedation for the general dentist for the phobic patient.

Although many central nervous depressants can be used as enteral sedation agents (e.g., barbiturates, chloral derivatives, and H1 blockers), the benzodiazepines have become the drugs of choice in providing phobic or anxious patients restful sleep the night prior to the appointment, and also as anxiolytics or moderate procedural sedatives.

As a drug class, benzodiazepines are extremely safe, and there is a wide margin between therapeutic and toxic doses. The use of enteral sedation using benzodiazepines to provide moderate sedation either by doses larger than those recommended or in multiple or stacked dosing techniques remains a paradigm unique to dentistry, and continues to be an evolving area, with the clinical practice moving ahead of an evidence-based scientific foundation.[37,38]

The benzodiazepines enhance the activity of the inhibitory neurotransmitter GABA by binding to the $GABA_A$ receptor subtype at a specific site distinct from that of the GABA site on the receptor. This enhanced GABA-induced activity facilitates chloride ion channel conductance, leading to hyperpolarization of the postsynaptic membrane and decreased neuronal excitability. This occurs largely within the cerebral cortex.[39,40] The clinical effects of the benzodiazepines useful for the phobic and anxious patient include anxiolytic/antipanic activity, induction of sleep, sedation, and memory impairment, hypnosis in higher doses, psychomotor impairment, and muscle relaxation. The potency and efficacy exhibited by the various benzodiazepines with regard to these and other characteristic effects depends upon their individual inherent affinity for the GABA receptor subtypes, as well as their degree of receptor binding.

Although all of the benzodiazepines have to one extent or another similar clinical properties and do have different receptor affinities that explain the differences in clinical doses, these potency differences are only quantitative in nature and do not reflect any qualitative differences in their neurochemical or neuroreceptor properties. The most popular oral benzodiazepines in dentistry are diazepam, triazolam, and lorazepam. These can be prescribed as sleeping aids for the anxious patient the night before surgery, as a premedicant prior to the appointment, or as a procedural sedative during the procedure.

As with all enteral medications, there are many pharmacokinetic factors that contribute to uptake and distribution of drugs that are beyond the control of the practitioner. First pass degradation may also decrease the amount of active compound arriving at the target organ, as well as factors surrounding the effects of the CYP3A enzyme system. For example, the sedative effects of midazolam are significantly decreased when CYP3A activity levels have been induced by a drug such as carbamazepine (Backman et al. 1996).[41] Significant drug interactions leading to prolonged activity may arise when benzodiazepines are combined with drugs that inhibit CYP3A enzyme activity, such as erythromycin, the azole antifungals ketoconazole, and fluconazole,[42,43] or grapefruit juice.[44,45] It is important to note that the lipophilicity of lorazepam is much less than either diazepam or midazolam, such that its onset is slower while its duration of action, both orally and intravenously, is much longer (6–10h), and patients must be warned of the dangers inherent in this extended action. Genetic variables can also lead to variations in patient response to the benzodiazepines. For example, one of the major pathways of diazepam metabolism is by the enzyme CYP2C19, which is polymorphically expressed in the liver. "Poor metabolizers," or those subjects lacking normal amounts of CYP2C19, such that they show significantly decreased metabolism of the prototype substrate S-mephenytoin, have been identified. The proportion of poor metabolizers in the population differs depending upon ethnic group, with estimates among Asian populations varying from 12% to 20%. In such patients, diazepam has been shown to be more slowly metabolized than subjects who are extensive metabolizers.[46]

Choosing an empirical oral dose may, at times, over or underdose a patient and titrating oral medications to desired effect is difficult. Most of the oral benzodiazepines have a longer clinical duration of action than is actually necessary for the dental appointment; see list in Table 5.1. Intelligent decisions surrounding the use of oral sedation not only includes a knowledge of the pharmacology of the drug and its rationale for use, but the fact that for some phobic patients, there will be failure if the patient is to remain in either minimal or moderate sedation for the duration of the appointment. A 2.5% of the patients will be hyporesponders, and 2.5% will be hyperresponders, and the dentist will have to understand how to manage both.[47]

One advantage of the benzodiazepines is that there is a specific antagonist available to reverse their effects. Flumazenil is a structural analog of the benzodiazepines that has a high affinity for the benzodiazepines receptor ligand. It has minimal intrinsic activity and thus acts as competitive antagonist to the benzodiazepine agonist. Posttreatment monitoring of the patient remains necessary even after the use of flumazenil, as resedation can occur, especially if the benzodiazepine used was long lasting.

Practitioners with advanced training may use the intravenous route for moderate sedation, but in both of these techniques, the benzodiazepines have become the most popular drugs to reduce anxiety, fear and apprehension. The intravenous route produces a much more rapid onset in the actions of benzodiazepines, and also allows the ability to titrate the drug

**Table 5.1**  Commonly used enteral benzodiazepines.

|  | Triazolam | Diazepam | Lorazepam |
|---|---|---|---|
| Metabolites | Insignificant | Yes | No |
| T$_{1/2}$ (h) | 1–6 | 20–100 | 10–20 |
| Onset (min) | 30–60 | 60–90 | 90–120 |
| Clinical effect (duration h) | 1–3 | 2–4 | 3–6 |

to effect. The most popular intravenous benzodiazepines used in dentistry are diazepam and midazolam. Diazepam is insoluble in water, and is formulated with propylene glycol, which may cause painful irritation on injection. Midazolam is water soluble, and both agents are lipid soluble and highly protein bound. As a sedative, midazolam is at least twice as potent as diazepam.

Nitrous oxide-oxygen sedation can be combined with either oral or intravenous techniques to provide the "fine tuning" to individualize the level of sedation.[48]

### Deep sedation/general anesthesia

There will be the occasional phobic patient in whom minimal or moderate sedation will not be potent enough to gain cooperation and produce an adequate amount of sedation. These patients will require referral to dental or medical anesthesia providers trained and competent to render the patient deeply sedated or unconscious via general anesthesia.

## SUMMARY

Local anesthesia remains the foundation of pain control in dentistry and is often the most stressful aspect of the dental experience. Newer techniques and drugs can reduce the pain and increase the efficacy of this approach. When behavioral techniques are not successfully in managing the phobic patient, the use of minimal and moderate sedation techniques can be safely used to reduce anxiety and gain cooperation safely and effectively by the trained dentist. They do, however, require advanced training and strict adherence to guidelines and an understanding of the pharmacological basis of what the drugs can and cannot do. Deep sedation and/or general anesthesia may be necessary to provide access to care in the most phobic patients when other techniques fail.

## REFERENCES

1.  Gatchel RJ, Ingersoll RD, Bowman L, et al. 1983. The prevalence of dental fear and avoidance: A recent survey study. *J Am Dent Assoc* 107:609–10.
2.  Milgrom P, Fiset L, Melnick S, et al. 1988. The prevalence and practice management consequences of dental fear in a major U.S. city. *J Am Dent Assoc* 116(6):641–7.
3.  Smith TA and Heaton LJ. 2003. Fear of dental care: Are we making progress? *J Am Dent Assoc* 134:1101–8.
4.  Maggirias J and Locker D. 2002. Psychological factors and perception of pain associated with dental treatment. *Community Dent Oral Epidemiol* 30(2):151–9.

5. Maggirias J and Locker D. 2002. Five-year incidence of dental anxiety in an adult population. *Community Dent Health* 19:173–9.

6. Eli I, Uziel N, Baht R, et al. 1997. Antecedents of dental anxiety: Learned responses versus personality traits. *Community Dent Oral Epidemiol* 25(3): 233–7.

7. Liem EB, Joiner TV, Tseuda K, et al. 2005. Increased sensitivity to thermal pain and reduced subcutaneous lidocaine efficacy in redheads. *Anesthesiology* 102(3):509–14.

8. Binkley CJ, Beacham A, Neace W, et al. 2009. Genetic variations associated with red hair color and fear of dental pain, anxiety regarding dental care and avoidance of dental care. *J Am Dent Assoc* 140(7):896–905.

9. Matsuura H. 1990. Analysis of systemic complications and deaths during treatment in Japan. *Anesth Prog* 36:219–28.

10. De St. Georges J. 2004. How dentists are judged by patients. *Dent Today* 23(8):96–9.

11. Friskopp J, Nilsson M, and Isacsson G. 2001. The anesthetic onset and duration of a new lidocaine/prilocaine gel intrapocket anesthetic (Oraqix®) for periodontal scaling/root planning. *J Clin Periodontol* 28(5):453–8.

12. Al-Melh MA and Andersson L. 2008. Reducing pain from palatal needle stick by topical anesthetics: A comparative study between two lidocaine/ prilocaine substances. *J Clin Dent*, 19(2):43–7.

13. Kosaraju A and Vandewalle KS. 2009. A comparison of a refrigerant and a topical anesthetic gel as preinjection anesthetics: A clinical evaluation. *J Am Dent Assoc* 140:68–72.

14. Malamed SF, Quinn CL, Torgersen RT, et al. 1989. Electronic dental anesthesia for restorative dentistry. *Anesth Prog* 36:195–7.

15. Yagiela, J. 2005. Safely easing the pain for your patients. *Dimens Dent Hyg* 3(5):20–2.

16. Hochman MN, Chiarello D, Hochman CB, et al. 1997. Computerized local anesthesia delivery vs. traditional syringe technique. *N Y State Dent J* 63:24–9.

17. Nicholson JW, Berry TG, et al. 2001. Pain perception and utility: A comparison of the syringe and computerized injection techniques. *Gen Dent* 49(2):167–72.

18. Malamed SF. 1982. The periodontal ligament (PDL) injection: An alternative to the inferior alveolar block. *Oral Surg* 53:117–21.

19. Hochman MN. 2007. Single-tooth anesthesia: Pressure-sensing technology provides innovative advancement in the field of dental local anesthesia. *Compendium* 28(4):186–93.

20. Coggins R, Reader A, Nist R, et al. 1996. Anesthetic efficacy of the intraosseous injection in maxillary and mandibular teeth. *Oral Surg Oral Med Oral Pathol Oral Radiol Endod* 81:634–41.

21. Parente SA, Anderson RW, Herman WW, et al. 1998. Anesthetic efficacy of the supplemental intraosseous injection for teeth with irreversible pulpitis. *J Endod* 24:826–8.

22. Hersh EV, Moore PA, Papas AS, et al. 2008. Soft tissue anesthesia recovery group: Reversal of soft tissue local anesthesia with phentolamine mesylate in adolescents and adults. *J Am Dent Assoc* 139(8):1080–93.

23. Laviola M, McGavin SK, Freer GA, et al. 2008. Randomized study of phentolamine mesylate for reversal of local anesthesia. *J Dent Res* 87:635–9.

24. Dionne RA, Yagiela JA, Cote C, et al. 2006. Balancing efficacy and safety in the use of oral sedation in dental outpatients. *J Am Dent Assoc* 173:502–13.

25. American Dental Association. 2007. *Survey of Current Issues in Dentistry: Surgical Dental Implants, Amalgam Restorations, and Sedation.* Chicago: American Dental Association, Survey Center.

26. Becker DE and Rosenberg M. 2008. Nitrous oxide and the inhalation anesthetics. *Anesth Prog* 55:124–31.

27. Clark, M and Brunick A. 2008. *Handbook of Nitrous Oxide and Oxygen Sedation*, 3rd edn. St. Louis, MO: Mosby/Elsevier.

28. Ramsey DS, Leonesio, RJ, and Whitney CW. 1992. Paradoxical effects of nitrous oxide on human memory. *Psychopharmacology* 106:370–2.

29. Berge TI. 1999. Acceptance and side effects of nitrous oxide oxygen sedation for oral surgical procedures. *Acta Odontol Scand* 57(4):201–3.

30. Veerkamp JS, Gruythusen RJ, Hoogstraten J, et al. 1995. Anxiety reduction with nitrous oxide: A permanent solution. *J Dent Child* 65:44–7.

31. Willumsen T and Vassend O. 2003. Effects of cognitive therapy, applied relaxation and nitrous oxide sedation. A five-year follow-up study of patients treated for dental fear. *Acta Odontol Scand* 61(2):93–7.

32. Dworkin SF, Chen AC, Schubert MM, et al. 1983. Analgesic effects of nitrous oxide with controlled painful stimuli. *J Am Dent Assoc* 107(4):581–5.

33. Robson JG and Davenport HT. 1962. The effects of white sound and music upon the superficial pain threshold. *Can J Anaesth* 9(2):105–8.

34. Anderson WD. 1980. The effectiveness of audio-nitrous oxide-oxygen sedation on dental behavior of a child. *J Pedod* 5:3–21.

35. Weinstein P and Nathan JE. 1988. The challenge of fearful and phobic children. *Den Clin North Am* 32:667–9.

36. Donaldson D, Quarnstrom FC, and Jastak JT. 1989. The combined effect of nitrous oxide and oxygen and electrical stimulation during restorative dental treatment. *J Am Dent Assoc* 118(6):733–6.

37. Dionne RA, Gordon SM, McCullagh LM, et al. 1998. Assessing the need for anesthesia and sedation in the general population. *J Am Dent Assoc* 129:167–73.

38. Jackson DL, Milgrom P, Heacox GA, et al. 2006. Pharmacokinetics and clinical effects of multidose sublingual triazolam in healthy volunteers. *J Clin Psychopharmacol* 26(1):4–8.

39. Greenblatt DJ. 1992. Pharmacology of benzodiazepine hypnotics. *J Clin Psychiatry* 53(Suppl):7–13.

40. Atack JR. 2003. Anxioselective compounds acting at the GABAA receptor benzodiazepine binding site. *Curr Drug Targets CNS Neurol Disord* 2:213–32.

41. Backman JT, Olkkola KT, Ojala M, et al. 1996. Concentrations and effects of oral midazolam are greatly reduced in patients treated with carbamazepine or phenytoin. *Epilepsia* 37:253–7.

42. Varhe A, Olkkola KT, and Neuvonen PJ. 1994. Oral triazolam is potentially hazardous to patients receiving systemic antimycotics ketoconazole or itraconazole. *Clin Pharmacol Ther* 56(6 Pt 1):601–7.

43. Wang JS and DeVane CL. 2003. Pharmacokinetics and drug interactions of the sedative hypnotics. *Psychopharmacol Bull* 37(1):10–29.

44. Bertold CW, Dionne RA, and Corey SE. 1997. Comparison of sublingually and orally administered triazolam for premedication before oral surgery. *Oral Surg Oral Med Oral Pathol Oral Radiol Endod* 84:119–24.

45. Flanagan D. 2005. Understanding the grapefruit drug interaction. *Gen Dent* 53:282–5.

46. Caraco Y, Tateishi T, and Wood AJ. 1995. Interethnic difference in omeprazole's inhibition of diazepam metabolism. *Clin Pharmacol Ther* 58:62–72.

47. Lu DP. 1981. Clinical investigation of relative indifference to pain among adolescent mental retardates. *ASDC J Dent Child* 48:285–8.

48. Jastak JT and Paravecchio R. 1975. An analysis of 1331 sedations using inhalation, intravenous or other techniques. *J Am Dent Assoc* 91:1242–9.

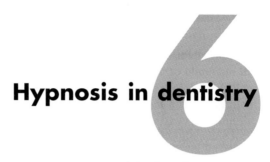

# Hypnosis in dentistry

Michael A. Gow

## INTRODUCTION

In the short time that it takes you to read this chapter, you will discover, as I did, some of the most powerful and practice-changing skills you can learn as a dentist.

You will discover some of the science behind hypnosis and also some hypnotic techniques that can be easily and effectively applied when managing anxious patients in a busy modern dental office.

This chapter will be an introduction for those who are new to dental hypnosis and will start a journey of exploration and expansion. For those who already know about hypnosis through previous training or reading, I hope it will introduce a few new concepts, techniques, and ideas, and perhaps also remind you about a few things that you have forgotten you knew.

Moss[1] defines *hypnodontics* as "that branch of dental science which deals with the application of controlled suggestion and hypnosis to the practice of dentistry."

This description from nearly 60 years ago identifies the fact that hypnosis in dentistry is far more than just the "formal" aspects and traditional ideas of hypnosis that most commonly come to mind.

In fact, the chapter from which the quote above is taken from, entitled "Hypnodontics Today," describes how suggestion plays a very important role in the dentist/patient relationship, from when the patient first "hears about the dentist at his bridge club" to the type of doorbell at the office, the appearance of the waiting room, the greeting of the dental assistant, the personal appearance of the dentist, the quality of his voice, his

*The Fearful Dental Patient: A Guide to Understanding and Managing.* Edited by Arthur A. Weiner
© 2011 Blackwell Publishing Ltd.

mannerisms—all of which are types of "suggestions." Gabor Filo (in Chapter 7 of Brown et al.[2]) offers "A Validation for Hypnosis in Dental Practice," addressing how hypnosis can be integrated into twenty-first century dentistry alongside rapidly advancing technology.

When studying hypnosis, practitioners are taught many techniques for effectively using suggestion, as well as other skills, such as rapport building, language, and communication skills, etc., that can then also be applied in everyday situations. Many who have trained in hypnosis and studied the work of Dr. Milton Erickson (see Rosen[3] and Rossi[4]) will tell you that the day-to-day "informal" uses of hypnotic principles are probably the most important clinical skills that you can ever learn and develop. Kirsch et al.[5] highlighted that "hypnotic and waking responses to the same suggestions are highly correlated, and the difference between them is relatively small." This concept has long been known; in fact, Stolzenburg[6] stated, "The practitioner who is competently trained in hypnosis will find that there is a diminished need for the use of hypnosis per se, with most of his patients." These techniques are especially invaluable in the initial therapeutic consultation with a fearful or phobic patient.

Kay Thompson once said, "My words are the chisels, the brushes used to attempt to reach the inner block of material, the canvas of the individual, modifying the story as the cues demand, and waiting for the message that change is ready, leaving the creation to be interpreted by the patient, the one who commissioned the vision in the beginning."[7]

Hypnosis is very effective in managing appropriate cases, and is often used most effectively when in combination with traditional techniques, complementing conscious sedation for example.

The "father of modern medical hypnosis" himself, Dr. James Braid, recognized his concept very early on and stated: "I consider the hypnotic mode of treating certain disorders is a most important ascertained fact, and a real solid addition to practical therapeutics, for there is a variety of cases in which it is really most successful, and to which it is most particularly adapted; and those are the very cases in which ordinary medical means are least successful, or altogether unavailing. Still, I repudiate the notion of holding up hypnotism as a panacea or universal remedy. As formerly remarked, I use *hypnotism ALONE only in a certain class of cases*, to which I consider it peculiarly adapted—and I use it *in conjunction with medical treatment, in some other cases*; but, *in the great majority of cases, I do not use hypnotism at all*, but depend entirely upon the efficacy of medical, moral, dietetic, and hygienic treatment, prescribing active medicines in such doses as are calculated to produce obvious effects" (emphasis added).[8]

## WHAT IS HYPNOSIS?

Hypnosis has been used for medical purposes in various guises for thousands of years. See Gauld[9] for a detailed history of hypnosis, and Chaves[10] for an overview of the history of hypnosis in dentistry. Certainly, Egyptians and Greeks are known to have gone to "Sleep Temples" to be healed by priests. Prior to the advent of reliable chemical anaesthesia, British medical surgeons such as Elliotson, Esdaile, and Braid pioneered the use of hypnotic techniques in controlling the pain and anxiety associated with medical surgery in the nineteenth century.[11,12] At this time, there was growing interest, and there were many theories such as "animal magnetism," or mesmerism. Dr. James Braid, a Scottish physician-surgeon working in Manchester, England, was the first to challenge these theories, and believed that the phenomena could be induced by suggestion and fixed mental concentration without the use of magnets. Braid,[12] who promoted his theories as early as 1841, ultimately adopted the term "hypnotism" (derived from *hypnos* or "*hupnos*," the Greek word for sleep). The terms *hypnotique, hypnotisme, hypnotiste* had previously been used by the French magnetist Baron Etienne Félix d'Henin de Cuvillers (1755–1841) around 1820, but Braid was the first to use the terms *hypnotism, hypnotize,* and *hypnotist* in English and to attribute the phenomena to psychology.[13] Braid himself, however, soon realised that "hypnotism" was quite different from his original sleep-based physiological theory, and came to favor the terms "neurohypnology," "braidism," or "monoideism" (mental concentration on a single idea) (p. 108).[13] "Hypnotism" and "hypnosis," however, were already popular terms and had become recognized across the world.

Over the years, there has been much debate as to how to define hypnosis and by what mechanisms it actually works. Essentially, hypnosis can be considered as either a mental state (state theory) or a set of attitudes and beliefs (nonstate theory). Some believe that hypnosis is an "altered state of consciousness" marked by changes in the way the brain functions. Others believe that hypnotized subjects are actively motivated to behave in a hypnotic manner and are not simply passively responding to hypnotic suggestions. There are many theories and models of hypnosis that are beyond the scope of this chapter; however, readers wishing to study these can easily find them in several books and resources (e.g., Lynn and Rhue,[14] Kirsch and Lynn,[15,16] Gruzelier,[17] Oakley,[18] Rossi,[19] Chapter 7 in Heap et al.,[20] Nash and Barnier,[21] and Brown and Oakley).

The American Psychological Association (APA) definition for hypnotism is:

> Hypnosis typically involves an introduction to the procedure during which the subject is told that suggestions for imaginative experiences will be presented. The hypnotic induction is an extended initial suggestion for using one's imagination, and may contain further elaborations of the introduction. A hypnotic procedure is used to encourage and evaluate responses to suggestions. When using hypnosis, one person (the subject) is guided by another (the hypnotist) to respond to suggestions for changes in subjective experience, alterations in perception, sensation, emotion, thought or behavior.[22]

The British Psychological Society (BPS)[23] definition is:

> The term "hypnosis" denotes an interaction between one person, the "hypnotist," and another person or people, the "subjects." In this interaction the hypnotist attempts to influence the subjects' perceptions, feelings, thinking and behaviour by asking them to concentrate on ideas and images that may evoke the intended effects. The verbal communications that the hypnotist uses to achieve these effects are termed "suggestions." Suggestions differ from everyday kinds of instructions in that they imply that a "successful" response is experienced by the subject as having a quality of involuntariness or effortlessness. Subjects may learn to go through the hypnotic procedures on their own, and this is termed "self-hypnosis."

A hypnotic subject is often said to be in a "trance," defined by Oakley[24] as "a particular frame of mind characterised by focused attention, dis-attention to extraneous stimuli, and absorption in some activity, image, thought or feeling." People can and do enter trance spontaneously every day, for example, when lost in thought, daydreaming, or absorbed in a book or listening to music, driving for long distances and not recalling the route taken, or being absorbed in meditation/relaxation procedures. Often in these examples, there will be a feeling of time distortion in that the passage of time is underestimated. We "dip" into these natural trances without being aware that it is going to happen. It is only after we have experienced these trances that we are aware of them.

With hypnosis, however, the subject knows that he or she is going to experience trance before it happens. Hypnotic procedures formalize the process of trance, intensify it, and allow it then to be a useful experience during which suggestions and therapeutic techniques can be utilized. Every experience of trance will differ, however: For many, being in trance may feel similar to the stage just before falling asleep, or when first awakening in the morning. An individual is conscious at these times but the brain is operating at a "lower frequency." When talking with patients, I often say that in some ways a hypnotic trance can be compared with being absorbed in a good book or film: "You become fully absorbed and if the storyline and suggestions are acceptable to your way of thinking, morals and belief system, they may change the way you think about certain things." Trance "depth" will fluctuate throughout the hypnotic experience, getting "deeper" and "lighter" at times.

## Requirements for hypnosis—some brief notes

Rapport and trust are essential for hypnosis to be effective (see Kane and Olness,[7] p. 530). If there is strong rapport and trust between hypnotist and patient, the intervention is far more likely to be successful.

Context and motivation are also essential (see Spiegel and Spiegel[25]). A patient must have motivation in order to overcome his or her problem.

Lack of motivation is one of the reasons why some smokers fail to quit, even when they have had hypnosis. I use this example to reassure patients who have concerns over "control," as it highlights that actually, the patients themselves maintain control of their actions and beliefs, allowing them freedom of will.

Expectation is also very important. "Many studies have shown that people respond they way they expect to respond and that changing those expectations changes the way they respond."[26]

It is worth noting that "hypnotizability" or "hypnotic suggestibility" is thought to have little importance on the efficacy of a hypnotic intervention (except for pain management/analgesia).[20] Most people are hypnotizable to some degree, but everyone differs in his or her responsiveness to hypnosis. There is some evidence which suggests that a person's "hypnotizability" is a fixed trait,[14] but other research suggests that a person can be "trained" to become more responsive to hypnosis.[27] If a person has been hypnotized before with success, this may be a positive indication that future hypnotic intervention also has potential to be successful. On the other hand, a previous failed experience with hypnosis may warn the clinician that there may be difficulties with, or perhaps issues to be resolved prior to, any hypnotic intervention.

Several hypnotizability scales exist that quantity hypnotizability.[20,28,29] Formal scales can be interesting, but are seldom used in clinical practice, as they can be time-consuming. Also, care also has to be taken to avoid decreasing a patient's expectations when employing such scales should a "low" score be recorded. It is thought that 30% of people will be able to experience a light trance, 50% a medium trance, and 20% a deep trance.

*Belief*, *context*, and *need* are also important factors in all hypnotic intervention. Ewin and Eimer[30] describe how hypnosis in emergency situations relies more on these factors rather than "hypnotizability" per se (see also Gow[31]).

## Contraindications

Each hypnosis case should be individually assessed. It is prudent for a practitioner considering hypnosis to ask patients if they have, or have ever been diagnosed with, a mood disorder or mental illness, are depressed, are under the care of a psychiatrist or specialist, are currently having suicidal thoughts or have ever had them. Screening questionnaires for anxiety and depression are useful tools when assessing patients for hypnosis—for example, the Hospital Anxiety and Depression Scale.[32] Extra care has to be taken if a subject has a history of mental illness, and appropriate referral should be considered. In some cases, hypnosis should be avoided. It would be wise for a dentist to consult with patients' physicians prior to embarking on hypnotic intervention. Dental practitioners using hypnosis should be aware that their use of hypnosis should be limited to dentistry. It is often appropriate to refer to a doctor or psychologist in cases where there are medical or psychological issues that would be inappropriate for a dentist to treat. Hypnosis is an adjunct to treatment or therapy and as such a dentist should only treat cases where there is a specific dental issue. It is often worth considering asking a patient if they have been hypnotized before, and if so, with what results.

### Myths and misconceptions dispelled

There are several common misconceptions and myths about hypnosis that it is important to dispel.[29] The information below refutes a few common myths and misconceptions.

*Amnesia:* Usually, patients will have full recollection, unless the hypnotist has chosen to elicit amnesia, and it has been deemed beneficial to block specific memories.

*Control:* During hypnosis, subjects are aware and in control. It is for this reason that people who deep down wish to continue smoking, for example, would find hypnosis ineffective in making them stop.

*Beliefs:* Subjects always keep their core morals and beliefs while hypnotized.

*Confidentiality:* Often, it is unnecessary for the hypnotist to know the exact details of the problem, so long as the subject is aware of them and the significance they may play to their treatment. Due to the confidential nature of the patient–hypnotist relationship, however, many people are surprised that they are happy to discuss issues that they may have never discussed before with anyone.

*Stuck in trance:* If tired, a patient may fall asleep; however, no one has ever been "stuck" indefinitely in trance. Occasionally, some patients will take a little longer than others to "come out" of trance. Someone who is hypnotized would return to full awareness naturally after a period of time even if unprompted.

*Unlocking lost memories:* Hypnosis can help to enhance memories, but once a memory is lost, it is lost forever. Care has to be taken not to elicit "false memories", whereby a person believes an event he or she has recalled while in trance to be true, when in fact it is either wholly or partly falsely constructed.

*Movement in trance:* It is important to know that it is OK to move during hypnosis. If someone has an itch, it may cause more distraction avoiding moving and scratching it. Long distance runners often experience trance while running. Patients are also able to easily talk while in trance.

*Therapy:* Hypnosis is never the therapy itself. Hypnosis is an adjunct to treatment or therapy. The hypnotist should be qualified in treating the specific condition that they are using hypnosis to treat.

*Lay hypnosis:* In the last century, valuable research has led to the rise in respectability for the use of clinical hypnosis, but there are currently few laws that control the practice of hypnosis. A quick look through the internet or the yellow/white pages highlights the large number of "lay" hypnotists, who may have seemingly impressive credentials. It is firmly held by most medical/dental/psychological hypnosis societies, however, that hypnosis should be only used by a practitioner who is qualified to be working in the specific field of its application.

*Stage hypnosis*: It is the view of many that hypnosis should never be used as a form of entertainment. Although hypnosis is very safe when practiced responsibly, there may be concerns regarding the safety and well-being of participants in some "stage hypnosis" shows.

# THE HYPNOSIS SESSION

Every clinician's technique and approach to hypnosis will vary to suit their personal style and the individual with whom they are working. Some clinicians prefer, or some cases lend themselves to a more direct approach, while an indirect approach may be indicated at other times. To understand the mechanics of hypnosis and what may be involved in a session, an understanding of certain techniques is helpful. Formal hypnosis sessions usually include use of the following techniques.

## Anchoring

"Anchoring" refers to the ability we all have to link or "anchor" an emotion, memory, etc. to a sight, sound, taste, feeling or smell. People set up their own "anchors" frequently—and often have anchors that were set up decades before being reactivated. Some anchors are negative (e.g., the sound of the dentist's drill, the sight of the white coat, the smell of the dentist's surgery). Other anchors are positive, for example, the noise at a football or soccer match, the smell of home baking, hugging a close friend or family member, etc.

A positive anchor should be set up before using hypnosis. The patient can then access positive emotions at any time in the future using a signal to themselves from themselves that other people would be totally unaware of. The positive anchor is reinforced during trance. Having a positive anchor set up before induction of hypnosis has the additional benefit that should the patient have an abreaction, the clinician has a technique that can reverse this and allow the patient to feel in a more positive frame of mind. An abreaction is when a patient responds unexpectedly during trance, releasing suppressed emotions and becomes upset. Most abreactions occur when the patient spontaneously regresses to a traumatic, unpleasant or upsetting memory. Although these are unusual, it is important that clinicians set up a positive anchor in order that they can lessen or reverse the negative response. Patients can often become emotionally aroused while working through the problem they have sought to resolve. This is controlled and expected in most cases, and can be part of the therapeutic process. An abreaction differs from this as it is unexpected and spontaneous.

There are several types of "self-anchors" that can be taught to patients; a simple example is, once a positive state is being experienced/remembered by the patients, to ask them to touch their thumb and either middle or index finger on their non-dominant hand. The patient is informed that "this is a private signal to yourself, from yourself and can be used at any time to bring back these positive feelings." The patient is instructed to strengthen this anchor by using it any time he or she has very positive experiences. This is very important as these instances are often more powerful anchors than the ones simply set by recalling previous positive memories and emotions.

## Anchoring a positive state (Figure 6.1)

(1)  Decide on a positive state you would like to be in (e.g., happy, confident, etc.)
(2)  Recall a specific occasion in the past when you have been in that state.
(3)  Recall it as vividly as you can remember all you could see, hear, smell, feel at that time.
(4)  Once you are experiencing that positive state, set an anchor to these feelings—for example, squeeze the tip of your thumb together with your middle or index finger on your "nondominant" hand.
(5)  Strengthen this anchor by setting it again any time in the future when you experience positive states. The more positive the experience, the more powerful the anchor will become.
(6)  Now you can re-access this state whenever it would benefit you by "firing" the anchor.

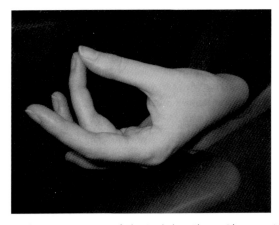

**Figure 6.1**  Anchoring. Courtesy of The Berkeley Clinic, Glasgow, UK.

## *Induction*

The hypnotic induction is the start of the formal process of hypnosis and allows the patient to enter a hypnotic trance. There are many induction techniques and the one selected should be one with which the clinician is confident and that is suitable for the patient.

## Induction technique example: Hand clasp induction technique (adapted from original technique taught by David Cheek; Figure 6.2)

> Clasp your hands together but keep the index fingers straight and separated by two or three centimeters.
>
> Stare at the space between the fingers. As you stare, you will become aware of the fingers wanting to move together. Perhaps you have already noticed that the room is becoming more and more blurry as you focus between the fingers. As the fingers move together, you will become aware of your eyes feeling more strained. You can allow your eyes to close, and your hands to drop comfortably to their lap when the tips of the index fingers finally meet. Just allow the fingers all the time they want. Sometimes they will move together quickly, sometimes it takes a few seconds.

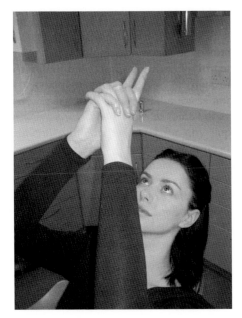

**Figure 6.2** Hand clasp induction technique. Courtesy of The Berkeley Clinic, Glasgow, UK.

(Due to the position of the hands and tendons, the subject would actively have to resist the natural tendency for the fingers to move together. If the fingers do not move together, it may be that the subject has some reservations about being hypnotized.)

## Deepening

A deepening technique is essentially any technique which "deepens" the patient's trance following the induction procedure. There are many techniques that can be employed as deepening techniques. Usually, it is unnecessary for the patient to be in deep trance for most dental hypnosis applications (perhaps with the exception of acute pain control). There are many techniques that aid relaxation and ultimately facilitate deepening. Progressive muscular relaxation was first described by Jacobson.[33] He understood that as muscular tension accompanies anxiety, anxiety can be reduced by learning how to relax muscular tension.

The "laughing place" (a variation of what is known as the safe place, special place, relaxing place, happy place, etc.) is a very effective deepening technique[34] (p. 55), and is also very useful in most hypnotherapy sessions. A deepening technique favored by the author is the "hands together" deepening technique, as it also ratifies to the patient that they are experiencing trance. The hands together technique is also an example of what is called an ideomotor response. This is a phenomenon whereby the subject experiences physical movement that is unconscious, and therefore appears to occur independent of conscious direction. It is worthy of note that the hypnotist should always watch the patient's breathing and deliver their suggestions on the outward breath.

## Deepening technique example: "Hands coming together" (Figure 6.3)

The subject's arms should be outstretched directly in front at shoulder width apart, with palms facing each other.

"I would like you to be aware that there is a natural tendency for your arms and hands to move together … . By thinking about this tendency … you can make it stronger and stronger and your hands will move closer and closer together … . Imagine that your hands are charged like two magnets … with the opposite poles facing each other … . And as you breathe in … and out … I wonder if you notice now, or will notice in a few moments … that your hands are beginning to draw a little closer together … like two magnets … closer and closer … . I don't know if the right hand will be more attracted to the left or if the left will be more attracted to the right … and, I don't know whether your hands will come together quickly or whether it will take a little longer … closer and closer … like two magnets …

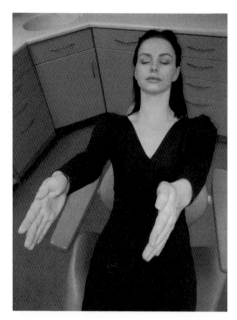

**Figure 6.3**  Hands together deepening technique. Courtesy of The Berkeley Clinic, Glasgow, UK.

closer and closer ... and like two magnets ... as your hands get closer and closer together...so the attraction between them will grow stronger ... closer and closer...closer still ... until they will soon meet ... I don't know which part of them will meet first ... but as they meet ... you will become twice as relaxed as you were before ... and so now as they are about to meet you can look forward to your hands drifting back down to a comfortable position ... I don't know whether they will feel more relaxed by your side or on your lap ... closer and closer just like two magnets until they finally touch ... (repeat relevant sections until the hands meet) ... and as your hands touch together ... and you feel so deeply relaxed ... allow them to find that comfortable position ... that's good ... now notice that all normal sensations and feelings have returned to your hands ... you may like to verify this by moving or wiggling your fingers ... feeling even more relaxed now than before ... deeply, deeply relaxed and comfortable.

## Ego strengthening

Ego-strengthening techniques are intended to improve the self-esteem, self-belief, and inner strength, etc., of the patient. Many believe that ego strengthening is among the most important techniques and suggestions that a therapist can use during a hypnotic intervention. Ego strengthening has been said to "stand as the bedrock upon which other hypnotic techniques are structured."[35]

### Ego strengthening example: "Calm, control and confident" script (adapted from original technique described by Craig et al.[36]; Figure 6.4)

This script assumes the patient is able to create mental images (i.e., is a "visualizer"), and should be tailored as required. The technique should be adapted to the patient's individual "Special Place," the following example uses a sandy beach. The triangle and words may be drawn on any object, with any object. Additional words may be included in the center of the triangle which are appropriate for the patient and their needs—for example, COPE, COURAGE, COMFORT, etc.

*Picture* yourself on your sandy beach. You can see the sand below your feet. ... When you can see this, just let me know by allowing your right index finger to move ... (*Prompt until finger moves. If it fails to move even following further prompting continue with:* "if you are unable to see this, relax because we are just going to consider some words.")

*Very good.* Now imagine that with a stick or a shell or perhaps just your finger you can draw a triangle in the sand ... —that's right, very good. Now around the triangle at its corners you will write some words...starting at the top...with the word ... CALM. *See* the letters as you spell out the word *C ... A ... L ... M ... . (Spell out the letters, pacing each letter with an outward breath)* Notice how the sand feels as you write the word *CALM* with the stick. Just *allow* yourself this feeling of CALM ... *enjoy* this feeling ... from now on feeling *calmer*

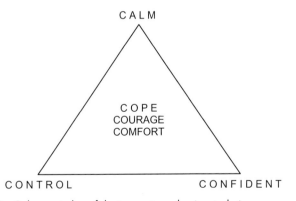

**Figure 6.4**  Calm control confident ego strengthening technique.

*and calmer* every day ... every day feeling *calmer and calmer*...more and more *calm* ... more *optimistic* ... these feelings of calmness *growing* and *increasing* ... *calmer* and *calmer* ... more *composed* ... more at *peace* ... *calm* ... C ... A ... L ... M. ...

Now choose one of the remaining corners of the triangle ... *or allow it to choose you* ... the corner by which you would like to *write* the second word. It's your *right* to *write* on the *left* or the *right*. To *write* on the *right* or the *left* is *right*. If it is the *left* corner then that's all *right* ... the *right* will be *left* for later ... but *right* now *you will write*, and so as you do so *you will feel more and more relaxed* as you *now write the word CONTROL* ... C ... O ... N ... T ... R ... O ... L ... (spell out the letters, pacing each letter with an outward breath) *CONTROL.* And so as you *write* the word control its *right* to *feel yourself more and more in control.*

As you become *calmer* ... more *composed* ... and more *confident* ... more able to *cope* ... you will find that you are *increasingly* able to ... *control* your own life ... each and every day from now on you will feel more and more in *control* ... more in control of your *circumstances* ... more in control of any *situation* ... more in *control of yourself.* You will *enjoy* this new found *control* ... this will allow you to *cope* with many situations ... in exactly the way you want to ... The final word ... to be written at the final corner is the word CONFIDENT.

*CONFIDENT* ... C ... O ... N ... F ... I ... D ... E ... N ... T ... (spell out the letters, pacing each letter with an outward breath) *Confident. Confident* to do the things that you *want* to do ... *every day* feeling more and more *confident* ... confident in *yourself* ... confident in you *abilities* ... confident in your *talents* ... confident that you can become CALM ... Confident that you are in *control*, confident that you can become more CONFIDENT.

Read these words to yourself again. These words that you have written which all begin with "C" ... and you will *now* begin to *see* ... and *feel* and *hear* what these words *really* mean: ... CALM ... CONTROL ... CONFIDENT ... *(pace with outward breaths.)*

*Feel* how *powerful* these words are: ... CALM ... CONTROL ... CONFIDENT ... .

## Diagnostic and therapeutic techniques

There are many techniques which are used in hypnosis that have a direct therapeutic intent, and variations of techniques that can be successfully employed for particular conditions.

As with every other aspect of medicine and dentistry, it is important that a correct diagnosis be made initially in order that an appropriate therapeutic intervention can then be delivered. Hypnoanalytical techniques such as "COMPISS," as described by Dabney Ewin[30,34] are valuable tools enabling hypnotherapists to be accurate in their diagnoses, thereby

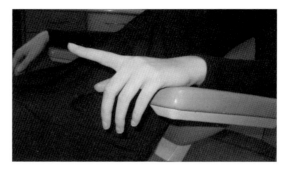

**Figure 6.5** Ideomotor signaling. Courtesy of The Berkeley Clinic, Glasgow, UK.

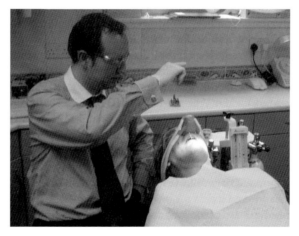

**Figure 6.6** Hypnosis complementing inhalation sedation.[49] Courtesy of The Berkeley Clinic, Glasgow, UK.

allowing them to select the most appropriate intervention. The COMPISS technique utilizes ideomotor signaling (see Figure 6.5), automatic motor responses given by the patient's fingers in direct response to questions the hypnotist poses to the patient's "unconscious." In the same way as we automatically nod our heads to indicate "yes" or "no," ideomotor signaling involves the movement of different fingers to indicate "yes" and "no" responses. Ewin's COMPISS technique assumes that most patients' problems will be influenced by one or more of the following categories: conflict, organ language, motivation, past experience, identification, self–punishment, and suggestion. Often more than one factor will be relevant in any particular problem being treated (Figure 6.6).

There are many therapeutic techniques which can be tailored to the patient's specific needs. Future pacing and reviewing techniques are examples of such techniques. Many more techniques can be sourced in books such as Hammond,[37] Fredericks,[38] Heap and Aravind,[39] Yapko,[29] Spiegel and Speigel,[25] Simons et al.,[40] and Brown.[2]

## Future pacing (also known as future rehearsal)

Future pacing techniques allow the patient to experience positive future changes. Patients' own words and goals are used to strengthen their future pacing (p. 56).[34] Future pacing is one of the most important therapeutic techniques in hypnosis. It increases expectation, belief, motivation, and confidence. Yapko[29] believes that it is important that the patient future paces into at least three different times in the future. Common techniques for future pacing include using imagery of TV screens, cinema screens, time machines, and mirrors. With these techniques, dental patients use future rehearsal to experience the positive feelings they will have when the treatment is finished and they have achieved their goals. Once these positive feelings have been elicited and anchored, the patient can "bring them back" to the present day.

## Regression, reliving, recalling: Techniques to resolve a traumatic experience

Regression/reliving/recalling techniques that can be used to go back to the time of a traumatic episode include techniques such as "Time Line," "Video Library," and "Single Memory Evaluation" (see Graham,[41] Heap and Aravind,[39] and Yapko[29]). For many patients, their dental phobia is the product of a single traumatic incident (or a series of similar events). A useful hypnotic approach is for the older, adult self to comfort the "younger" self, hug it, and reassure it that it is in fact the living proof that it survived the event and that everything will be OK soon. It is sometimes helpful for the patient to review the incident in hypnosis and to gather together any positive learnings from the experience. In some cases, rescripting some of the outcome of the earlier event may be helpful, perhaps using skills and strategies that were not available to the individual at the time, but are now. It is important to work with the earliest traumatic event to ensure that the phobia can be effectively treated and overcome in the long term. Obviously, due care must be taken when using these techniques, and the hypnotist should be prepared to cope with any abreaction encountered.

## Posthypnotic suggestions

"Posthypnotic suggestions are those given to the client while he or she is in hypnosis that encourage particular thoughts, behaviors, or feelings he or she is to have in some other future context" (p. 255).[29] Posthypnotic suggestions allow the patient to carry new possibilities and changes into future situations where they can take effect. Posthypnotic suggestions can therefore often allow future treatment to be carried out more quickly and in a relaxed manner. This can often mean that any time spent in the initial "therapy" is soon repaid by facilitating faster future treatment sessions.

## Safeguards and ethical blocks

Safeguards and "ethical blocks" are essentially posthypnotic suggestions that protect the patient from being hypnotized at inappropriate times or by inappropriate people.

Example script: "In the future, you will find it easier to go into trance at appropriate and safe times for you to do so, and with your full knowledge and consent. You will only allow yourself to be hypnotized during your self-hypnosis sessions, or with the guidance of a medical doctor, dentist, psychologist, or other appropriate professional who is trained in using hypnosis."

## Reversal/arousal/reorientation

Traditional "reverse counting" techniques are often disliked by patients as it assumes that they will respond and reorientate exactly in time with the counting. A more permissive and gentle way would be the following example script:[42]

> And now it is time to fully return to the present moment. Back fully
>     present in your physical body.
> Any strange sensations … totally disappearing.
> Your muscle tone returns to normal.
> Your co-ordination returns to normal.
> And this will happen each time you come out of trance.
> BRIGHT. ALERT, and WIDE AWAKE.
> When you are ready … OPEN YOUR EYES.
> Well done.

## Self-hypnosis

Self-hypnosis is also known as autohypnosis, and is a self-induced form of hypnosis. Patients can carry out specific exercises as taught by the hypnotist and make use of self-suggestions. Self–hypnosis is an important aspect of hypnosis.

# HYPNOSIS IN DENTISTRY—"HYPNODONTICS"

The uses of hypnosis in dentistry include:[43]

- gagging (during procedures or denture/appliance intolerance);
- para-functional habits, for example, bruxism, tongue-thrusting;

- TMJ dysfunction;
- modification of other unwanted oral habits (e.g., thumbsucking, nail-biting);
- salivation control;
- bleeding control;
- smoking cessation;
- improved compliance with oral hygiene regimes;
- treatment of anxiety/stress-related recurrent aphthous stomatitis;
- reduction of symptoms of burning mouth syndrome;
- acute pain control;
- chronic facial pain;
- psycho-somatic facial pain;
- anxiety management/relaxation;
- complementing conscious sedation-(inhalation/intravenous/oral);
- alternative to conscious sedation; and
- phobia management (specific phobias, e.g., general dental, needle, dental needle, blood, drill, amalgam).

The spectrum of applications of hypnosis in dentistry is surprisingly wide, and the literature in these applications is ever growing. There are many reference books that go into these applications in detail. Simons et al.[40] and Brown,[2] for example, are especially useful resources for dentists. Hypnosis has been shown to be of benefit in improving oral hygiene,[44] such as reducing the symptoms of burning mouth syndrome and TMJ dysfunction,[39] smoking cessation,[45,46] oral ulceration,[36] and other problems. Detailed analysis of every application of hypnosis in dentistry is beyond the scope of this chapter, but it is worth considering gagging, bruxism, and pain in more detail.

Bassi et al.[47] presented a useful paper that reviews literature on gagging from 1940 to 2002. They highlight the multifactoral etiology, observing that there seem to be two main categories: the somatogenic group, in which gagging is induced by physical stimuli of "trigger zones," and the psychogenic group, in which gagging is induced by psychological stimuli. It may be difficult to differentiate between the two groups, as a physical stimulus may provoke gagging of psychogenic origin. Milgrom et al.[48] believe that the problem may be best viewed as a psycho-physiological reaction that has become overlearned. Patients who have a strong gag response may be more anxious in general of dental treatment. Hypnosis has been demonstrated to be effective in helping patients with strong gag reflexes to accept dental treatment[49] and to tolerate appliances such as dentures.[50] Robb and Crothers[51] explain that the permanent reduction of the gag reflex can be approached in three main ways using hypnosis:

(1) *Hypnosis as an adjunct to desensitization*: For example, the authors say, "Using hypnosis as a way of producing pleasant emotions and sensations when the plate is inserted will help to reduce the reflex and

ultimately extinguish it in a susceptible patient." This approach is the basis of the recommendations of Barsby.[50]

(2)  *Actively engaging patients in their own treatment* by encouraging them to see the benefits of their treatment (e.g., health, appearance), and to view overcoming the problem as a positive achievement.

(3)  *Uncovering circumstances that caused the reflex to develop.* This can be a useful technique and may reveal a previous event which has led to the current inappropriately strong gag reflex. Obviously, care must be taken when using such techniques, as the patient may reexperience traumatic memories of, for example, sexual abuse. There may also be the possibility of creating a "false memory" of a previous trauma. Should uncovering techniques begin to reveal a history that the practitioner feels is beyond his or her expertise, it is appropriate to refer the patient to an appropriately trained and competent practitioner.

Hypnosis is increasingly used in the management of the inappropriate gag response. It is likely that this success is at least in part due to the possible psychogenic nature of the etiology. It would seem that hypnosis is most beneficial when used in conjunction with other techniques. For example, if the problem is with gagging during a dental procedure, hypnosis may be of most use in combination with relaxation, distraction, and breathing techniques. Advising the patient to practice swallowing with the mouth open at home, while breathing in a calm and steady manner can aid with desensitization as well. This desensitization exercise can be further added to by having the patient repeat this while holding water in the mouth (the swallow reflex can be activated without actually swallowing the contents of the mouth). In the case of denture intolerance, an intervention as described by Barsby[50] whereby hypnosis is integrated into treatment, including desensitization with plastic discs and latterly training bases, would be the likely approach of choice.

As Gastone[52] writes, "With the possibility that psychological and personality aspects may be important in the etiology, there is a growing reputation for hypnosis being a beneficial adjunct in the treatment of bruxism." The first systematic study on hypnosis and bruxism was by Mulligan and Clark,[53] who used an EMG to record the masseter muscle activity. Half of the subjects (3 out of 6) showed a significant decrease in EMG activity. One subject reported no improvement, four a reduction, and one complete resolution. A pilot study by Clarke and Reynolds[54] also demonstrated a reduction in EMG recordings of the activity of the masseter muscle. Subjects indicated improvement both immediately following treatment and over the long term. A pilot study by Gow (in preparation for publication,[55] cited in Simons et al.[40]) demonstrated that compared with a control group, hypnotic intervention significantly improved the bruxism habit in the opinion of the experimental group, and that this was confirmed by a significant decrease in masseter EMG activity. Several techniques and suggestions were used, including a variation of the original[56] clenched-fist technique.[57]

Clarke[58] reports an estimated success rate of 75–80%, concluding that bruxism is a problem which demands a variety, and sometimes combinations, of treatments. Certainly, Somer[59] and Gow[60] also highlight the importance of considering multiple etiological factors when treating bruxism. Hypnosis should be considered if a patient's bruxism is thought to be influenced by stress, anxiety, conflict, or other psychological issues.

Hypnosis can be considered as a management option for patients with xerostomia (dry mouth due to lack, or perceived lack, of saliva) that is symptomatic only, that is, psychogenic or related to anxiety, nervousness, or depression. It may play a role in improving patient symptoms, and potentially even in increasing the volume of saliva produced. Self-hypnosis may allow patients to control these factors themselves. Obviously every effort should be made to identify and treat the underlying cause(s) of a patient's xerostomia. Conversely, most dentists have experienced difficulty in controlling patient salivation (e.g., while placing a child's fissure sealants), despite the nurse's best efforts with the suction. Self-hypnosis may then help patients reduce excessive salivation themselves at subsequent dental visits. Frost[61] suggests that the dentist should say: "Before you open your mouth, I want you to swallow hard three times. This will leave your mouth dry and free from saliva. As you then open your mouth, it will remain dry and saliva will cease to flow into it until treatment is finished."

Other references include Gow,[62] Sector,[63] Spanos et al.,[64] and Winer et al.[65]

Early reports of surgery using hypnosis for analgesia often noted that there seemed to be little bleeding, and that healing was rapid. Tuckey[66] found that the smaller arteries and capillaries were "almost invariably contracted in hypnosis, so that even deep wounds tended to produce little or no haemorrhage." The exact mechanisms of hypnosis in bleeding control remain subject to some debate. However, it is accepted that some degree of bleeding control is certainly achievable by some subjects using hypnotic techniques and suggestions. We know that emotions and mental processes influence the vasomotor system (e.g., fear causes pallor; embarrassment causes blushing). An early study by Forel[67] found that local flushing could be induced by simple suggestion. It is also well known that one of the indicators of anxiety is increased perspiration of the palms of the hands, which is due to capillary dilation, followed by a drop in temperature. Reduction in anxiety (e.g., with hypnosis) results in constriction of capillaries, dry palms, and a rise in local temperature. It would seem to follow that reduction in anxiety should therefore also constrict capillaries and small blood vessels in and around an extraction socket, thereby reducing postoperative bleeding or arresting hemorrhage. Blood pressure and pulse rate also influence bleeding and can likewise be reduced by suggestions of relaxation and calmness, or increased by suggestions of excitement and agitation. It therefore stands to reason that some amount of control of postextraction bleeding must be possible by influencing these factors.

(Other references include Newman,[68] Chaves et al.,[69] Enqvist et al.,[70] and Gow.[71])

The simple suggestions and techniques outlined below may be given with or without formal hypnotic induction.[71]

To control hemorrhaging following extraction:

- "Visualize the blood in the extraction socket as water coming from a tap which could be turned off."
- "Visualize constricting and collapsing blood vessels in the involved area for as long as necessary."
- "Visualize mentally suturing the sides of the wound" (perhaps suggest the image of the "blood vessels being tied with a magic thread").
- Suggestions of coldness at extraction site.
- Basic relaxation techniques will reduce bleeding by reducing pulse, blood pressure, etc.

To prevent alveolar osteitis (dry socket) following extraction:

- "Visualize blood in the extraction socket as water coming from a tap which could be turned on."
- "Visualize dilating and opening blood vessels in the involved area for as long as necessary."
- Suggestions of warmth at site to increase bleeding.
- Stimulating visualization to increase bleeding (e.g. active imagery such as running or cycling) to increase pulse, blood pressure, etc.

An application of hypnosis that gains much interest from the medical professions and in research is that of pain control. The first reported use of hypnosis for acute pain control during a dental extraction was in 1836 when Oudet, a Parisian physician, extracted a tooth from a hypnotized patient.[24] With the advent of more reliable chemical anesthetics, however, the medical and dental professions understandably focused on researching and developing these techniques. But there are cases even in today's dentistry when it is not possible or feasible to use traditional pharmacological techniques for pain control, as when an alternative to local anesthetics and/or sedation is needed for a patient with an allergy or an unusual reaction to local anesthetics or sedation, or there is a complicated medical history, or the patient has requested it, based on research and education.

Gow and Friel,[72,73] in a televised case, demonstrated for the first time that it is possible to extract teeth using hypnosis in place of local anesthetics, and then to place immediate dental implants. A similar case[74] demonstrated an internal sinus lift and implant placement with hypnosis in place of local anesthetics.

There are many different suggestions and techniques which can be used in pain management, for example, "Comfort Dials" (Gow and Friel[73]), and "Glove Anaesthesia" (Auld in Battino and South,[75] Chapter 16), which can be employed in such cases. There is now a plethora of research that is establishing an impressive and growing evidence base in the field of pain control. Patterson and Jensen[76] concluded that "Hypnosis has a reliable and significant impact on acute procedural pain and chronic pain conditions." Montgomery et al.[77] highlighted the evidence base for hypnosis in acute and chronic pain management for a number of conditions in a meta-analysis of 18 studies, indicating a moderate to large hypnoanalgesic effect. The exact mechanisms of how hypnosis actually works in pain control is only now in the twenty-first century becoming more understood, with an increase in neuroimaging studies, such as those carried out by Derbyshire et al.[78,79] The former study "identified brain areas directly involved in the generation of pain using hypnotic suggestion to create an experience of pain in the absence of any noxious stimulus. In contrast with imagined pain, functional magnetic resonance imaging (fMRI) revealed significant changes during this hypnotically induced pain experience within the thalamus and anterior isualise, insula, prefrontal, and parietal cortices. These findings compare well with the activation patterns during pain from nociceptive sources and provide the first direct experimental evidence in humans linking specific neural activity with the immediate generation of a pain experience."

## Dental anxiety and phobia management

When considering the most appropriate management technique for any patient, it is essential that all options be fully considered and discussed. There are basically two treatment plans to construct with the patient. One is the plan for the dental treatment, and the second is the treatment plan for what can be done to reduce the patient's anxiety to allow the treatment to take place. Consideration must be given to safety, simplicity, analgesia, amnesia, acceptability, compatibility, and cost. Patients usually like the idea of amnesia of their treatment, but it should be highlighted to them that the use of sedation or general anesthetics only may be unable to help them overcome their phobia in the long term (as they may not remember any positive experience). Often, simple behavioral approaches, communication skills, and rapport techniques will go a long way in combination with the chosen approach.[80] Hypnosis can be used to overcome dental phobias including general dental, needle, dental needle, blood, drill, and amalgam phobia (see Baker and Boas,[81] Finklestein,[82] and Gow[31,43,83–85]). In preparation for dental treatment, hypnosis can be used to uncover the reason why the phobia developed, resolve feelings about previous bad experiences, engage the patient in the treatment by using future rehearsal techniques, act as an adjunct to desensitization techniques, and overcome embarrassment or other issues. During dental treatment, hypnosis and suggestion can be used to complement local anesthetics by reducing levels of anxiety and pain. As the majority of dental patients have their treatment carried out using local anesthetics alone, this is an area in which a dentist

trained in hypnosis could use "informal" hypnotic techniques and suggestion on a day-to-day basis.

## Patient testimony

I hadn't been to the dentist for nearly 10 years and was in desperate
need of treatment. It wasn't really a problem for the first 4 or 5 years.
However, the last few years this fear had been really getting me
down and it was starting to affect my life, especially over the past
year. About 3 years ago one of my pre-molars had broken and I just
assured myself that I would make an appointment to see the dentist
'soon' but at the same time knew I just couldn't bring myself to do
this. Looking back now, it was like I was trapped in this fear and was
embarrassed about my teeth, and couldn't possibly let a dentist look
in my mouth, but knew I needed treatment and it was inevitable that
one day I would have to get some. However, taking that first step to
even make an appointment just seemed impossible to me and there
was no way I could do it without help. I began searching websites
for information about dental phobias and found a wealth of information. I came across a website by Mike Gow, a dentist who practices
hypnotherapy for patients with dental phobias who had helped a
number of people. I then decided that I had to contact Mike and that
he would be able to help me overcome my fear. It took me a while
to pluck up the courage to do this, but eventually I did. I contacted
Mike and just talking to him initially on the phone was so much
easier than I had first anticipated. He arranged for me to meet him
and just have a chat about my fears and what he could do to help.
There was no pressure at all to look at my teeth, and he made
me feel at ease straightaway and I found him very approachable.
I couldn't believe I was so calm talking to a dentist! Before this even
the mention of the word 'dentist' would send me into a panic.

At my second visit I had hypnotherapy, which was unbelievable
and helped enormously. The session was recorded and I then lis-
tened to the CD the night before each appointment. I was also taught
techniques which helped me to relax when I felt over-anxious. By the
third visit I felt ready to have treatment, and throughout this Mike
assured me that if at any time I felt uneasy or scared to let him know
and he would stop immediately, but I'm glad to say this never hap-
pened and after this each time became easier. I still get a little anxious
before an appointment but probably no more than the average person
now. I have now had all my treatment and have accomplished my
goals. I have even booked an appointment for my 6 months check-up!
I can honestly say that overcoming this phobia has been so much
easier than I thought it would be and it really is all down to the
sympathetic, understanding, supportive and friendly approach.

## Complementing conscious sedation

A recent book by Lang and Laser[80] describes the use of rapid rapport, language, suggestion and hypnotic techniques to improve day-to-day interactions and communication with patients and reduce anxiety and pain. Hypnosis can certainly be used to complement conscious sedation.[49,86-88] Without behavioral intervention, a sedated patient can often still be difficult to manage. The advantages of positive suggestion with inhalation sedation have long been known and practiced. It has been demonstrated that nitrous oxide does in fact increase suggestibility.[89] Treatment that combines hypnotic techniques and suggestions with sedation is often quicker, helps the patient learn coping skills while fostering trust, expectation, motivation, and rapport, as well as removing some of the dependency on the sedation.[87] Less sedative is often required and recovery and healing times are faster.[88]

Other advantages of combining sedation and hypnosis include:

- Reduction in anxiety, blood pressure, heart rate, etc.
- A technique called "glove anesthesia" can create altered sensation in a hand or arm prior to IV cannulation.
- Suggestions can be used to promote vasodilaton of a vein prior to IV cannulation.
- Relaxation and breathing techniques work synergistically with inhalation sedation.
- Hypnotic time distortion can allow longer cases to seem shorter to the patient.
- Specific suggestions can be given to control pain, bleeding and gagging.
- Specific suggestions, especially with IV sedation, can be given to create amnesia or enhance recall as appropriate.
- Posthypnotic suggestions can be given to promote comfort and healing after the treatment.

# "INFORMAL" HYPNOTIC TECHNIQUES IN DAY-TO-DAY DENTAL PRACTICE

It is often commented by delegates at conferences that "if you pick up one or two gold nuggets, it was worth going."

The following random selection of "gold nuggets" for your consideration are a few techniques that are based in hypnotic principles and can be immediately applied directly in your dental office—even without formal training in hypnosis! Some of these techniques have aspects of neurolinguistic programming (NLP). NLP models do not have strong empirical evidence; however, some NLP techniques can be very useful in practice (see Faulkner[90]).

## Communication

Excellent communication is essential between all staff and patients. Most patient complaints are due to communication breakdown or misunderstanding. Be aware of the impact of the language that you use, and avoid emotive words with anxious patients. For example, replace the word "pain" with "pressure," "drill" with "handpiece," "waiting room" with "lounge," and so on (see Gow[91] and Yapko[29]). Even when we remain silent, we are communicating. Nonverbal communication can account for a large proportion of a message. In 1971, Mehrabian[92] proposed his 7%, 38%, 55% rule, suggesting what proportion of communication is conferred by words, tone, and body language. (This is often misquoted, however, so it is important to note that he was referring to particular cases of expressing feelings or attitudes rather than to every communication.)

## Rapport

Rapport is a feeling of comfort with another or others. A good rapport between all staff and the patient is extremely important in ensuring that the patient is totally at ease. The opportunity to build rapport begins as soon as a new patient contacts the practice, and continues with patients you may have been treating for years.

*Rapport building with mirroring* (see Lang and Laser[80]): Rapport can be improved by subtly mirroring something about the other person. For example it is possible to mirror movement, posture, facial expressions, angle of head, position of arms, hands, legs and feet, speed and rhythm of breathing. You can even mirror the sound of the patient's voice: rhythm, pitch, volume, timbre, and speed. This technique can even be used over the telephone.

*Handshake rapid rapport technique:* Allow other person to "lead" the handshake. Mirror the position of how they hold the handshake, mirror the strength of the grip, and the movement. Also, subtly mirror the position of the person's body/gait, nod of head, and tone/pace of voice during the handshake (see Faulkner et al.[90]).

*"Name" rapid rapport technique:* Rapid rapport can be achieved by then asking patients what their friends call them. By asking this you are finding out what they like to be called (e.g., rapport is often destroyed by calling for someone William, if he is only ever called Bill). With this technique, you are also effectively asking for permission to be their friend!

## Positive language[29,80,91]

I am now going to let you in on a secret that could change your professional (and personal) life forever. I am going to share with you what is probably the most powerful, practice changing skill I have learned when studying hypnosis. It is very simple, easy to do once you get the hang of it, and it can be used by every dentist in his or her day-to-day work and personal life. The secret is simply using the power of positive language and suggestion. To demonstrate how negative language and suggestion can have the opposite effect to that intended, consider the following:

> Whatever you choose to think about right now—just don't think about elephants. Don't think about an elephant that you have seen before perhaps in a zoo, a circus, on safari or even on TV. Certainly don't think about African or Indian elephants and how their ears are different shapes and sizes. Don't even think about soft toy elephants, and that they are often either blue or pink. Don't think about wooden carvings or ornaments of elephants. Try not to remember even looking at a picture or photograph you have seen of an elephant. Whatever you think about—just don't think about elephants right now." Despite these instructions, what are you thinking about? To "not" think about something, you have to think about it! Imagine now what happens if you say things to a patient such as "Don't worry, this won't hurt," "Don't cry," or "This won't take long." Despite your best intentions to reassure them, what do you think will be going through that patient's mind, especially if they are anxious? It is a valuable skill to train yourself to avoid using negatives—and equally important to encourage your coworkers to follow suit!

## "What can I do to help you?"

The first thing a dentist should ask any patient is "What can I do to help you?" The patient will probably then tell you about what he or she considers the most important dental problem. Invite patients to prioritize their treatment (e.g., pain, cosmetic, function).

You should ensure at this point that the information you get is actually framed positively—that is, a "positive goal" rather than a problem: "What would you like to change?" or "where would you like to be?" or "So, what you really want is to be out of pain." The patient's answer should be positive rather than retrospective, for example: "I would like to have nice looking, healthy, strong white teeth."

If the patient requires a lot of treatment, or has requested cosmetic treatment, ask them why he or she has decided to do something about seeking this treatment now, rather than last year, for example. (This may help you understand and be aware of any ongoing barriers to them having treatment now—fear/finances, etc.) When planning the treatment, tackle the main issue the patient first presented with, if possible. This will increase compliance, trust, and rapport. Once a good solid treatment plan has been made (and is appropriate) the actual dentistry will be much easier.

## Distraction during local anesthetics

The following distraction technique can be useful when placing local anesthetics with a patient who is anxious with needles. This "eyes open" technique was described by Gow[43] as part of a dental needle desensitization protocol.

Just before the needle is inserted, most people will have their eyes closed. The needle should be positioned close to the mucosa and the patient asked to open their eyes, or, if his or her eyes are already open, asked to keep eyes open. Verbalization such as "I wonder if you would open your eyes right now" should then be given. Occasionally, patients need to hear more of the following verbalization before opening their eyes. What is important is that the needle is gently inserted a couple of millimeters into the mucosa simultaneously to the eyes opening. As the eyes fully open, the solution should be slowly infiltrated and the needle gently advanced while the verbalization continues: "In much the same way as blind people say that their other senses are heightened, if you keep your eyes closed your brain will attempt to gain more information from other sources. With your eyes open, and by listening to what I am saying, your brain has to process more information, and everything can be more comfortable, that's great, well done, only 10 seconds now 9, 8, 7, 6, 5, 4, 3, 2, 1, 0, well done!" The verbalization should be paced to the speed of the injection. It is often useful to give the patient a countdown from 10 to zero when the procedure is nearing completion. It is possible that this verbalization acts only as a distraction while the anesthetic is being delivered, but it is my experience that most people seem happy to accept the theory and find it useful.

## AN ANCHORING TECHNIQUE FOR CHILD DENTAL PATIENTS—"THE HIGH FIVE ANCHOR"

The "high five anchor" is a technique I developed and have used with a lot of success over the years. It is most effective with prepubescent children, as older children may be less responsive to the idea of "high fives" with their dentist! A "high five" is essentially an "anchor" that most parents teach their children at an early age. Even very young, pre-verbal children do it!

At the child's first visit, ensure that rapport is built, and that the child feels safe and happy. This can take a while, and sometimes means postponing even looking at the patient's teeth on this visit in order that rapport can be developed. At the end of the rapport-building session, when the child is in a positive mood/state, say "Give me five!" and present your hand. When they hit your hand, say to the child, "Come on—hit me harder—do it as hard as you can—so hard that it will make my hand sting!" When the child repeats the anchor, this time doing it harder, he or she will tend to be smiling. The dentist should, with a smile, "play act" that in fact it really did hurt by smiling and saying "Ouch—that was excellent!" (Note to practitioner: Sometimes it does actually hurt!) The child then leaves the session in a very positive mood and an anchor has been set.

When the child returns in the future for a check up or for dental treatment, the anchor can be used to bring back, very quickly, that positive state. As soon as the child walks in the door, present your hand and say something along the lines of "Hi there! Give me five! I bet you can't do it harder than you did last time!" The child's mood/state changes very quickly (often from a negative emotion—fear/anxiety/etc.) to that same state of trust/happiness, etc. that had been built at the last session. As soon as the child "gives five," re-enact the game of smiling and saying "Ouch!" before quickly saying, "excellent—now jump up on the chair and if you "give me five" we can get (e.g.) this tooth fixed." Strengthen the "high five" anchor again at the end of the treatment, and praise the child for how well he or she has done, and how easy the treatment was.

## The illusion of choice

A "bind" or an "illusion of choice" is a very useful technique. It is known that if someone asks if you would like a cup of tea, for example, then you have a basic "yes" or "no" response. If you were asked if you would like a cup of tea or a cup of coffee, you are more likely to choose one or the other rather than decline. In a similar vein the child, can be informed that he or she has a choice between "filling a" and "filling b." This "illusion of choice" is extremely effective, especially with children. This also rapidly gains consent for the treatment you wish to carry out at that visit, and increasing compliance. For more information on "binds," and "double binds" see texts such as Hammond,[37] p. 34, and Yapko.[29]

# CONCLUSIONS

Gow and Canning[93] demonstrated that out of 154 dentists in British Columbia, Canada, 38% would consider using hypnosis (if they had appropriate training), and 14% already used it for anxiety management. However, 0% of 90 randomly selected members of the public reported ever having knowingly experienced hypnosis at the dentist. Thirty-eight percent of the 90 reported that they would be willing to try hypnosis if they had the option. This highlights the fact that there is a growing interest by dentists in hypnosis, and also a growing demand by patients who more and more seem to be seeking nonpharmacological interventions for medical and dental problems. This is certainly an increasing demand that the dental profession must be able to meet.

The twentieth century saw a huge amount of research into hypnosis, with some of the earliest scientific studies using statistical and experimental analysis starting as early as 1933.[94] In the twenty-first century, there is now an increasing rise in the understanding and acceptance by the dental profession, as well as demand by the public for dental hypnosis.[93,95] With solid support in the evidence base, which is essential in modern medicine, the dental profession must sit up and take note that a valuable yet underused tool exists that can be effectively integrated into the modern dental office. The principles of hypnosis, rapport, language, and communication should be taught in every dental school. This would be of huge benefit to the dental profession, and ultimately result in happier, better cared-for patients. Over 150 years ago, Dr. James Braid recognized that hypnosis should have a place in mainstream medicine. This understanding has been reinforced over the decades by a number of very successful clinicians. For those dentists who have already come to this understanding, it has changed their clinical practice, making life as a dentist easier, more satisfying, and more enjoyable. Hypnosis is very much a part of mainstream medicine and dentistry, and as more and more practitioners become aware of its clinical uses and the science continues to provide the evidence that demonstrates the neurophysiological processes by which it works, twenty-first-century dentistry is going to enjoy some exciting changes in patient care.

## SUGGESTED HYPNOSIS SOCIETIES, TRAINING PATHWAYS, AND CONTACTS FOR DENTISTS

*International:* International Society of Hypnosis, www.ish-web.org

*Europe:* European Society of Hypnosis, www.esh-hypnosis.eu

*United States:* American Society of Clinical Hypnosis, www.asch.net

Society for Clinical & Experimental Hypnosis, www.sceh.us

*United Kingdom:* The British Society of Clinical and Academic Hypnosis, www.bscah.com

The British Society of Medical and Dental Hypnosis (Scotland), www.bsmdhscotland.com

The Royal Society of Medicine-Hypnosis and Psychosomatic Medicine Section, www.rsm.ac.uk

The Hypnosis Unit UK, www.hypnosisunituk.com

## REFERENCES

1.  Moss AA. 1953. *Hypnodontics or Hypnotism in Dentistry*. Brooklyn, NY: Dental Items of Interest Publishing Company.
2.  Brown DC (ed.). 2009. *Advances in the Use of Hypnosis for Medicine, Dentistry and Pain Prevention/Management*. Bethel, CT: Crown House Publishing Ltd.
3.  Rosen S. 1991. *My Voice Will Go With You: The Teaching Tales of Milton H. Erickson, M.D.* New York: W.W. Norton & Company.
4.  Rossi EL, Ryan MO, and Sharp FA (eds.). 1998. *Healing In Hypnosis—The Seminars, Workshops and Lectures of Milton H Erickson Vol. 1*. London: Free Association Books.

5. Kirsch I, Mazzoni G, and Montgomery GH. 2007. Remembrance of hypnosis past. *Am J Clin Hypn* 49(3):171–8.
6. Stolzenber J. 1961. Technique in conditioning and hypnosis for control of gagging. *Int J Clin Exp Hypn* 9:97–104.
7. Kane S and Olness K (eds.). 2004. *The Art of Therapeutic Communication. The Collected Works of Kay F. Thompson.* Carmarthen, UK: Crown House Publishing.
8. Braid J. 1852. *Magic, Witchcraft, Animal Magnetism, Hypnotism, and Electro-Biology, Etc.* London: John Churchill, pp. 90–1.
9. Gauld, A. 1992. *History of Hypnotism.* Cambridge: Cambridge University Press.
10. Chaves JF. 1997. Hypnosis in dentistry: Historical overview and current appraisal. In: Mehrstedt M and Wikstrom PO (eds.), *Hypnosis in Dentistry: Hypnosis International Monographs 3.* Munich: MEG Stiftung, pp. 5–23.
11. Esdaile J. 1846. *Mesmerism in India, and Its Practical Application in Surgery and Medicine.* London: Longman, Brown, Green, and Longmans, 1846.
12. Braid J. 1847. Facts and observations as to the relative value of mesmeric and hypnotic coma, and ethereal narcotism, for the mitigation or entire prevention of pain during surgical operations. *Med Times* 15(385):381–2; 16(387):10–1.
13. Gravitz MA and Gerton MI. 1984. Origins of the term hypnotism prior to braid. *Am J Clin Hypn* 27(2):107–10.
14. Lynn S and Rhue J (eds.). 1991. *Theories of Hypnosis: Current Models and Perspectives.* New York: Guilford.
15. Kirsch I and Lynn SJ. 1995. The altered state of hypnosis. *Am Psychol* 50(10):846–58.
16. Kirsch I and Lynn SJ. 1998. Dissociation theories of hypnosis. *Psychol Bull* 123:100–15.
17. Gruzelier JH. 1998. A working model of the neuropsychopysiology of hypnosis: A review of evidence. *Contemp Hypn* 15(1):5–23.
18. Oakley DA. 1999. Hypnosis and consciousness: A structural model. *Contemp Hypn* 16:215–23.
19. Rossi EL. 2000. In search of a deep psychobiology of hypnosis: Visionary hypotheses for a new millennium. *Am J Clin Hyp* 42(3–4):178–207.
20. Heap M, Brown RJ, and Oakley DA. 2004. *The Highly Hypnotizable Person: Theoretical, Experimental and Clinical Issues.* Hove, UK: Brunner-Routledge.
21. Nash MR and Barnier AJ (eds.). 2008. *The Oxford Theory, Research and Practice.* Oxford: Oxford university Press.
22. Green JP, Barabasz AF, Barrett D, et al. 2005. Forging ahead: The 2003 APA Division 30 definition of hypnosis. *Int J Clin Exp Hypn* 53(3):259–264.
23. The British Psychological Society. 2001. *The Nature of Hypnosis.* A report prepared by a working party at the request of the Professional Affairs Board of The British Psychological Society. The British Psychological Society, March 2001.
24. Oakley DA. 2001. The use of hypnosis in dentistry. *Dentistry* 6:14–5.

25. Speigel H and Speigel D. 2004. *Trance & Treatment. Clinical Uses of Hypnosis*, 2nd edn. London: American Psychiatric Publishing, Inc.

26. Kirsch I. 2001. The altered states of hypnosis. *Soc Res* 68:795–807.

27. Spanos NP. 1986. Hypnosis and the modification of hypnotic susceptibility: A social psychological perspective. In P. Naish (ed.), *What Is Hypnosis?* Philadelphia: Open University Press, pp. 85–120.

28. Kirsch I, Capafons A, Cardena-Bulena E, et al. 1999. *Clinical Hypnosis and Self-Regulation: Cognitive-Behavioural Perspectives.* Washington, DC: American Psychological Association.

29. Yapko M. 2003. *Trancework: An Introduction to the Practice of Clinical Hypnosis*, 3rd edn. New York: Brunner-Routledge.

30. Ewin DM and Eimer BN. 2006. *Ideomotor Signals for Rapid Hypnoanalysis.* Springfield, IL: Thomas Books.

31. Gow MA. 2006. Emergency extraction. *Contemp Hypn* 23(2):83–91.

32. Zigmond AS and Snaith RP. 1983. The Hospital Anxiety and Depression Scale. *Acta Psychiatr Scand* 67(6): 361–70.

33. Jacobson E. 1938. *Progressive Relaxation.* Chicago: University of Chicago Press.

34. Ewin DM. 2009. 101 *Things I Wish I'd Known When I Started Using Hypnosis.* Crown House Publishing Ltd.

35. McNeal S and Frederick C. 1993. Inner strength and other techniques for ego strengthening. *Am J Clin Hyp* 35(3):170–8.

36. Craig S, Fairful-Smith GW, and Ferguson MM. 1982. *The Treatment of Apthous Stomatitis and Lichen Planus with Hypnotherapy.* Paper presented at the Ninth International Congress of Hypnosis and Psychosomatic Medicine, Glasgow, August.

37. Hammond C (ed.). 1990. *Handbook of Hypnotic Suggestions and Metaphors.* An American Society of Clinical Hypnosis book. New York, London: WW Norton & Co.

38. Fredericks LE. 2001. *The Use of Hypnosis in Surgery and Anaesthesiology. Psychological Preparation of the Surgical Patient.* Springfield, IL: Charles C. Thomas Publisher Ltd.

39. Heap M, and Arivand KK. 2002. *Hartland's Medical and Dental Hypnosis*, 4th edn. London: Churchill Livingston/Harcourt Health Sciences.

40. Simons D, Potter C, Temple G. 2007. *Hypnosis and Communication in Dental Practice*, 1st edn. Surrey, U.K: Quintessence Publishing Co., Ltd.

41. Graham G. 1987. *It's a Bit of a Mouthful.* Blaydon upon Tyne, UK: Real Options Press.

42. MacKinnnon H. 2010. *The British Society of Medical and Dental Hypnosis Training Module Workbook.* Glasgow: BSMDH (Scotland).

43. Gow MA. 2008. Hypnosis at work. *Dentistry* 9(16):30.

44. Kelly M, McKinty H, and Carr R. 1988. Utilization of hypnosis to promote compliance with routine dental flossing. *Am J Clin Hypn* 43(1):41–52.

45. Law M and Tang JL. 1995. An analysis of the effectiveness of interventions intended to help people stop smoking. *Arch Intern Med* 155:1933–41.

46. Green JP and Lynn SJ. 2000. Hypnosis and suggestion-based approaches to smoking cessation: An examination of the evidence. *Int J Clin Exp Hypn* 48:195–224.

47. Bassi GS, Humphries GM, and Longman LP. 2004.The etiology and management of gagging: a review of the literature. *J Prosthet Dent* 91: 459–467.

48. Milgrom P, Weinstein P, and Getz T. 1995. *Treating Fearful Dental Patients: A Patient Management Handbook*, 2nd edn. Seattle: University of Washington, Continuing Dental Education.

49. Gow MA and Newlands J. 2009. Combating the hypersensitive gag reflex. *Dentistry Scotland* February:27–38.

50. Barsby M. 1997 Hypnosis in the management of denture intolerance. *Hypnosis International Monographs* No. 3: Hypnosis in Dentistry, pp. 71–8.

51. Robb ND and Crothers AJR. 1996. Sedation in dentistry, part 2: Management of the gagging patient. *Dent Update* 23:182–6.

52. Gastone L (1983) Indications for the use of hypnosis in the treatment of bruxism in relation to its relation to its psychosomatic nature. *Minerva Med* 30;74(51–52):2975–8.

53. Mulligan R and Clark GT. 1979. Effects of hypnosis on the treatment of bruxism. Abstract No. 926. *IADR Program & Abstracts* 23:58.

54. Clarke JH and Reynolds PJ. 1991. Suggestive hypnotherapy for nocturnal bruxism: A pilot study. *Am J Clin Hypn* 33(4):248–53.

55. Gow MA. Hypnosis in managing sleep bruxism—A pilot study. In preparation for publication.

56. Stein C. 1963. Clenched fist as a hypnobehavioural procedure. *Am J Clin Hypn* 2:113–9.

57. Gow MA. 2006. Managing sleep bruxism with hypnosis—A case study. *Dentistry Scotland* September:24–5.

58. Clarke JH. 1997. The role of hypnosis in treating bruxism. *Hypnosis International Monographs* No. 3, pp. 79–85.

59. Somer E. 1991. Hypnotherapy in the treatment of the chronic nocturnal use of a dental splint prescribed for bruxism. *Int J Clin Exp Hypn* 39(3):145–54.

60. Gow MA. 2008. Introducing a patient questionnaire for investigating the aetiology of bruxism. *Dentistry* 9(1):74–8.

61. Frost TW. 1959. *Hypnosis in General Dental Practice*. London: Henry Kimptom.

62. Gow MA. 2007. Dental hypnosis and suggestion in controlling patient salivation. *Scottish Dentist* September–October(88):36–7.

63. Secter II. 1990. Control of Salivation. In: Hammond DC (ed.), *Handbook of Hypnotic Suggestions and Metaphors*. An American Society of Clinical Hypnosis book. New York, London: WW Norton & Co.

64. Spanos NP, Brice P, and Gabora NJ. 1992. Suggested imagery and salivation in hypnotic and non-hypnotic subjects. *Contemp Hypn* 9:105–11.

65. Winer RA, Chauncey HH, and Barber TX. 1965. The influences of verbal or symbolic stimuli on salivary gland secretion. *Ann N Y Acad Sci* 131:864–83.

66. Tuckey CL. 1921. *Treatment by Hypnotism and Suggestion*. London: Bailliere, Tindall and Cox.

67. Forel A. 1949. *Hypnotism*. New York: Allied.

68. Newman M. 1971. Hypnotic handling of the chronic bleeder in extraction: a case report. *Am J Clin Hypn* 14(2):126–7.

69. Chaves, JF, Whilden D, and Roller N. 1979. Hypnosis in dental behavioural science: control of surgical and post-surgical bleeding. In: Ingersoll BD and McCutcheon WR (eds.), *Clinical Research in Behavioural Dentistry. Proceedings of the Second National Conference on Behavioural Dentistry.* Morgantown, WV: West Virginia School of Dentistry.

70. Enqvist B, von Konow L, and Bystedt H. 1995. Pre- and perioperative suggestion in maxillofacial surgery: effects on blood loss and recovery. *Int J Clin Exp Hypn* 43(3):284–94.

71. Gow MA. 2007. Dental hypnosis and suggestion in post-extraction bleeding control. *Scottish Dentist* May–June(86):33–4.

72. Gow MA and Friel PJ. 2008. Dental extractions, immediate placement and temporisation of dental implants in the aesthetic zone. Michael A. Gow and Philip J. Friel present a case featured on BBC television using hypnosis in place of local anesthetics—A world first in dental practice. Part 1 of 2. *Dentistry* 9(4) (March).

73. Gow MA and Friel PJ. 2008. Dental extractions, immediate placement and temporisation of dental implants in the aesthetic zone. Michael A. Gow and Philip J. Friel present a case featured on BBC television using hypnosis in place of local anesthetics—A world first in dental practice. Part 2 of 2. *Dentistry* 9(5) (March).

74. Gow MA and Faqir A. 2008. Internal sinus lift and placement of an osseointegrated implant using hypnosis as the sole method of pain control—A first in dental practice. *Implant Dentistry Today* 2(1):31–7.

75. Battino R and South TL. 1999. *Ericksonian Approaches. A Comprehensive Manual*. Bethel, CT: Crown House Publishing Ltd.

76. Patterson DR and Jensen MP. 2003. Hypnosis and clinical pain. *Psychol Bull* 129(4):495–521.

77. Montgomery GH, DuHamel KN, and Redd WH. 2000. A meta-analysis of hypnotically induced analgesia: How effective is hypnosis? *Int J Clin Exp Hypn* 48:138–53.

78. Derbyshire SWG, Whalley MG, Stenger VA, et al. 2004. Cerebral activation during hypnotically induced and imagined pain. *Neuroimage* 23:392–401.

79. Derbyshire SWG, Whalley MG, and Oakley DA. 2009. Fibromyalgia pain and its modulation by hypnotic and non-hypnotic suggestion: An fMRI analysis. *Eur J Pain* 13:542–50.

80. Lang E and Laser E. 2009. *Patient Sedation without Medication Rapid Rapport and Quick Hypnotic Techniques*. Victoria, BC: Trafford Publishing.

81.  Baker S and Boas F. 1983. The partial reformulation of a traumatic memory of a dental phobia during trance: A case study. *Int J Clinical and Exp Hypn* 31:14–8.

82.  Finklestein S. 1991. Hypnotically assisted preparation of the anxious patint for medical and dental treatment. *Am J Clin Hypn* 33(3):187–91.

83.  Gow MA. 2002. Treating dental needle phobia with hypnosis. *Aust J Clin Exp Hypn* 30(2):198–202.

84.  Gow MA. 2003. Management of dental needle phobia using hypnosis, relaxation and desensitisation techniques: A clinical case report. *J Soc Advan Anaesth Dent* 20(2 S12.3):14.

85.  Gow MA. 2006. Hypnosis with a blind 55 year old female with dental phobia requiring periodontal treatment and extraction. *Contemp Hypnosis* 23(2):92–100.

86.  Dyas R. 2001. Augmenting intravenous sedation with hypnosis, a controlled retrospective study. *Contemp Hypn* 18(3):128–34.

87.  Gow MA. 2010. Alternative/complementary anxiety management-hypnosis. *J Soc Advan Anaesth Dent* 26:46–8.

88.  Spencer Brown M. 2004. *A Comparative Study of the Use of Intravenous Sedation Alone and in Combination with Hypnosis on Sedation Levels and Recovery Rates in Anxious Dental Patients.* Research dissertation submitted in partial fulfillment of the requirements of the MSc in Applied Hypnosis, Department of Psychology, University College London.

89.  Whalley MG and Brooks GB. 2009. Enhancement of suggestibility and imaginative ability with nitrous oxide. *Psychopharmacology* 203:745–52.

90.  Faulkner C, McDonald R, and Hallbom T. 2003. *NLP: The New Technology of Achievement.* Kansas City, MO: Nightingale Conant.

91.  Gow MA. 2008. Are you positive? *Dentistry* 9(18):23–25.

92.  Mehrabian. 1971. *Silent Messages,* 1st edn. Belmont, CA: Wadsworth.

93.  Gow MA and Canning G. 1998. Dental anxiety and its management in Vancouver B.C. Canada. *Elective Project; Behavioural Science* 27: 1998, Glasgow Dental Hospital & School Library.

94.  Hull CL. 1933. *Hypnosis and Suggestibility: An Experimental Approach.* New York: Crown House Publishing.

95.  Gow MA. 2006. Hypnodontics—Hypnosis in dentistry. *Scottish Dentist* May–June 2006(80):43.

# Management of complicated, high-risk patients with psychiatric comorbidities

Kelly M. Wawrzyniak and Ronald J. Kulich

## INTRODUCTION

The dental practitioner is likely to encounter complicated patients throughout his or her career regardless of clinical setting or specialty. Experiences with complicated patients range from a difficult clinical relationship to a treatment-resistant case, or even a patient with significant medico-legal risk. Patients with psychiatric comorbidities are among the most demanding in these ways. This chapter reviews common psychiatric diagnoses that are encountered with the complicated patient. An awareness of diagnostic criteria, screening, effective management, and referral likely improves dental outcomes and offers the patient optimal care.

## OVERVIEW: BEHAVIORAL SCIENCE AND THE COMPLICATED PATIENT

Psychiatric disorders are as common in primary care dentistry as they are in general medical practice, with some reports suggesting that as many as one out of four patients present with mediating mental health issues.[1] With the expanding role of dentistry in health care, there is an increased awareness that the general dentist must take on the responsibility to assess, refer, and manage complicated patients. Indeed, the practicing dentist makes contact with a regular patient more frequently than other healthcare providers, a status that places dentistry in a unique position to positively impact public health.

*The Fearful Dental Patient: A Guide to Understanding and Managing.* Edited by Arthur A. Weiner
© 2011 Blackwell Publishing Ltd.

Within dental practices, self-reported depression is second in frequency only to hypertension.[1,2] Substance abuse, anxiety, anorexia nervosa, bulimia nervosa, insomnia, bipolar disorder, and posttraumatic stress disorder follow in frequency of reports. Anxiety disorders are also particularly common in general practice. With the volume of a typical dental practice, the general clinician may see at least one patient with an anxiety disorder per day, and only one out of four receiving proper mental health care. Patients with these untreated disorders are likely to be less compliant, miss follow-up appointments, and have poorer outcome over a range of dental treatments.[3]

Some clinicians may elect to forgo a comprehensive medical and psychosocial assessment within their practice, based in the belief that an effort of this sort is not within their domain of responsibility. Indeed, some clinicians intentionally avoid asking difficult questions where mental health issues are concerned. The dentist may also fail to collect data from other sources, for example, primary care, other subspecialists, or family members, in part because of his or her own discomfort with asking sensitive questions. However, this approach may do a disservice to the patient as well as expose the clinician to medico-legal risks as dentistry continues to have an expanded role in the healthcare field.

## POSTTRAUMATIC STRESS DISORDER

Anxiety disorders can interfere with both the professional relationship and adherence to dental treatment. Of these, none can compromise care as much as posttraumatic stress disorder (PTSD).[4,5] Dental-related phobia, panic disorder, and generalized anxiety disorders are also commonly encountered, while treatments for the related symptoms are addressed at greater length in other chapters of this book.

For a diagnosis of PTSD, there are two criteria for an event to be considered traumatic: (1) the event must involve actual or threatened death, serious injury, or a threat to the physical integrity of the person or others, and (2) the person experiencing or witnessing the event must respond with intense fear, helplessness, or horror.[6] Common precipitating traumatic events include physical or sexual assault, natural disasters, and motor vehicle accidents. Some have argued that particular dental or medical procedures might be considered sufficient to precipitate PTSD, though data appear to offer little support for this. It is more likely that dental or medical procedures "trigger" an anxiety response that has been generalized from an earlier traumatic event.

The PTSD patient also shows a persistent reexperiencing of the event, that is, "flashbacks." This can take the form of intrusive thoughts, dreams of the event, reliving of the event, and an intense psychological or physiological response to cues that resemble aspects of the event (p. 468).[6] Although symptoms typically begin within the first 3 months of the traumatic event, there are cases when the onset of symptoms may be delayed months to years after the time of the event.[6]

To deal with the distressing reexperiencing of the event, the person may display a number of avoidance and "numbing" behaviors. Patients may avoid conversations about their trauma and make concerted attempts to avoid situations that evoke memories of the trauma. Hence, dental settings may be particularly problematic for patients with PTSD if the sounds, smells, tastes, or other cues are related to the traumatic event. Often, aspects of the traumatic event become generalized for the patient; the traumatic event did not have to occur in a dental setting for aspects of the dental office to evoke memories of the trauma. These patients may have difficulty falling or staying asleep, increased irritability and anger outbursts, concentration problems, and an exaggerated startle response. Depression is a common comorbid condition, and some patients attempt to ameliorate symptoms with alcohol or other substances. Sometimes those with PTSD cannot maintain employment, housing, or relationships with family.

Awareness of PTSD is particularly important given the growing populations of veterans who have experienced combat or torture, are victims of physical and psychological abuse, survivors of disasters, such as Hurricane Katrina, and refugees exposed to terrorism or war. These patients may be at higher risk for developing PTSD.[5] PTSD can occur at any age and the severity, duration, and proximity of a person's exposure to the traumatic event are significant factors influencing the development of this disorder.[6] The lifetime prevalence of PTSD is estimated at 8–14%,[6] and even higher estimates for U.S. veterans.[7] PTSD is estimated to be the fourth most common psychiatric illness in the United States.[8] Most notably, co-occurrence of PTSD and domestic violence is quite high, with more than 80% of domestic violence patients suffering from the disorder. This should be of special importance, as many states require that all healthcare providers review basic abuse and violence risk issues for their patients.

PTSD can be followed by the development of pain conditions, such as chronic orofacial pain. Estimated prevalence of PTSD in orofacial pain populations is 15% compared with an average estimate of 10% in the general population, while some report even higher numbers.[9] Some investigators have also suggested that permanent central processing changes may occur at the level of the brain when the trauma occurs. To date, the data appear to support the notion that trauma-induced vulnerability in the central nervous system may be a precursor to the development of a treatment resistant pain problem, while genetic factors also may play some role.[8] Given the above prevalence with persistent facial pain, PTSD symptoms should be considered in the differential diagnosis of patients who present with significant head or facial pain.

The general dentist might not observe the patient's flashbacks or avoidance behaviors. However, the dentist can be aware of common symptoms, including a phobic response associated with any devices placed in the mouth, or even a panic attack associated with observing the dentist with a mask. In contrast to a simple dental phobia, these patients present with severe anxiety and other psychiatric comorbidities. Hence, management by simple relaxation or desensitization techniques within the dental office would likely be ineffective as a sole focus of treatment. As a result, identification of PTSD for referral and collaboration with other providers remains important. During the clinical interaction with the patient, the dentist may be able to notice the signs of elevated anxiety, including insomnia, poor concentration, heightened startle response, hypervigilance for danger, and irritability.[10] The medical and psychiatric history also may reveal a history of PTSD, and the dentist has an obligation to query the patient with respect to any precipitants and triggers that might occur in the dental setting. A patient presenting with a complicated regimen of psychiatric medications may offer a similar cue for the dentist to proceed with a more in-depth assessment of the patient's symptoms.

After recognizing the presence of a PTSD diagnosis, the dentist should convey his or her empathy and understanding of the patient's symptoms. Assurance and query about potential triggers should be direct with the patient, while some patients may be reluctant to discuss such triggers. Where possible, a family member can be included in the assessment.[8] Communication with the patient's mental health provider also may assist with patient adherence. In cases where the patient has no mental health provider in place, referral should be considered. While not as simple as the management of dental phobias, anxiety management techniques that maximize the patient's control and reduce anxiety around the treatment setting offer the best options. In some cases, premedication for particular dental procedures can be considered, while care should be taken to coordinate such pharmacotherapy management strategies with the patient's other treating providers.

## Other anxiety disorders

While posttraumatic stress disorder can present a challenging diagnosis for primary dentist, most clinicians have a certain level of comfort in managing the patient with more *generalized anxiety*.[11] As anxiety becomes severe or reaches the level of a psychiatric disorder, commonly associated symptoms include autonomic arousal and increased somatic complaints, such as chest pain. The patient may also report diagnoses of the stress-related medical disorders, such as irritable bowel syndrome.[11] As with PTSD, common comorbidities can include major depressive disorder and substance use disorders,[11] and the dentist should assess for their presence.

Panic attacks can be common with any anxiety disorder, while a specific psychiatric diagnosis of *"panic disorder"* also may be present. Approximately one-third of the population will experience a panic attack in the course of his or her life.[12] A panic attack is the abrupt onset and escalation of a number of somatic and cognitive symptoms that usually peak within

**Table 7.1**  Symptoms of panic attack.

| Possible cognitive symptoms | Possible somatic symptoms |
| --- | --- |
| Fear of losing control or going crazy<br>Fear of dying | Palpitations/accelerated heart rate<br>Sweating<br>Trembling/shaking<br>Shortness of breath<br>Feeling of choking<br>Chest pain/discomfort<br>Nausea<br>Dizziness/feeling faint<br>Derealization/depersonalization<br>Paresthesias<br>Chills or hot flushes |

Source: APA.[6]

10 min.[6] A list of these symptoms is presented in Table 7.1, and a minimum of four must be present.

After the experience of recurrent and unexpected panic attacks, the patient must also experience persistent concern about a forthcoming attack, worry about the implications of the attack, or display significant changes in behavior related to the attacks.[6] Hence, the patient becomes anxious "about being anxious." Panic disorder can co-occur with agoraphobia, a strong fear of public or open places, which can lead to seclusion in the home.[6,12] The worry that an unexpected panic attack will occur in a shopping center, grocery store, or at a dental office can lead one to avoid these places.

Depending upon the individual, a person with panic disorder may avoid coming to the dental office, or avoid returning if a panic episode occurs in the context of his or her dental care. However, the patient may feel less worry in coming to the appointments than elsewhere if he or she believes that there would be available assistance if an attack were to happen at the clinic. The patient with panic disorder may premedicate or employ other nonpharmacological strategies to ease the anxiety prior to coming to the dental appointment.[13] With a proper assessment of the patient early in the treatment process, the dentist can adequately prepare the patient for their return visit with such strategies.

Patients with specific *dental-related phobias* are rarely seen in psychiatric settings, and are often managed solely by the practicing dentist. These patients are often less impaired than those with other anxiety disorders outlined above.[14] A specific phobia is a persistent fear that is excessive or unreasonable, and that is cued by the presence or anticipation of the specific object or situation. Exposure to the situation invariably provokes an immediate anxiety response, which may include many of the somatic symptoms described in panic. In contrast to the panic attack, the person with a phobia does recognize that the fear is excessive or unreasonable,

**Table 7.2** Common dental phobias.

Needles, injections (trypanophobia)
Instruments (appearance, sounds)
Objects in the mouth, sharp objects, and instruments (aichmophobia)
Odors associated with dental office and treatment
Prone position
Masks
Small rooms (claustrophobia)
Social settings, medical settings
Members of the same/opposite sex
Gagging or vomiting or just dentists

and the object or situation is avoided. Dental-related anxiety is a significant problem for both patients and practitioners,[15] and the prevalence of severe dental phobia is estimated between 8 and 15%.[15]

For patients with dental-related phobia, it is important to know what aspect of a dental visit is the distressing part. The assessment is the same as with more severe anxiety disorders, while management may be easier for the practicing dentist. Common dental phobias are listed in Table 7.2.

Strategies for management of dental phobia are outlined elsewhere in this book, while the mainstay of treatment involves behavioral and pharmacologic strategies.[16,17] These aim to reduce the patient's pre-visit anticipatory anxiety, as well as instituting desensitization procedures that reduce anxiety within the dental setting once the patient's specific fears are identified.

Operant conditioning principles also are paramount for success. For example, a patient presenting with a panic attack while in the dental chair should *not* be managed by an abrupt cancellation of the appointment. The act of leaving the dental setting would then result in the reduction of the patient's anxiety, thereby reinforcing "escape" or avoidance behavior. Alternatively, the dentist is advised to keep the patient *within* the setting, for example, the dental chair, employ anxiety management strategies, and only discharge the patient *after* the anxiety subsides. Otherwise, the dentist would successfully reinforce the patient's phobia and avoidance response.

# MAJOR DEPRESSIVE DISORDER AND RELATED MOOD DISORDERS

When considering healthy mood, there is a neutral baseline from which we all experience periods of time above and below. The range of these peaks and valleys, however, is limited for most individuals. For some patients, the depth of depression and related symptoms are sufficiently severe that they meet criteria for a diagnosis of a *major depressive disorder* (MDD). Severe depression is typically marked by a sense of hopelessness

**Table 7.3**  Symptoms of major depressive episode.

|  | Cognitive/emotional | Behavioral |
|---|---|---|
| Must have one or both of these symptoms | Depressed mood most of the day<br>Diminished interest or pleasure in activities |  |
| Can have any of these symptoms for at least five total | Feelings of worthlessness/ excessive guilt<br>Difficulty concentrating<br>Thoughts of death or suicide | Psychomotor agitation or slowing<br>Insomnia/hypersomnia<br>Fatigue/ loss of energy<br>Significant weight change |

Source: APA.[6]

about the future. Without any hope, motivation is lost, and life looks very bleak.[6] The common cognitive and behavioral symptoms of a major depressive episode are listed in Table 7.3. While a depressive episode can be difficult to distinguish from the typical responses to life events, such as bereavement or substance use, failure to recognize a major depression carries the risk of high patient morbidity, with as many as 13% of patients committing suicide. Risk of suicide is of particular concern, and more completed suicides occur for those aged 65 or older, and among men.[18,19]

The *bipolar depressive disorders*, type I and type II, are considered variants of a major depressive disorder. Bipolar depression criteria includes periods of depression that alternate with periods of mania.[20] As with any other psychiatric disorders noted above, these patients can lead normal, productive lives with appropriate pharmacotherapy and other adjunctive non-medication approaches. While bipolar symptoms may vary from person to person, manic episodes are generally characterized by extreme irritability, feeling unusually "high" or overly optimistic. Patients may speak rapidly, that is, present with "pressured speech." They may maintain extreme energy despite minimal sleep. They may have periods of grandiose beliefs about their abilities or powers, have extreme spending sprees, and act out in impulsive ways with notably impaired judgment. In more severe cases, delusions or hallucinations may be present. When symptoms of mania are less severe, the term "hypomania" is used. Differential diagnosis often includes ruling out substance use or other medical factors impacting the patient's mental status, including particular pharmacological agents that can place the bipolar patient at greater risk for a manic episode. Some of these possible precipitants for the at-risk patient are listed in Table 7.4.

While the practicing dentist should not be expected to diagnose the patient with a major depression, bipolar disorder or manic episode, recognizing these symptoms remains a critical role within the dentist's scope of practice. Since the range of pharmacotherapy approaches employed by the dentist is expanding, the possible psychiatric consequences of those

**Table 7.4** Common substances that trigger episodes of mania in bipolar disorder.

Alcohol
Bronchodilators
Caffeine
Cocaine
Corticosteroids
Dopamine agonists
Interferon
Hallucinogens
Pseudophedrine
Stimulants
Tricyclic and other antidepressants

medications in the at-risk patient must be recognized. As noted, the dentist also sees the patient at a greater frequency than many other healthcare providers, and readily becomes familiar with the patient's history and typical demeanor. For the long-term patient, changes in mental status may alert the dentist, allowing for cross-communication with the patient's primary care physician or mental health provider. In many patients who develop depression, reports of medically unexplained somatic symptoms, such as pain or sleep disruption, precede reports of cognitive or emotional symptoms.[21] The dentist should not hesitate to review the common symptoms of major depression noted above with patients. In the rare cases where the patient admits to suicidal ideation with a plan, the dentist also has an obligation to immediately refer the patient to an emergency facility for full assessment and care. If the dentist feels that there is an impending risk of harm, disclosure of the patient's status to other treatment professionals, the patient's family, or legal authorities does *not* place the dentist at legal risk.

## CHRONIC PAIN DISORDER AND RELATED SOMATOFORM DISORDERS

Patients with *temporomandibular disorders* have higher rates of psychiatric comorbidities than the general population, and they can be notoriously difficult to manage in a general dental setting.[22] The era of narrowly assessing the patient's occlusion, palpating muscles, and examining joint mobility has passed and falls below the standard of care with such complicated patients. While the practicing dentist can manage chronic pain conditions, there often is a requirement of co-management with other disciplines.

The history of *orofacial pain* management mirrors the early beginnings of care for other persistent pain conditions. In the historical context, headache, trigeminal neuralgia, atypical pain, temporomandibular disorders, and countless other complex disabling disorders have never ceased to ignite controversy among practitioners. For temporomandibular disorders, treatments have ranged across disciplines and include interventional approaches, biofeedback and cognitive therapy, physical therapy and chiropractic interventions, pharmacotherapy, various complementary medicine approaches, oral occlusal appliance therapies, and surgical approaches. Evidence-based reviews have offered some guidance, usually with a recommendation of conservative management. Long-term management, preventing harm to the patient, reducing pain, and assessing/treating comorbid conditions is the mainstay of patient care, often requiring the expertise of multiple disciplines.

With respect to the common psychological comorbidities in the chronic orofacial pain patient, the practicing dentist must recognize that many of the symptoms are bidirectional, that is, the psychological and pain symptoms can each influence the other set. The existence of persistent pain surely can precipitate psychological symptoms, such as anxiety, depression, insomnia, and family/work disruption. In turn, psychosocial factors such as depression, somatoform disorders, PSTDs, and litigation/disability can precipitate or greatly contribute to the development of a treatment resistant facial pain condition. The dualist view, which suggests that the patient's symptoms are either "physical" or "psychological," has been gradually abandoned with the advent of a biopsychosocial model of pain. More recent functional imaging studies also support the argument that the pain is quite "real," at least at the level of the brain. Medical and psychiatric comorbidities remain common, and both have a complex role in chronic orofacial pain.

In a sample of 1,060 patients diagnosed with temporomandibular disorders, medical comorbidities were present along with psychiatric conditions.[22] Psychiatric conditions, including mood and anxiety disorders, were reported by over 35% of their sample, while other investigations reveal that more than 50% of chronic pain patients develop a major depression within 2–5 years of the onset of pain.[23] While virtually all chronic orofacial pain patients also present with anxiety symptoms, approximately 80% have functional sleep disorders that are frequently secondary to depression, anxiety, poor sleep habits, and somatic overconcern. The presence of pain site in a location other than the head and face decreases the likelihood for a patient's recovery threefold.

Common pharmacological agents also complicate the picture, where side effects may create iatrogenic problems. The use of chronic opioid therapy in dental practice has become increasingly controversial, where issues of adherence to the regimen, dependence, addiction, and illegal diversion of the medications have arisen.

Disability is particularly common with this population, as persistent pain contributes to work-related disability at a greater rate than any other medical or psychiatric condition. A significant compromising factor in ability to function is the patient's beliefs about which type of care might work best. Patients preferring passive approaches, that is, providers taking the active role in administering the intervention, have much poorer outcomes than those who prefer active, self-directed approaches to treat-

**Table 7.5** Typical statement suggestive of catastrophizing.

I worry constantly about when the facial pain will end!
I am sure these dentists have missed something serious!
I know that this medication would not be strong enough.
I am having more pain; I know I have harmed my jaw!
I am certain that there is nothing I can do to feel better.
The pain surely will get worse if I even speak.
I keep thinking about the pain
I will never fall asleep, the pain is just too bad!

ment.[24] Hence, the adherent, dependent patient who relies on the dentist to just "fix the problem" may have the worse outcome.

A patient's chronic orofacial pain can have substantive secondary effects on the family. Family members of pain patients suffer with considerably higher rates of stress-related symptoms than the general population. Medical and dental costs to the patient and society also are daunting, exceeding most other chronic conditions. In brief, chronic orofacial pain disorders result in a plethora of costs to the patient, family, and society.

Research on the dynamics of pain perception and experience has identified specific cognitive, affective, and behavioral constructs with a significant role in chronic pain. Currently accepted psychological factors that impact the subjective reports of pain include perceived emotional distress, disability, and the widely researched construct of "catastrophizing."[25] Recent studies suggest that having the patient "catastrophize" may actually cause changes at the brain level and increase inflammation.[26] Table 7.5 illustrates typical "catastrophizing" statements by the patient in pain.

Operant and reinforcement factors also may play a role with patients who experience persistent facial pain. Due to fear of pain or injury, the patient may restrict use of the jaw or limit neck movements. The immediate consequence of restricted movement is a reduction of pain. However, further inactivity and restriction of movement follows, and the patient becomes progressively impaired.

In addition to common dental interventions, biobehavioral treatments for temporomandibular disorders are well established in the evidence-based literature. Cognitive behavioral therapy, relaxation training-based treatments, biofeedback, and adjunctive use of individual and group approaches have been employed with success for more than 25 years, while interdisciplinary treatments appear to be most effective with the very complex patients.[27,28]

Assessment of the chronic orofacial pain patient necessarily requires a multimodal approach. Any patient presenting with a persistent pain condition lasting more than 3 months typically presents with the array of psychosocial comorbidities noted above. When the patient appears overly complicated, collaboration with other professionals or treatment within a multidisciplinary setting should be considered.

## Other somatoform disorders

The DSM IV-TR psychiatric diagnostic classification system distinguishes between a chronic pain disorder where the patient might show marked somatic concern and the patient with a true *"somatization disorder."* With respect to somatization disorder, the patient presents with multiple somatic symptoms (not only pain), and symptoms often have unclear etiology. Symptoms typically start prior to age 30, with the patient seeking out multiple healthcare providers over many years. The patient may have multiple concurrent treatment providers, with a lifelong list of disabling somatic complaints that, according to the patient, have challenged the best of their practitioners. Hence, in addition to temporomandibular and facial pain, the patient may present with complaints across all physical systems including vague neurological symptoms, gastrointestinal complaints, sexual and reproductive complaints, all of which have been shown to have negative medical findings. In cases where medical or dental diagnoses are established, the level of complaints typically exceeded the level of objective findings. In other cases, patients may eventually develop iatrogenic conditions resulting from their prior treatments, for example, multiple abdominal exploratory surgeries resulting in scar tissue or other damage, or in the case of dentistry, multiple tooth extractions with unclear past diagnoses. Secondary effects from chronic medication use may also complicate the patient's status. Muscle disuse or muscle spasm from inactivity further compromises the medical and dental picture.

The classic patient with somatization disorder is best illustrated by the case of Alice James, sister of the famous nineteenth-century writer Henry James. She traveled the world with her famous brother, often being introduced on stage to a host of curious medical providers as "a collection of symptoms." Her disability and marked somatic concern persisted through much of her life, confounding physician after physician. She viewed herself as helpless and chronically incapacitated by her symptoms. This is underscored by her only published article in an otherwise prolific family of writers. She authored the article under the pseudonym, "the invalid." Her comfort was only achieved late in life; only upon learning that she had a diagnosis of breast cancer; she finally achieved a credible diagnosis. As with many patients suffering from somatization disorder, the search to validate their suffering can appear endless, leaving their dental providers frustrated by there seemingly impotent treatment efforts.

From the standpoint of the primary care dentist, the most helpful role to have with for the patient with somatization disorder is similar to that of the primary care physician. Regularly scheduled appointments in which the dentist conducts a routine examination in an effort to address the patient's concerns may offer the patient assurance. These are best conducted on a strict schedule so the patient does not have to "be sick" to arrange a crisis visit. Referrals to dental subspecialists should occur with great care, lest the patient be subject to unnecessary procedures. Where possible, treatment is directed toward self-care through educating the patient on the use of consistent health behaviors to manage symptoms.

As patients with somatization disorder may develop significant anxiety and affective symptoms due to their plight, collaboration with primary care and mental health providers often is necessary. Of course, the standard of care for these patients should be as thorough as for any complex dental patient, despite the patient's impaired self-report that continues to hamper the diagnostic process. Bearing this in mind, the dentist should be cautioned that the patient with somatization disorder can develop medical and dental problems that do have clear etiology often masked by the enormity of their complaints.

*Body dysmorphic disorder* is another condition that may be more common among patients seen by cosmetic dentistry, while other dental subspecialists may see large numbers of these patients as well.[29,30] These patients have a distorted perception of their relatively normal appearance and develop a preoccupation with these perceived defects to the point of spending many hours of the day looking at the mirror and concerned about being severely deformed.[31] They may seek surgical procedures to correct the perceived defect in appearance, though they are rarely satisfied.[15,32] This preoccupation is often associated with significant anxiety and depression. Functioning is often impaired, while the presentation is different from what is seen with the somatization disorder patient. In the case of body dysmorphic disorder, the patient may be secretive about the level of their concern and their suffering may go unrecognized by the clinician. Despite the best efforts of the dentist and numerous procedures, the smile or the teeth are "not quite right ... damaged ... ugly in some way...."

The above somatoform disorders are necessarily distinguished from factitious disorders or malingering, where the patient makes a *conscious* attempt to deceive the dentist. A small number of patients may engage in conscious deception for purposes such as acquisition of opioids or validation of a legal disability claim. However, even in cases where deception is present, the patient may still have very legitimate dental or psychiatric pathology. Dentists, physicians, and even mental health providers are among the least capable of identifying those patients who choose to consciously deceive the clinician.

# SCHIZOPHRENIA

While a review of all psychiatric disorders within dentistry is beyond the scope of this chapter, the major psychiatric disorder of *schizophrenia* is among the more challenging for the primary dentist. As a result, this tends to be a largely underserved population. There are five subtypes of this disorder: paranoid, disorganized, catatonic, undifferentiated, and residual. While each has its own criteria, characteristic symptoms include delusions and hallucinations, disorganized speech, disorganized or catatonic behavior, and negative symptoms, such as flat affect or avolition. This generally is a chronic illness with social and occupational dysfunction. Prevalence is reported as 0.5–1.5%, with onset usually in late teens to the mid-30s. First-degree relatives of those with schizophrenia are at 10 times the risk of developing this disorder. Onset can be abrupt or insidious, with symptoms including social withdrawal, loss of interest in school or work interest, deterioration of hygiene, unusual behavior, and angry outbursts. Differential diagnosis must consider other medical condition, as well as drug-induced conditions.

If a diagnosis of schizophrenia is established, the dentist may have a special and important role. Friedlander,[33] a recognized author from the dental management perspective, comments that "dentists cognizant of the signs and symptoms … are likely to feel more secure in treating patients … and more confident when obtaining advice (from collaborating providers). Dentists usually can provide a full range of services to such patients, can enhance these patients' self-esteem and can contribute to the psychotherapeutic aspect of management." Patients with a schizophrenia diagnosis often require more intense care in areas such as periodontal treatment, dental restoration, and extractions. Conventional psychopharmacological approaches have particular impact, as they can introduce risk for salivation problems, oral ulcerations, and infections. Pharmacotherapeutic efforts to control thought disorder symptoms may impact jaw muscles or impair the gag reflex. Acute dystonias, pseudoparkinsonias, and tardive dyskinesia may be present. There are some case reports in the literature on oral self-injury in patients with thought disorders such as schizophrenia, where the patient's delusions and hallucinations led to the belief that tooth extraction or other injury was necessary. Patients with paranoid type delusions may display a fearful, suspicious, and distrustful relationship with the dentist. Important considerations for the dentist who is managing a patient with schizophrenia are listed in Table 7.6.

**Table 7.6** Managing the patient with schizophrenia.

Confer with the psychiatrist or psychiatric nurse regarding pharmacotherapy risks
Review pharmacotherapy regimen with the patient
Assess adherence to treatment on an ongoing basis
Schedule more frequent routine appointments with the patient
Inquire about comorbidities including recent toxicology tests
Confer with family members or primary caretakers
Rehearse written, simple treatment plans with the patient and family
Establish a long-term professional relationship with the patient and family
Consider fixed as opposed to removable appliances and prosthodontics
Provide referral for early onset of symptoms or new deterioration in mental status
Work toward understanding the patient's ongoing treatments

Source: Friedlander and Marder.[33]

Friedlander and Marder[33] offer a template for patient management that one might expect from the patient's pharmacotherapy regimen. A primary dentist would be rewarded for working with this relatively underserved population, with certain appreciation from the patient and their family.

## PERSONALITY DISORDERS

Disorders of personality are significant disruptions in a person's ability to interact with others, and are more extreme than personality "traits" and "styles" that impact, but typically do not impair, functioning. The dental patient with a personality disorder often presents with communication issues that severely interfere in personal relationships and occupational roles.[34] As a patient presenting to a general dental practice, he or she may report few relationships at all, a general disinterest in relationships, or many tumultuous relationships. The patient's ability to build rapport and a professional relationship will feel either too difficult or too easy, depending upon the personality disorder, but all will present with significant distress during the course of the interactions. Diagnostically, personality disorders are considered stable, enduring maladaptive patterns of thoughts and behaviors, often having their inception in adolescence and early adulthood. Prevalence estimates range from 0.5% to 3% in the general population. Two of the 10 personality disorders will be reviewed below as they present significant complications in dental practice.

*Dependent personality disorder* is among the most frequently reported in mental health clinics, while patients with this diagnosis frequently appear in general dental practices as well. People with this disorder have an excessive need to be taken care of, that appears submissive and clinging with fear of separation from those with whom they interact. They may overly rely upon the dentist for assurance with each examination or procedure, responding by frequent calling for advice and guidance. These people also seek reassurance and advice from others, prefer family members and healthcare personnel to hold the responsibility in major areas of their life, and fear the loss of support and approval from significant others in their life. With such self-doubt and feelings of worthlessness, people with dependent personality disorder may be at increased risk of mood, anxiety, and adjustment disorders.[6] Within a dental practice, they may attend visits reliably, while report feeling rejected and abandoned if the dental office reschedules or asks the patient to follow with another colleague in the office. These patients find it difficult to make simple dental care decisions without an excessive amount of advice and reassurance from the dentist. They may ask the dentist to assume responsibility in areas where self-care should be occurring, and have great difficulty in expressing disagreement with the dentist. Efforts to encourage independence should be made, as well as the scheduling of regular appointments with structured guidelines for between-session contacts.

One dentist relates a case where the patient would send more than 30 emails per month, inquiring about aspects of her care. She was reliable with her treatments, but could never be assured with respect to the smallest detail of her care. She refused to have contact with other clinicians in the practice. A phone call to her internist revealed that her communication style was the same with him, while her contacts "dropped off" when the "new dentist" became more involved in her care. Management included direct discussion with the patient where it was agreed that all emails would be reviewed within an allotted monthly appointment, emergencies would be handled by any clinician covering the practice, and the patient would accept a referral for counseling around issues of anxiety and family stressors. While the patient's overall style of interaction failed to change, her situation became manageable within the group practice. The patient was able to adhere to the structured treatment plan, as she valued to dentist–patient relationship. The outcome might be less positive with the following diagnosis.

*Borderline personality disorder* (BPD) is a highly researched, discussed and often feared diagnosis by healthcare providers.[34] Patients with this disorder may initially idealize the dentist, for example, "you're the best, no one in the past could handle these problems … I read your resume and I'm so impressed…." However, interactions with the patient may ultimately feel manipulative after an initial period of effusive praise. Complaints about earlier providers are common, as well as complaints about other individuals in the patient's family on whom the patient blames his or her life dilemmas. The patient with BPD laments that he or she has been treated poorly by most providers who preceded the new clinician, and may comment on occasions of taking legal action against prior doctors. In many cases, there are efforts by the patient to cross boundaries, encouraging the dentist to reach outside of his or her area of expertise. The patient also may ask the dentist to intervene with another provider, for example, "the other doctor will write the hydrocodone if you just call him and just say it's OK…." Crossing boundaries may include request for special financial and fee arrangements, demands for services not initially agreed to, and bursts of anger when the dentist or other staff belatedly attempts to set limits on care. In some cases, the patient may attempt to cross personal boundaries by introducing social or sexual requests, another common area where licensing board complaints are generated. Overall, this disorder is marked by a pervasive pattern of instability of relationships, self-image, and emotions, and marked by impulsivity.[6] Specific diagnostic criteria for a borderline personality disorder diagnosis are outlined in Table 7.7.

In the dental clinic, these patients often can be initially identified by their interactions or various battles with support staff. Hence, all members of the practice should have clear direction with respect to management of the patient. The initial interactions with the patient can be very seductive, and it is easy for even the seasoned clinician to be pulled into the dramatic and manipulative relationship. There will eventually be a point in time

**Table 7.7**   Borderline personality disorder diagnostic criteria.

A diagnosis requires the patient have at least five of the following
  Frantic efforts to avoid real or imagined abandonment (by the dentist)
  Pattern of unstable, intense relationships that alternate between extreme
    idealization and devaluation
  Identity disturbance: unstable self-image
  Impulsivity in behaviors that are potentially self-damaging (spending, sex,
    substance use)
  Emotional instability
  Chronic feelings of emptiness
  Recurrent suicidal behavior, gestures, or threats; or self-mutilating behavior
  Inappropriate, intense anger or difficulty controlling anger
  Transient, stress-related paranoid thoughts or severe dissociative symptoms

Source: APA.[6]

**Table 7.8**   Managing the patient with borderline personality disorder.

Be cognizant of the new patient who excessively idealizes the dentist
Set limits early in treatment, decline tasks that are not within the scope of your expertise
Avoid crossing professional boundaries under any circumstances
Document interactions in detail, even uncomfortable interactions
Provide written treatment instructions, with a copy in the dental record
Be aware of psychiatric comorbidities (substance use, depression, suicidal behavior)
Communicate with co-treating clinicians early in the patient's care
Seek a second opinion
Meet with the family or spouse to clarify treatment plans
Follow a clear plan for patient discharge where necessary

where the real or imagined abandonment occurs in the patient's point of view, and he or she will shift from idealizing the clinician to extreme devaluation and anger. In order to prevent the anticipated abandonment, this patient may threaten suicide in order to elicit "help" and commitment to staying with her or him.

Communication with earlier clinicians is the first step in management of the patient with borderline personality disorder, as those providers may give the dentist critical insight into the patient's history. While all patients deserve access to quality dental care, a practice can decline to treat the patient if the patient fails to adhere to a specific treatment pain or declines to give the dentist access to other concurrent or past providers. Mental health treatment approaches range from medications, to individual psychotherapy, to day treatment programs that use a group format. From the dentist's perspective, the mainstay of management includes early recognition of this patient and the establishment of clear boundaries and expectations.[34] A patient with this diagnosis is considered a high risk from a medico-legal standpoint, and thorough documentation is especially paramount. Important considerations for the dentist who is managing health care for these patients are outlined in Table 7.8.

# SUBSTANCE USE DISORDERS

*Substance use disorders* not only affect your professional relationship with the patient, but can create dental complications. Research points to increased periodontal disease, poor outcomes from surgery, diminished adherence to treatment plans, and inaccurate self-reporting among these patients.[35-37] Oral manifestations of particular substance abuse are well documented elsewhere and beyond the scope of this chapter, substance abuse and substance dependence can co-occur with other mental health disorders, often as a means of coping with the psychiatric symptoms. It is important to distinguish when psychiatric symptoms are a product of substance abuse and substance dependence versus when substance abuse co-occurs with the presence of psychiatric symptoms. A variety of psychiatric symptoms can occur due to intoxication from a substance, during withdrawal from the drug, or be persistent effects of its use. Possible psychiatric effects during these phases include delirium, dementia, psychotic disorder, mood disorder, anxiety disorder, sexual dysfunction, and sleep disorder.[6] Diagnostic criteria for both substance dependence and substance use disorder are outlined in Table 7.9.

The implications of chronic substance abuse and dependence include orofacial, systemic, and behavioral consequences. Turner and colleagues[38] found that 58% of a cohort of drug users received dental care in a 2-year period. Those receiving both care from a psychiatrist and antidepressant medication showed two-thirds higher adjusted odds of receiving dental care than those with neither form of treatment. Having consistent mental or medical healthcare increased subsequent use of dental services.[38] Milgrom and colleagues[36] confirm that with appropriate substance abuse

**Table 7.9** Substance disorders diagnostic criteria.

| Substance dependence: at least 3 | Substance use disorder: at least 1 |
| --- | --- |
| Tolerance (need for increased amounts of substance to achieve desired effect) | Impaired ability to fulfill obligations at work, home, or school |
| Withdrawal symptoms | Recurrent substance-related legal problems |
| Substance used in larger amounts or over longer periods of time than intended | Recurrent use in situations in which it is physically hazardous |
| Persistent desire or unsuccessful efforts to cut down | Continued use despite substance-related social problems |
| Much time spent in activities related to obtaining, using, or recovering from substance | |
| Social or occupational activities impaired or given up | |
| Continued use despite substance-related physical or psychological problems | |

Source: APA.[6]

treatment, dental anxiety and adherence to treatment improved. In addition to the improved treatment outcomes, a thorough assessment of substance use decreases the risk for both the patient and the dentist when pharmacotherapy is used. Drug–drug interactions and liver damage from long-term substance abuse can place the patient at physical risk, while prescribing opioid medications for a recovered substance abuser can place the patient at behavioral risk for relapse of the addiction.

An increasing area of attention within dental medicine has been the use of opioid therapy with chronic pain. Some states report that dentists have been among those with the greatest number of prescriptions written for long-acting opioids. Prescribing practices have caught the attention of state licensing boards, with some states enacting guidelines for prescribing. This response by governing authorities has occurred from the standpoint of concerns about both patient addiction and diversion (selling to others) of the medications by patients. As noted above, complex chronic orofacial pain conditions necessarily require interdisciplinary treatment, and sole dental practitioners are unlikely to be successful at managing these patients with only opioid therapy. Again, more thorough psychosocial assessment can help determine early on in treatment if the pain problem is complex and requires a treatment team.

Healthcare providers are notoriously poor at effective screening of patients with substance use disorders, while their obligation to assess is not negated by this dilemma.[39] Brief standardized questionnaires or specific items imbedded in the initial dental practice screening forms may help. A useful brief screening tool is the CAGE comprised of four questions answered with "yes" or "no," two of which account for 81 percent of the variance for predicting substance abuse:[40] (1) In the last year, have you ever drunk or used drugs more than you intended to? and (2) Have you felt that you needed to cut down on your drinking or drug use in the last year? Obtaining an exact quantity and frequency of substance use, when the patient is willing to disclose this information, is imperative for your clinical notes. Descriptions of "socially," "once in a while," or "only on the weekends" is not helpful in determining substance use disorders or changes over time. The presence of a family member or significant other can assist with any assessment, as it does with any of the psychiatric diagnoses discussed above. In a patient well known to the dental practice, other red flags for substance abuse can include deterioration in personal appearance and hygiene, job loss, or significant disruption in major relationships. Other possible cues to substance abuse include the development of particular medical disorders, for example, abnormal liver function, and gastrointestinal complaints. Curiously, "smelling alcohol" on the patient breath is a factor that is not reliably assessed by most clinicians, and the other factors noted above may be much more predictive of a substance use problem. Upon identifying a potential substance problem, appropriate referral is in order. This might include providing the patient with specific resources, or contacting the primary care physician to do so.

# EATING DISORDERS

Many *eating disorders* are first observed by the general dentist. Given the prevalence and risks associated with these disorders, the primary dentist is placed in a unique position in the healthcare field. Unfortunately, only 18% of clinicians refer patients for treatment, with 1 in 10 patients actually receiving care.[41] Mortality rates are 12 times higher than all other causes of death for 15–24-year-old females. Aside from direct morbidity, women with eating disorders have a higher sensitivity to muscle palpation, show temporomandibular signs and symptoms, and suffer from depression and anxiety.[42] An extra-oral symptom of note in some cases is parotid gland enlargement.[43] For those who induce vomiting in these disorders, the dentist can notice enamel erosion that differs from that due to other means, while there is mixed evidence regarding increased prevalence of dental caries and periodontal disease in these patients.[43] There also may be scarring or calluses on the dorsum of the hand from contact with the teeth if the patient uses this form of induction of vomiting.

*Anorexia nervosa* is marked by an intense fear of gaining weight or becoming overweight despite being underweight, and weight can drop to below normal range. There may be a yellowing of the skin and a light downy hair that presents on the body. In postmenarcheal women, amenorrhea can occur. There can be some significant general medical conditions with the reduction in weight, malnutrition, and vomiting and laxative use. *Bulimia* nervosa is marked by recurrent episodes of binge eating characterized by eating an excessively large amount of food in a discrete period of time and a sense of lack of control over the eating. After binge eating, there is a compensatory behavior in order to prevent weight gain, including vomiting, use of laxatives, fasting, or excessive exercise. These patients may appear within normal weight range and to have stable weight. However, their self-evaluation is unduly influenced by body shape and weight.

As with other psychiatric disorders, the primary care dentist must first identify the condition, refer, and co-manage the patient with relevant mental health and medical providers.

# GENERAL MANAGEMENT RECOMMENDATIONS

It may be useful to review your new patient information forms to include questions regarding substance use, medications including psychotropic medications, and history of treatment with a psychiatrist, psychologist, or other counselor. These are some relatively benign mental health-related questions that, when interspersed with other health history, increase disclosure of this information. Reviewing the patient's current and past medications, their prescribers, and purpose of use can reveal significant mental health history not otherwise shared. To the extent that you incorporate these psychiatric questions into the routine health history assessment, the less stigmatizing and more normalizing it will feel for patients to disclose this information to you. It is when patients feel singled out upon questioning or have the belief that their psychiatric history is separate and unrelated to dental history that this information is withheld.

Contacting the current mental health clinician can be cost-effective and evade medico-legal risks. Having a conversation with this clinician can summarize the current status of the psychiatric disorder, health history, and substance use history. There may also be a concern regarding informed consent and the patient's ability to participate in the appropriate treatment plan. The mental health clinician may be able to give an opinion on the patient's mental status, cognitive abilities, and overall level of functioning and ability to perform activities of daily living.

The primary dentist can also provide some significant information to the mental health clinician based upon your observations and interaction with the patient and your dental exam. The oral consequences of psychotropic medications are numerous and are seen with selective serotonin reuptake inhibitors, conventional and atypical antipsychotics, mood stabilizers, and tricyclic antidepressants.

If a patient discloses suicidal intentions or appears to have broken from reality into delusion or dissociation, he or she needs to go to the nearest emergency room for evaluation. For those patients who appear to have psychiatric symptoms but no mental health clinician is available, a referral to seek one may be imperative. If the primary dentist does not have access to mental health clinicians near the practice, a call to the primary care clinician can be useful in mobilizing resources for the patient. Having resources of clinicians in the area can be helpful for the dental treatment plan with the patient in a number of ways. In addition to treating the underlying or comorbid psychiatric disorder, psychologists are trained in motivational theory and interventions, health behavior changes, and cognitive behavioral coping to help patients adhere to and follow through with the recommended treatment plan (see list containing a summary of recommendations in Table 7.10).

**Table 7.10**  Summary of recommendations for managing the complicated patient.

Thoroughly review symptoms
   Thoroughly review medications, including psychopharmacological agents
Assess the association between symptoms and specific events or situations
Involve family members and significant others in assessments and interventions
Observe the patient
Seek other sources of information, including records and other healthcare providers
Assess for comorbid disorders and symptoms
Consider adjunctive behavioral treatments
Encourage consolidation of care
Consider interdisciplinary referral
Consult, consult, consult
Document, document, document

# REFERENCES

1.  Woods CD. 2003. Self-reported mental illness in a dental school clinic population. *J Dent Educ* 67(5):500–4.
2.  Yap AU, Tan KB, Chua EK, et al. 2002. Depression and somatization in patients with temporomandibular disorders. *J Prosthet Dent* 88(5): 479–84.
3.  Dumitrescu AL. 2006. Psychological perspectives on the pathogenesis of periodontal disease. *Rom J Intern Med* 44(3):241–60.
4.  Friedlander AH, Mills MJ, and Wittlin BJ. 1987. Dental management considerations for the patient with post-traumatic stress disorder. *Oral Surg Oral Med Oral Pathol Oral Radiol Endod* 63(6):669–73.
5.  Wright EF, Thompson RL, and Paunovich ED. 2004. Post-traumatic stress disorder: Considerations for dentistry. *Quintessence Int* 35(3):206–10.
6.  American Psychiatric Association. 2000. *Diagnostic and Statistical Manual of Mental Disorders*, 4th edn., text rev. American Psychiatric Association, Washington, DC.
7.  Gibson C. 2008. Approaches to PTSD in the dental setting. *Office of Dentistry Homeless Veterans Dental Program Newsletter* 10(1):2–3, 8.
8.  Friedlander AH, Friedlander IK, and Marder SR. 2004. Posttraumatic stress disorder: Psychopathology, medical management, and dental implications. *Oral Surg Oral Med Oral Pathol Oral Radiol Endod* 97:5–11.
9.  DeLeeuw R, Bertoli E, Schmidt JE, et al. 2005.Prevalence of post-traumatic stress disorder symptoms in orofacial pain patients. *Oral Surg Oral Med Oral Pathol Oral Radiol Endod* 99(5):558–68.
10.  Keane TM and Barlow DH. 2002. Posttraumatic stress disorder. In: Barlow DH (ed.), *Anxiety and Its Disorders: The Nature and Treatment of Anxiety and Panic*, 2nd edn. New York: The Guilford Press, pp. 418–53.
11.  Roemer L, Orsillo SM and Barlow DH. 2002. Gereralized anxiety disorder. In: Barlow DH (ed.), *Anxiety and Its Disorders: The Nature and Treatment of Anxiety and Panic*, 2nd edn. New York: The Guilford Press, pp. 477–515.
12.  White KS and Barlow DH. 2002. Panic disorder and agoraphobia. In: Barlow DH (ed.), *Anxiety and Its Disorders: The Nature and Treatment of Anxiety and Panic*, 2nd edn. New York: The Guilford Press, pp. 328–79.
13.  Friedlander AH, Marder SR, Sung EC, et al. 2004. Panic disorder: Psychopathology, medical management and dental implications. *J Am Dent Assoc* 135:771–8.
14.  Antony MM and Barlow DH. 2002. Specific phobias. In: Barlow DH (ed.), *Anxiety and Its Disorders: The Nature and Treatment of Anxiety and Panic*, 2nd edn. New York: The Guilford Press, pp. 380–417.
15.  Feinmann C and Harrison S. 1997. Liaison psychiatry and psychology in dentistry. *J Psychosom Res* 43(5):467–76.
16.  Berggren U. 2001. Long-term management of the fearful adult patient using behavior modification and other modalities. *J Dent Educ* 65(12):1357–68.

17. Rafique S, Banerjee, A, and Fiske J. 2008. Management of the petrified dental patient. *Dent Update* 35(3);196–8, 201–2, 204.

18. Friedlander AH and Mahler, ME. 2001. Major depressive disorder: Psychopathology, medical management and dental implications. *J Am Dent Assoc* 132:629–38.

19. Friedlander AH and Norman DC. 2002. Late-life depression: Psychopathology, medical interventions, and dental implications. *Oral Surg Oral Med Oral Pathol Oral Radiol Endod* 94(4):404–12.

20. Friedlander AH, Friedlander IK, and Marder SR. 2002. Bipolar I disorder: Psychopathology, medical management and dental implications. *J Am Dent Assoc* 133:1209–17.

21. Simon GE, VonKorff M, Piccinelli M, et al. 1999. An international study of the relation between somatic symptoms and depression. *N Engl J Med* 341(18), 1329–35.

22. Burris JL, Evans DR, and Carlson CR. 2010. Psychological correlates of medical comorbidities in patients with temporomandibular disorders. *J Am Dent Assoc* 141:22–31.

23. Polatin PB and Mayer TG. 1996. Occupational disorders and the management of chronic pain. *Orthop Clin North Am* 27(4):881–90.

24. Mellegard M, Grossi G, and Soares JJF. 2001. A comparative study of coping among women with fibromyalgia, neck/shoulder and back pain. *Int J Behav Med* 8(2):103–15.

25. Keefe FJ, Rumble ME, Scipio CD, et al. 2004. Psychological aspects of persistent pain: Current state of the science. *J Pain* 5(4):195–211.

26. Edwards RR, Kronfli T, Haythornthwaite JA, et al. 2008. Association of catastrophizing with interleukin-6 responses to acute pain. *Pain* 140(1):134–44.

27. Turner JA, Mancl L, and Aaron LA. 2006. Short- and long-term efficacy of brief cognitive-behavioral therapy for patients with chronic temporomandibular disorder pain: A randomized, controlled trial. *Pain* 121(3):181–94.

28. Orlando B, Manfredini D, Salvetti G, et al. 2007. Evaluation of the effectiveness of biobehavioral therapy in the treatment of temporomandibular disorders: A literature review. *Behav Med* 33(3):101–18.

29. Vulnik NCC, Rosenberg A, Plooij JM, et al. 2008. Body dysmorphic disorder screening in maxillofacial outpatients presenting for orthognathic surgery. *Int J Oral Maxillofac Surg* 37(11):985–91.

30. Hepburn S and Cunningham S. 2006. Body dysmorphic disorder in adult orthodontic patients. *Am J Orthod Dentofacial Orthop* 130(5):569–74.

31. Phillips KA. 2004. Body dysmorphic disorder: recognizing and treating imagined ugliness. *World Psychiatry* 3(1):12–17.

32. Phillips KA, Grant J, Siniscalchi J, et al. 2001. Surgical and nonpsychiatric medical treatment of patients with body dysmorphic disorder. *Psychosomatics* 42:504–10.

33. Friedlander AH and Marder SR. 2002. The psychopathology, medical management, and dental implications of schizophrenia. *J Am Dent Assoc* 133(5):603–10.

34. Sperry L. 2003. *Handbook of Diagnosis and Treatment of DSM-IV-TR Personality Disorders*, 2nd edn. New York: Brenner-Routledge.

35. Amaral CS, Luiz RR, and Leao AT. 2008. The relationship between alcohol and periodontal disease. *J Periodontol* 79(6):993–8.

36. Milgrom P, Weinstein P, Roy-Byrne P, et al. 1993. Dental fear treatment outcomes for substance use disorder patients. *Spec Care Dentistry* 13(4):139–42.

37. Friedlander AH, Marder SR, Psiegna JR, et al. 2003. Alcohol abuse and dependence. *J Am Dent Assoc* 134:731–40.

38. Turner BJ, Laine C, Cohen A, et al. 2002. Effect of medical drug abuse, and mental health care on receipt of dental care by drug users. *J Subst Abuse Treat* 23:239–46.

39. The National Center on Addiction and Substance Abuse. 2000. Missed opportunity: National survey of primary care physicians and patients on substance abuse, Published report. The National Center on Addiction and Substance Abuse, New York, NY.

40. Brown RL, Leonard T, Saunders LA, et al. 1997. A two item screening test for alcohol and other drug problems. *J Family Pract* 44(2):151–60.

41. DeBate RD, Plichta SB, Tedesco LA, et al. 2006. Integration of oral health-care and mental health services: Dental hygienists' readiness and capacity for secondary prevention of eating disorders. *J Behav Health Serv Res* 33(1):113–25.

42. Emodi-Perlman A, Yoffe T, Rosenberg N, et al. 2008. Prevalence of psychologic, dental and temporomandibular signs and symptoms among chronic eating disorders patients: A comparative control study. *J Orofac Pain* 22(3):201–8.

43. Robb ND and Smith BGN. 1996. Anorexia and bulimia nervosa (the eating disorders): Conditions of interest to the dental practitioner. *J Dent* 24(1–2):7–16.

# 8

# Understanding and managing the fearful and anxious child

## Laura Camacho-Castro

## INTRODUCTION

The foundation of practicing dentistry for children and adolescents is the ability to guide them through the completion of any dental procedure successfully and to create and promote a positive attitude toward dentistry, with emphasis on the prevention of dental disease.

Dentists and dental health practitioners have a challenging task when providing care to young patients given the wide variability of factors that take place in the dental setting, factors that will have some bearing on the way dental care is delivered to the pediatric patients.

Dental treatment for children involves a complex relationship between the dentist, the child and the parent. Unlike providing care for adults, treating children includes the participation of one or both parents; as a result, the ultimate decision regarding on how a child will be treated dentally must be done collaboratively by the parent and the dentist.

Once the caretaker is informed and has decided to carry on with the dental treatment suggested by the clinician an informed consent must be obtained.[1]

Informed consent is the legal process that protects the patient's right not to be treated in any way without the parents' permission.

The parents must be informed beforehand on the potential manner that the child's behavior will be handled by the staff and the dentist; caretakers must provide verbal and written authorization before any type of behavior management technique is used with their children. The practitioner must

---

*The Fearful Dental Patient: A Guide to Understanding and Managing.* Edited by Arthur A. Weiner
© 2011 Blackwell Publishing Ltd.

make sure that the parents have a clear understanding of the specific technique to be utilized during the dental treatment.

In other words, an informed consent implies that the parents are aware of the type of treatment, consequences, and alternatives pertaining to the treatment and the risks involved.

The same process of obtaining informed consent applies to the clinician who treat adolescents; occasionally, these older children will present unaccompanied by a parent for dental care, and the dentist and the office staff will be under the assumption that it is appropriate to deliver any dental treatment because the patient agrees. Many times, the parent will not be in agreement with the treatment, and the dentist will be facing a difficult dilemma. It is advised that only noninvasive and limited procedures be performed in these circumstances.

The multiple variables that may influence the manner that dental treatment is granted to the pediatric patients may include one or a combination of two or more factors. For instance, individual personality of parent or child, socioeconomic factors, type of dental procedure, clinician and parent relationship, a history of an unpleasant dental experience by parent or the child, language barriers, diverse ethnic and cultural backgrounds, and many more.

The successful emotionally uneventful completion of dental treatment in pediatric patients is an important part of any practice dedicated to treat children.

Furthermore, pediatric patients who are anxious and fearful may become uncooperative and difficult to treat dentally; therefore, it is imperative for the clinician to have the necessary tools to select the appropriate approach in these unique clinical scenarios.

In order to offer and complete dental treatment in anxious and fearful children, dentists are trained to use and implement a variety of management techniques to deal and resolve these difficult behaviors.

## WHAT IS NEW IN BEHAVIOR MANAGEMENT?

The American Academy of Pediatric Dentistry (AAPD) sponsored two consensus conferences on behavior management over the past two decades, and after an extensive review of literature, it was concluded that numerous clinical studies exist about behavior management, and that multiple surveys and opinions have been written on the subject of behavior management techniques in the field of pediatric dentistry. Most of these documents are opinion based, and there is minimal evidence derived from clinical studies on techniques used to control undesirable behaviors.

Many questions remain regarding the efficiency and effectiveness of clinical protocols associated with behavior management.[2]

A recent survey of the American Board of Pediatric Dentistry Diplomates on parenting and its effects on practice indicated that children's behaviors have changes for the worse over the last 10 years. Children cry more and demonstrate more disruptive behaviors while being treated.[3] Parents, on the other hand, have become more permissive and overprotective.

The old adage "the doctor knows best" is not longer true; absolute trust is no longer part of the dentist–parent relationship. A parent expects that a pediatric dentist can administer local anesthesia to crying, difficult-to-manage child only because she/he is a "pediatric dentist."

In today's litigious society, the ability to recruit, justify, and perform scientifically sound clinical studies is more limited. In addition, these potential studies are highly regimented and regulated by institutional review boards, and frequently present significant barriers to the efficiency of performing these studies. Parenting and child-rearing skills and other societal forces are changing and possibly interfering with the enlistment of children into clinical studies has been mentioned.[3]

In a study done by Eaton, 55 parents were examined in their attitude toward current behavior management techniques used in pediatric dentistry, and it was found that a modified hierarchy of acceptability is emerging in behavior management techniques, and that the aggressive physical management techniques appear to be less favorably accepted; however, the pharmacological techniques are increasing in acceptance over time.[4]

Today's dentists enjoy many advantages compared with their predecessors. The dental settings are designed to be children friendly. Contemporary materials, advances in technology and staff, who are trained to serve children, supplement the ambiance. Yet the mission of a pediatric dentist remains the same as it was a generation ago: to perform quality dental procedures on children and adolescents whose behavior may range from cooperative to aggressive, to defiant and anxious or fearful.[5]

The general public has become suspicious of science and science-based professions while demanding all the benefits of scientific discovery. This Western culture demonstrates diminished respect for and is less trustful of professionals. The multimedia exposure influences the general public, and people question professionals' intelligence, ethicsand safety of care.[6]

Today's parents reflect the changes in society. The traditional parent role included setting boundaries, maintaining discipline, and teaching respect for others have become obsolete. These parenting styles have affected adversely the behavior of children and adolescents in the dental office.[2]

Some of the behavior managements techniques used and taught in dental schools are now perceived negatively by parents.[7]

Many parents now attempt to dictate the treatment approach; however, the vast majority of these parents lack the scientific background to understand what dentists do. Many of the parents will demand for their child to be sedated or to be placed under general anesthesia for procedures that clearly can be managed without anything else than with the appropriate of behavior management technique.

In recent years, we have seen a significant increase of the interest in "better" parenting. One possible explanation might come from the more and more complex issues in raising children in today's society. Certain child-rearing issues faced in the 1950s or 1960s have been replaced with more difficult to deal with factors such as drug use, suicide, violence and teen pregnancy.[5]

According to a survey done by Casamassimo of board-certified pediatric dentists, they believe that parenting styles have changed during their professional lifetime, and that parents today are less likely to set boundaries on their children's behavior. The survey also showed that parents are more likely to accept their children's disrespect and are more overprotective. These perceptions are difficult to confirm; however, we can examine some of these changes in parenting styles from looking at trends in society and how these trends impact parenting styles.[3,8]

Members of families are influenced by other members within the same family, and children's behavior will be impacted by a variety of factors within the same family, community, and the changing society.

Parenting styles are influenced by popular advice from friends, grandparents, and the media. Parents are looking for advice on how to respond to specific behaviors on the Internet without following any scientific background.

Another important factor that impacts children's behavior in today's society is that parents are spending less time with their children and more time working to provide for their basic needs. Women are now part of the workforce, and more and more women are the main breadwinners in the family, and at the same time they are expected to be mothers, wives, and housekeepers.

Another difference in today's families is that men are now increasingly involved in household chores and find themselves caring for their children and sharing housekeeping responsibilities more as well.

Another factor that impacts the families nowadays is that we are under an increasing financial stress. When both parents work and share the financial responsibilities of the family, parents will be exposed to routine stressors, such as dealing with a sick child at home and missing a day's work pay, rush hour traffic, school issues, deadlines to meet, etc.

Among other factors that definitely will change our style as clinicians is that our society is multicultural and is presently composed of many different ethnicities with their own particular parenting styles. By 2050, it is projected that 50% of the population will be composed by groups that now we consider minorities.[9] In respect to certain behavior management techniques, what might be acceptable for some ethnic backgrounds might not be for others, hence it is the dentist's responsibility to assure that parents are well informed on how their children will be managed during the dental appointments.

In 2004, the American Academy of Pediatric Dentistry conducted a "Behavior Management Conference" addressing specific issues and seeking input from attendees regarding current behavior techniques used in their practices. The purpose of the conferences was to discuss the appropriateness and effectiveness of current behavior management techniques, the scientific support for those techniques, and the role of the pediatric dentist in managing the difficult child.[10]

The assembled panel of this conference consisted of pediatric dentists, an attorney, child psychologists, parents, and a specialist in early childhood education and a pediatrician.

The recommended actions from the participants included a need for improvement in communicative methods with parents and other family members. It is important to mention that behavior management "begins" with the parent's initial call to the office. The common saying on first impression applies here. Methods of communication with parents that are simple, succinct, and compassionate will likely lead to better dental experiences for the parent, the child, and the pediatric dentist.

Also, it was noted that it is necessary to seek further discussion and information on the impact that changing attitudes towards behavior management may have on the accessibility of treatment.[10]

Regarding patient care, it is important to note that not every dental appointment can be a positive experience for every child, and that is not possible that the dentist can instill a positive attitude in every child either. Some behavior management techniques, particularly the "tell–show–do" technique are the tools most likely to enable the dentist to lead the child to a positive dental attitude.[10]

Parents and patients should be treated with respect, and at the same time we as clinicians will expect to be treated in the same manner. The pediatric dentist should attempt to determine the parents' expectations for every visit, and, when necessary, help them establish realistic expectations. Parents should be involved in treatment decision to certain extent and with the clinician's guidance.

In reality, no pediatric dentist uses a "pure" technique; behavior management comes with experience, and children have their own individual personalities and will respond differently to the different behavior techniques.[10]

The term "difficult" child refers to a noncompliant child. Children who are uncooperative usually are because of specific behavioral issues, such as ADD or a psychological, mental, or a systemic disorder, or because of anxiety and fear due to a wide variety of factors.

The pediatric dentist's responsibility lies primarily with the second group, children who are anxious or fearful.

The definition of a "difficult" child may also include children whose parents often have a difficult interaction with the dentist.

Some instances of difficult parents might be parents who are overprotective, anxious themselves and transmit their fears and anxieties to their children, parents who do not comply with the basic dental needs of their children, or parents who show overall neglect toward them.[10,11]

As mentioned earlier, working with children and adolescents is different than working with adults.

Children are not just "small adults," and like adults, they are not all alike. Children are experiencing rapid changes in the area of physical, intellect, social, and psychological areas, among others. The rates at which these areas develop vary with each child. It is important for the clinician to understand these areas in order to deal with these children and their parents in the dental setting.

For example, a 2-year-old child is referred as being in the precooperative stage due to its inability to comply with dental treatment.

Since each child needs to be viewed as an individual, the behavior should be expected to be different for each child. However, there are certain norms related to a particular age group, and it is only meant to help the clinician understand the development of each child at that particular chronological age.

## BIRTH TO TWO YEARS OLD

Children at this age are completely dependent from their parents and possess very limited ability to understand and tolerate dental procedures; effective communication is also very limited due to their developmental stage (see Figure 8.1).

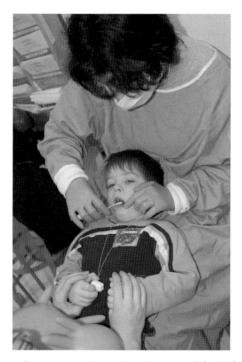

**Figure 8.1**   Knee-to-knee examination position. Parent and dentist face each other with knees touching; the child faces the parent and parent restrains the child's legs and hands.

Simple dental procedures can be performed with the parent's assistance, such as dental examinations, cleanings, and fluoride applications.

Dental treatment that requires more cooperation from the child often needs to be done under minimal sedation or in the case of extensive multiple dental disease, these children will require full mouth rehabilitation under general anesthesia.

The clinician must obtain the necessary information from the caretaker about their child social behavior and proceed accordingly.

Whenever these children need to be examined, a knee-to-knee method is suggested. The child faces the parent and the head of the child rests on the lap of the dentist; this allows the dentist to explain what it is seen during the examination to the parent at the same time.

At this age group, the "unknown" is generally the factor that will cause the fear and anxiety in these children.

## TWO YEARS OLD

At this age, the vocabulary development varies greatly, and it depends vastly on their social development. Thus, communication with this age group poses a challenge.

Social behavior at this age varies greatly as well; some children will display extrovert social interaction while others will desperately "cling" to the parent when the clinician attempts to interact with them.

In any case, regardless of their individual personality, these children are categorized as being in the "precooperative" stage. They usually are self-centered, do not like to share, and they play alone. Parents should always accompany the child during dental procedures and offer physical and emotional comfort.

These children can sit on the dental chair by themselves with the parent in close proximity, or, holding their hand, keeping eye contact, or if deemed necessary, the children in this age group can still sit on the parent's lap for simple dental procedures. Communication and coaching skills are important for the dentist of any age of patient, but are absolutely essential in dentistry for the preschool child.[12]

Sedation methods are often needed for procedures that will require more time and cooperation from the patient.

Fear and anxiety stems from their developmental immaturity and the difficulty in communicating with them.

## THREE TO SIX YEARS OLD—THE PRESCHOOL AGE

These children develop and mature socially at this age; they are less ego-centric and enjoy their personal achievements at home and in school.

Children at this age like to please and look for compliments from adults. They learn rapidly on how to listen and follow simple commands.

In school, they participate well in small groups with the same age children and become empathetic toward other children. They will feel at ease by having the parent close by and will constantly look for approval when they are praised by the dentist when they do a "good job."

At this age, they have conquered the fear of parental separation and will behave well on their own. They are becoming less dependent from the parent, especially when they are well established in a school setting. Some children will develop fears and anxieties related to all these multiple transitions, and can become defiant, introverted and have some mood changes that in most cases will be temporary.

## SIX TO TWELVE YEARS OLD

By this age, children are well established in school and in their social circles; they enjoy having friends and feel independent from parents (see Figure 8.2). Differences among boys and girls become evident, and behavior management language needs to be used accordingly. Boys do not like to demonstrate fear and will attempt to repress those feelings. Girls might behave opposite demonstrating exacerbated manifestations of anxiety and fear sometimes.

Communication between the dentist and the child now is easier, since these children will inquire openly about specific procedures and how "it" will feel. The children should be encouraged to express their feelings by asking "open" questions and avoiding questions that will require just a "yes" or a "no" answer.

It is important to note that the dentist must always be as honest as possible when explaining a procedure so that the dentist–child relationship

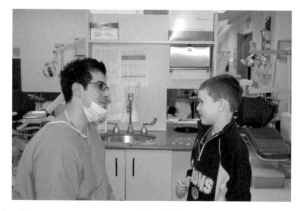

**Figure 8.2** Dentist communicating with a child positioning himself at the same eye level to gain his attention.

will not be undermined. Once the trust is damaged, it is extremely difficult to attain it again. Children at this age group should be confident to remain without the parent in the operatory for dental treatment. This scenario makes the rapport between dentist and child closer and easier and without any parental influences. Parents should be always informed ahead of time about the clinician's advice to remain in the waiting area while the child is being treated. However, if parental presence does not influence the behavior negatively, the parent can stay in the operatory as a silent and passive observer.

## THE TEENAGE YEARS—ADOLESCENCE

Teenagers are often a challenge to deal with, not only as dental patients, but as individuals as well. The teenagers are not children anymore and they are not young adults quite yet; patients at this age can be rebellious and defiant and outspoken; however, some adolescents can be withdrawn and display passive aggressive behaviors. The key with teenagers is to keep in mind the countless changes they are undergoing in their life; coping with peer pressure, rapid social changes, school work, exposure to drugs and violence.

Reinforcing the basic standards of care in a nonreprimanding manner works best with most of these children. Being truthful, tolerant, and flexible will make the dental appointments easier to handle for the adolescent, the parent, and the dentist.

Fears and anxieties in these children originate from a multiple sources. Many teenagers will become needle-phobic due to unfavorable past dental experiences or be predisposed to anxiety and fear related to dental pain. The adolescent patients will benefit greatly with the use of minimal sedation like nitrous oxide/oxygen inhalation procedure when indicated.

## WHEN DOES FEAR OR ANXIETY FIRST DEVELOP IN CHILDREN?

There is no clear explanation to this question. The etiology of dental fear in children is multifactorial.[13,14]

In children who do not behave well on the dental chair, it is useful to evaluate the cause for the negative behavior if possible. The parent is the best source to collect information regarding the health history and also the social history of the child. The assessment of the potential behavior of the child is performed by analyzing the child's temperament before any dental treatment is performed. This information will assist the dentist to scrutinize the parent concerning their child's temperament.

It has been proven that children will progress through the same sequence of cognitive stages and once they have mastered one they will continue to the next stage. Also, researchers have suggested that children possess a characteristic temperament, and that this will remain to certain extent for their rest of their life.

Children's temperament is a good predictor on how the child will behave during the dental appointment.[15]

Pinkham explained that there are different types of fears discussed by children about their dental experience.

These are, in summary, real fears, such as the fear of the needle or the fear that is acquired by a previous bad dental experience by the child or by any other person close to the child.

The second type would be the theorized fear, also called the "Freudian" fear, where the mouth being a pleasure center will be invaded by the dentist and creates an intense anxiety reaction by the patient.

The third category of fear is the potential fear; an example of this type of fear, which is triggered by the dentist or the dental assistant's insecurities and the impact these have on the patient, is, for instance, young inexperienced clinicians will increase behavioral problems on children who sense the clinician's lack of competence. The lack of effective communication, "rushed" dental procedures, inattentiveness with the child will also have this negative behavior results.

The fourth type includes the fear of the unknown or fear of potential bodily harm, strangers, or, in younger patients, the anxiety that arises when a child is separated from the parent. These last groups of fears have a biogenic origin, meaning that they are not learned but acquired. They are protective in nature, their origin is early in life, and they evolve as the child matures and becomes older.

In any instance, the clinician must analyze if these fears can be managed by the traditional behavior management techniques alone or if the child has important underlying factors that should be consider.[16]

Children who are acutely or chronically ill, children with a history of abuse or neglect, and children who are mentally or emotionally challenged will likely require pharmacologic management for dental treatment.

Regardless of the behavior management technique performed by the dentist, the decision pertaining on which technique to be used is a complex decision process that must weigh the benefit and risk for the child. The dentist serves as an expert about dental care; the legal guardian shares the decision whether to treat or not to treat and will decide the strategy for execution of the proposed dental treatment.

# BASIC BEHAVIOR MANAGEMENT TECHNIQUES

## Voice control

It is a controlled modification of the clinician's voice to influence the behavior of the child. The objective is to gain and maintain the attention of the patient, avoid negative behavior, and establish the adult–child role in the clinical setting. When using voice control, the dentist must be aware that when communicating with a child, the words being used must be used at an age-appropriate level, using terms that the child will understand and using commands that the child will understand and able to follow easily. Changing the tone of voice will keep the child's attention, the tones of the voice will praise the positive behavior, and others will discourage the negative behavior to progress.

This technique can be used at any age.

## Positive reinforcement

Praising the child for being well behaved will reinforce good behavior. This technique includes not only the verbal praise by the dentist, but also from the staff and the parent.

The core principle of this technique is that children and adolescents will respond better to immediate rewards. The initial and any thereafter positive behavior should be reinforced, and once the desirable behavior has been attained and children have learned, the reinforcers should be used with measure and only occasionally in order to maintain their value.

These reinforcers consist in social and nonsocial. Examples of social reinforcers are a pat on the shoulder, a big clap for the young child, a smile, and the verbal praise.

The nonsocial reinforcers are material things offered at an age-appropriate level, like stickers, toys, or money.

It can be used in all ages.

## Tell–show–do

The tell–show–do (TSD) technique was introduced in 1959 by Addelstone, and from then on, it has been widely used as one of the most effective behavior management techniques in children.

TSD is promoted as the hallmark of behavior management in pediatric dentistry.[2]

The TSD technique is a sequential technique that shapes the behavior of the child by using a series of approximations, and is a technique that should be used not only by the dentist, but also by the staff.

This technique requires good communication skills by the clinician, and includes some of the techniques described above. It involves "*telling*" what the procedure will be, "*showing*" how it will be done, and finally "*doing*" it. The tell–show–do technique involves the visual, auditory, olfactory, and tactile senses of the procedure in a carefully, non-threatening manner (Figure 8.3a–c).

It is highly effective at any age.

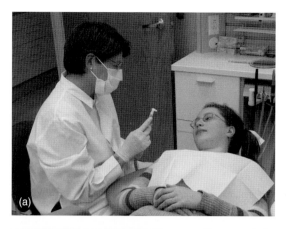

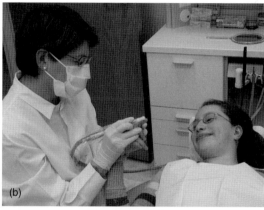

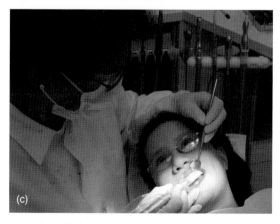

**Figure 8.3** Examples of behavior management modality Tell–Show–Do. (a) Dentist "telling" the patient about the procedure. (b) Dentist "showing" the procedure. (c) Dentist "doing" the procedure.

## Distraction

The distraction technique is diverting the patient's attention from what it could be perceived as an unpleasant procedure. This technique is particularly useful in children who have a strong gag reflex. The distraction methods can be used by the dentist and the staff using their creative imagination. For example, if a young child is gagging when alginate impressions are being taken, the operator can distract the child by asking the patient to move their right foot, or to "wiggle" their left toe, or by trying to make a noise "like a cat."

For older children and teenagers, breathing exercises are very useful distraction techniques in order to decrease anxiety or the gag reflex during certain procedures, such as impressions or radiographic procedures.

It also can be used at any age.

## Modeling

The modeling technique is a behavioral method that provides an example or a demonstration on how to do a procedure.

The modeling technique can be a tape in which a child is being treated by the dentist and at the same time the different steps are explained at an age-appropriate level. The film is then shown to children who may benefit by watching how a dental appointment is being conducted. The purpose is for the patient to imitate or reproduce the behavior displayed by the child in the film.

The modeling technique may include also an actual patient demonstration where a child is being treated and another child is watching the procedure. The purpose is for the observant child to imitate the positive behavior of the child being treated.

The modeling technique can be used for younger children and has not been proven to be effective in all cases, particularly in children who are anxious or fearful. In fact, researchers have questioned the value of the audiovisual aids for the behavior modification in children.

# SHOULD THE PARENT REMAIN IN THE OPERATORY?

There is a very broad range of opinions from pediatric dentists about allowing the parent to remain in the operatory. Parents have an important role in how their child will behave during the dental appointment.[17,18]

Parental presence can be beneficial and sometimes detrimental toward the behavior of their children.

In younger children, the parent's presence can be used to gain cooperation from the patient by decreasing the anxiety and fear to the unknown.

Ultimately, it is the clinician's decision to determine if the rapport with the child will be undermined by the parent's presence and hinder the

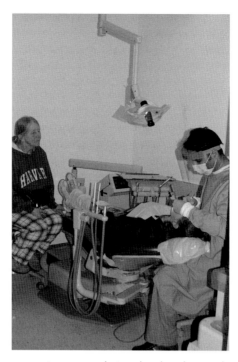

**Figure 8.4**   The parent is present during the dental procedure and becomes a "silent" observer as instructed by the dentist.

completion of treatment. On the other hand, parental presence might be beneficial and may assist for the child to behave favorably.

Parents who demand being present must be guided by the clinician on what is expected from them to allow the dentist to establish a good rapport with the child.

A survey completed by pediatric dentists showed that practitioners with more years of practice allow a lesser number of parents during treatment versus recent graduates or pediatric dentistry residents.[19] As the clinician gains confidence with years of experience, it is easier to transmit that confidence to parents who will not mind remaining in the waiting area, understanding that the child will be fine without them during treatment (Figure 8.4).

# PHARMACOLOGICAL MANAGEMENT OF BEHAVIOR PROBLEMS

The vast majority of pediatric patients can be successfully managed with the traditional behavior management techniques. However, in some cases, the use of pharmacological methods is necessary in order to treat patients unable to cooperate on the dental chair.

Behavior management techniques are many and sometimes controversial. They vary in the style of delivery, as the number of practitioners who use the techniques.[20]

The diversity of these techniques, the way they are used by the clinicians is also influenced by the training programs that teach their use.[21]

One technique that does not change and has remained consistent throughout the years is the pharmacological management of children with behavior problems.

Pharmacological management of pediatric patients can be divided into two main categories:

(1)   sedation; and
(2)   general anesthesia.

The question arises: When should we opt to use pharmacological methods to treat a child?

There are numerous important factors to consider, and that will assist the clinician to decide whether to use sedation or general anesthesia, and the clinician must weigh the risk-benefit ratio evaluating each patient individually. For example, what is the extent of the dental needs? The number of appointments needed and whether the child is healthy or medically compromised will impact the decision to either treat the child in-office using sedation or using general anesthesia in a hospital setting.

Is there any increased health risk using sedation procedures compared with the use of general anesthesia?

If there are any complications with the pharmacological procedure, will the clinician be able to "rescue" the child?

Cost and third-party reimbursements also play an important factor that will influence the parents' and the dentist's decision on how the patient will be treated.

The risks involved using pharmacological ways to treat children may vary; the most severe are brain damage and death. These complications are most commonly caused by airway compromise and respiratory complications.[2]

Minor risks include nausea, vomiting, and paradoxical and defiant behaviors.

Children who are medically compromised pose a greater risk than healthy children; therefore, a thorough review of the medical history and an updated physical examination is mandatory before any kind of pharmacological management is performed.

The airway evaluation is imperative and must include the evaluation of tonsil size; enlarged tonsils will increase the complications of airway problems during sedation procedures, and the awareness of their status will help the clinician anticipate increased risks with the procedure and be prepared accordingly.

On the other hand, general anesthesia for a healthy, fearful, and anxious child is extremely safe. It can be performed in the dental office or in a hospital.

Children who need extensive dental work and multiple appointments or children who pose a greater risk for complications with sedation are good candidates for general anesthesia.

Children with special needs or medically compromised patients should be treated in a hospital setting and admitted for observation if deemed necessary.

Behavior management is based on scientific principles; its implementation requires an understanding of these principles. Behavior management is more than pure science and requires skills in communication and general experience by the clinician; listening to the patient and parent with genuine compassion and patience will help the dentist comprehend their fears and anxieties, thus making the provision of dental care acceptable by the parent and the pediatric patient.

## SUGGESTED READING

Addelstone HK. 1959. Child patient training. *Fortn Rev Chic Dent Soc* 38:7–9, 27–9.

Garcia Coll C and Pachter LM. 2002. Ethnic and minority parenting. In: Bornstein MH (ed.), *Handbook of Parenting*, Vol. 4, 2nd edn. Mahwah, NJ: Lawrence Erlbaum Associates, pp. 1–20.

Harper DC and Alessandro DM. 2004. The child voice: Understanding the contexts of children and families today. *Pediatr Dent* 26(2):114–20.

Hulbert A. 2003. *Raising America: Experts, Parents, and a Century of Advice about Children*. New York: Alfred Knopf.

Nathan JE. 1989. Management of the difficult child. A survey of pediatric dentists' use of restraints, sedation and general anesthesia. *J Dent Child* 56: 293–301.

Pinkham J, Casamassimo P, Fields HW, et al. 2005. *Pediatric Dentistry Infancy through Adolescence*, 4th edn. St Louis, MO: Mosby Elsevier, pp. 394–412, Chapter 23.

Reference Manual. 2009–2010. *American Academy of Pediatric Dentistry, Definitions, Oral Health Policies, and Clinical* Guidelines, pp. 125–31.

Repetti RL, Wood J. 1997. Effects of daily stress at work on mothers' interactions with preschoolers. *J Fam Psychol* 11:90–108.

Wright GZ, Starkey PE, and Gardner D. 1983. *Managing Children's Behavior in the Dental Office*. St. Louis, MO: C.V. Mosby Company.

# REFERENCES

1. St Clair T. 1995. Informed consent in pediatric dentistry. A comprehensive over review. *Pediatr Dent* 17(2):90–7.
2. Wilson S and Cody WE. 2005. An analysis of behavior management papers published in the pediatric dentistry literature. *Pediatr Dent* 27(4):331–8.
3. Casamassimo PS, Wilson S, and Gross L. 2002. Effects of changing US parenting styles on dental practice: Perceptions of Diplomates of the American Board of Pediatric Dentistry presented to the College of Diplomates of the American Board of Pediatric Dentistry, 16th Annual Session, Atlanta, GA. *Pediatr Dent* 24:18–22.
4. Eaton JJ, McTigue DJ, Fields H Jr, et al. 2005. Attitudes of contemporary parents toward behavior management techniques used in pediatric dentistry. *Pediatr Dent* 27(2):107–13.
5. Sheller B. 2004. Challenges of managing child behavior in the 21st century dental setting. *Pediatric Dentistry* 26(2):111–3.
6. Ecenbarger W. 1997. How honest are dentists? *Readers Digest*, February, pp. 50–6.
7. Lawrence SM, McTigue DJ, Wilson S, et al. 1991. Parental attitudes towards behavior management techniques used in pediatric dentistry. *Pediatr Dent* 13:151–55.
8. Long N. 2004. The changing nature of parenting in America. *Pediatr Dent* 26(2):121–4.
9. Garcia Coll C and Pachter LM. 2002. Ethnic and minority parenting. In: Bornstein MH (ed.), *Handbook of Parenting*, Vol. 4, 2nd edn. Mahwah, NJ: Lawrence Erlbaum Associates, pp. 1–20.
10. Adair S. 2004. Behavior Management Conference Panel I report—Rationale for behavior management techniques in pediatric dentistry. *Pediatr Dent* 26(2):167–70.
11. Baier K, Milgrom P, Russell S, et al. 2004. Children's fears and behavior in private pediatric dentistry practices. *Pediatr Dent* 26(4):316–21.
12. Chambers DW. 1977. Behavior management techniques for pediatric dentists: An embarrassment of riches. *ASDC J Dent Child* 44(1):30–4.
13. Chellapah NK, Vignehsa H, Milgrom P, et al. 1990. Prevalence of dental anxiety and fear in children in Singapore. *Community Dent Oral Epidemiol* 18:269–71.
14. Klingberg G, Berggren U, Carlsson SG, et al. 1995. Child dental fear: Cause-related factors and clinical effects. *Eur J Oral Sc* 103:4103–12.
15. Radis FG, Wilson S, Griffen AL, et al. 1994. Temperament as a predictor of behavior during initial dental examination in children. *Pediatr Dent* 16:122–7.
16. Pinkham JR. 1995. Personality development, managing behavior of the cooperative preschool child. *Dent Clin North Am* 39(4):771–87.
17. Pinkham JR. 1990. Behavior themes in dentistry. *J Dent Child* 57:38–45.

18. Pinkham, JR. 1991. An analysis of the phenomenon of increased parental participation during the child's dental experience. *J Dent Child* 58: 458–63.

19. Cipes MH and Miraglia M. 1985. Pedodontists' attitudes toward parental presence during children's dental visits. *J Dent Child* 53:341–3.

20. McKnight-Hanes C, Myers DR, Dushku JC, et al. 1991. The use of behavior management techniques by dentists across practitioner type, age and geographic region. *Pediatr Dent* 15:267–71.

21. Nathan JE. 1989. Management of the difficult child. A survey of pediatric dentists' use of restraints, sedation and general anesthesia. *J Dent Child* 56:293–301.

# The geriatric patient: psychophysiological factors associated with aging and dental anxiety

Arthur A. Weiner and Kathryn Ragalis

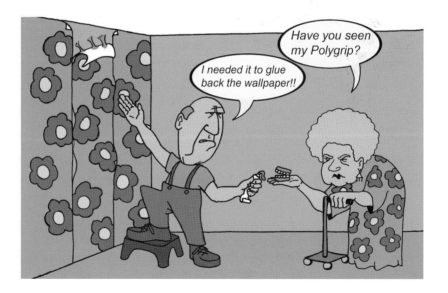

## INTRODUCTION

The world's population is increasing at an annual rate of 1.2%, while the population of individuals over the age of 65 is increasing at a rate of 2.3%.[1] Today, approximately 600 million people are over the age of 65, and that

*The Fearful Dental Patient: A Guide to Understanding and Managing.* Edited by Arthur A. Weiner
© 2011 Blackwell Publishing Ltd.

number is expected to double by 2025.[2] By 2050, it is estimated that there will be 2 billion elderly individuals, 80% of them living in developing countries. Those over 80 years of age will make up 20% of the world's population.[3] The growing number of elderly people represents an enormous challenge to health providers in all countries. People are living longer, thanks in part to advancements in scientific research, medicine and technology. The elderly population ranges from those who are very healthy, vibrant, and living independently to those who are medically compromised with numerous physical and psychological problems that influence their ability to care for themselves.

Age and the risk factors associated with chronic diseases are also common to most oral diseases. The World Oral Health Report 2003[4] stressed that oral health is an integral component of general health, and an important component of the quality of life (QoL). The relationship between oral and general health becomes more evident as age increases. General and associated oral health conditions directly affect the QoL, manner and lifestyle. The many physiological and psycho-social changes associated with aging can have profound effects upon quality of life in later years.

This chapter reviews the major changes associated with aging with a focus upon the psycho-social aspects of aging, and provides strategies for effectively managing the older dental patient. The process of aging is a slow, progressive decline in the physiologic reserve, such that the person loses some of the ability to adapt and becomes more vulnerable to minor changes and stresses.[5]

# UNDERSTANDING THE CHANGES ASSOCIATED WITH AGING

## Culture ethnicity and sociodemographic factors influencing age and oral health-related quality of life

Worldwide increases on life expectancy make the issues of cultural and ethnic differences in the aging experience an important consideration today, more than in previous times. People born in developed countries today can expect to live some four decades longer than their counterparts born at the beginning of the twentieth century. The reduction of the number of young people entering the world's population, due to decreases in the fertility rate combined with increased and better medical care, which has increased longevity, has led to an increase in the ratio of older people in the world's population.[6]

Ethnic and cultural minorities begin old age with a variety of disadvantages. They are more likely to be associated with poorer health, do not score well in physical and cognitive function tests, report greater number of medical conditions, and on the whole are less wealthy and possess incomplete and poorer health insurance. They may also be less educated, have labored over more difficult occupations, and have had with lesser amounts of medical care in their early childhood days.

The relevance of culture and ethnicity for the aged can sometimes be seen in the variations of treatment and respect of the aged person. In developing countries, esteem and respect for the elderly is greatly visible, while in well-established and developed countries, reports of neglect and the uncertain status of the elderly are increasing. Also, in developing countries, many of the young individuals travel to the larger cities seeking employment, thus reducing the availability of family caregivers.

Ethnic and cultural groups also vary in their dedication to providing family care. African Americans sanction the primacy of family care over white Americans, and are less likely to utilize long-term facilities for their aged such as nursing homes. Similarly, Latinos and Latinas, delay placing their elderly into long-term care facilities relative to white individuals. According to Alpert,[6] ethnic and racial minorities are less likely to take advantage of preventive health services, such as required vaccination and prescreening test for a variety of diseases.[7,8] In 2006, Makhija et al. noted that dentate and edentulous individuals, African Americans, those with less than a 6th grade education, and people earning less than $16,000/year, particularly when, combined with transportation difficulties, were more likely to have decreases in their oral health-related quality of life (OHRQoL). In the dentate group (those with dentition), transportation, race education, and income were associated with decreased OHRQol, while in the non-dentate group (endentulous) only race and education were the major factors.[9,10] This is not meant to infer that other variables were not as important for the edentulous person. In a study in the United Kingdom in 2001, McGrath and Bedi[11] found that the OHRQoL was affected by age, employment status and ethnicity. Many times access to and use of dental care by older edentulous individuals is far less than for those individuals that have dentition.

Thus, cultural and socio-economic factors may play important roles in the ultimate oral health of elders.

## Physiological changes associated with aging[12–18]

The process of aging involves a progressive decline in physiological function, often leading to decreased function and increased susceptibility to minor changes and stresses.[5] However, the aging process varies tremendously among individuals, so it is important to avoid stereotyping or "ageism." Chronologic age and functional age are often very different.

In general, the aging process may involve overall decreasing vigor and energy accompanied by:

- sensory impairment (declines in hearing, sight, smell and taste);
- lower vital capacity;
- slower nerve conductivity;
- decreased number and function of muscle cells (in association with decreased activity); and
- declines in organ system function.

## Changes in muscle and tissue function

There is a steady decline in the efficiency of all physiological mechanisms with age, becoming more rapid after the mid-sixties. The generalized loss of muscle mass can make chewing, swallowing and speaking difficult, a problem common to edentulous patients. Sagging facial muscles adversely contribute to the patient's ability to adapt to dentures, hindering ability to chew, swallow, and speak. The amount of subcutaneous fat declines, and the skin becomes less elastic as individuals age. The lining of the oral cavity also becomes more friable with age.

Basal metabolic rate decreases and may be associated with increased weight because fewer calories are utilized each day due to reduced activity, especially for individuals aged 65 and older. Malnutrition is often seen, secondary to a disease condition or as a result of factors associated with aging.

## Changes in cardiovascular functioning

Cardiovascular functioning declines with age as blood flow to the central and peripheral vessels decreases. Although the heart may pump harder, it achieves less, resulting in decreased cardiac output. Arterial walls rigidify, myocardial contractions lessen, and peripheral resistance declines. Atrial fibrillation is often seen with increased age; many individuals suffer from coronary artery disease and hypertension. The treatment of cardiovascular diseases often has an impact on oral health and dental treatment, for example, some medications have side effects causing xerostomia and orthostatic hypotension. The decline in peripheral blood flow is also associated with a loss of skin tone.

## Intestinal changes

Intestinal tone and decline in digestion and absorption can lead to the constipation and abdominal discomfort common with elders. Misuse of laxatives can result in potassium depletion. The unpleasant feeling of constipation can lead to the avoidance of proper eating, leading to malnutrition.

## Bone changes

Bone physiology also changes with age, with bone resorption exceeding deposition, resulting in a net loss of bone mass. There is a progressive decrease in overall skeletal mass, often leading to osteoporosis and bone fractures. Severe bone loss results in vertebral fractures, low back pain, a stooped position, and subsequent loss of height.

## Kidney changes

Decreases in renal function can have far-reaching effects, especially dehydration. Decline in the ability to recognize thirst with age may result in decreased water consumption. The associated dehydration can cause changes such as skin wrinkling, collapse and wrinkling of facial tissues, and diminished tear production, resulting in dry eyes. Loss of total body water directly affects drug therapy, necessitating constant adjustments in dosage. Severe dehydration can be fatal. Bladder muscles also weaken with age, often leading to incontinence.

## Sensory changes

Decreased ability to smell foods combined with the reduced action of the taste buds is a contributing factor to malnutrition in the aged population.

Loss of sight and hearing frequently occurs with aging and can affect an individual's overall attitude, increasing fears and anxiety often leading to improper sleep habits. Accumulation of wax and exfoliation of surface tissue cells in the ear canals may interfere with hearing. Hearing loss sometimes can be associated with imbalance and ability to communicate properly due to failure to hear completely what is being communicated. The eyelids are often affected, and droop due to loss of elasticity.

## Visual impairments

Impairment of vision in the form of macular degeneration, cataracts retinal detachment, and glaucoma are some of the chronic eye disorders affecting the older person. Blindness may be associated with diabetes retinopathy, trachoma, and leprosy, according to Schembri and Fiske.[19] Visual impairment can alter an older person's ability to maintain oral health, and to recognize the early signs of dental disease, such as bleeding when brushing, loss of a filling, or detecting a small cavity. The degree of periodontal disease may be higher because of the difficulty of attaining adequate oral hygiene owing to a diminished ability to see if gums are bleeding or plaque and stain have been sufficiently removed. For visually impaired elderly individuals, particularly those in residential homes, the risk of root caries is exceptionally high due to poor plaque control, diets high in refined carbohydrates, and xerostomia, usually the result of medications.

## Changes in the immune system

With age, the immune system becomes less effective and less protective against infections. There is a decline in T cell function and production, impairing the ability to resist infection. Wound healing and repair is also influenced by aging, often slowing as age increases. The result is increased susceptibility to infection.

### Reproductive changes

Reproductive systems also change with age in both males and females, but are more obvious in the female, in association with menopause. Menopausal symptoms can interfe with sleep and daily activities. The occurrence of hot flashes during dental appointments may cause a patient to feel uncomfortable and embarrassed leading to increased anxiety and even avoidance.[13] Oral changes occurring in postmenopausal woman may include:

- insufficient saliva and the resulting increased risk for dental caries;
- taste alterations;
- atrophic gingivitis;
- increased periodontitis; and
- jaw osteoporosis (this can be a contraindication to dental implant placement).

## Oral changes associated with aging

### Oral changes

The oral changes associated with aging are many. Defoliation of the tongue, with subsequent decline in taste bud function, often results in decreased ability to taste foods. Gingival recession and the prevalence of periodontitis seem to correlate strongly with advancing age. Gingival recession with subsequent exposure of root surfaces is common, and may be partially related to inadequate blood flow. Cardiovascular diseases, such as stroke and coronary heart disease, are associated with tooth loss and severe periodontal disease.[12]

### Teeth

Increase in dental caries, including root surface caries, is common in the elderly, in association with xerostomia. Broken teeth and lost restorations are also frequent findings. Tooth loss can lead to many problems, including migration of adjacent teeth, malposed teeth, and malocclusions. Food may become trapped in spaces, which also may cause difficulty with chewing and swallowing as well as leading to periodontal problems. Temporomandibular joint dysfunction may follow due to malocclusion and drifting, as well as loss of teeth. After years of habits, such as bruxism, teeth may be severely worn, unaesthetic, and fractured.

### Periodontium

Improvements in health care, longevity, and social conditions have led to people living longer and having an associated increase in periodontal disease expectancy. Aging itself, however, does not cause a significant loss of periodontal attachment in the healthy elderly individual.[20] The effects of aging are based on biomolecular changes of the cells of the periodontium that accelerate bone loss in elderly with periodontitis. These effects may be associated with:

- alterations in differentiations and proliferations of osteoblasts and osteoclasts;
- increase in periodontal cell response to oral microbiota and mechanical stress; and
- systemic endocrine alterations in elderly individuals.

Chronic infection inherent in periodontitis may also be associated with cardiovascular events.[21–24]

Periodontal conditions have been related to carotid calcifications in the elderly.[25] In one study, cardiovascular disease, diabetes and rheumatoid disease were all significantly correlated to the number of teeth lost.[26] Edentulous individuals also appear to be at a greater risk of coronary heart disease and premature death.[27]

## *Xerostomia and root caries*

Xerostomia, a condition of decreased salivation, in association with dryness of the tissues of the oral cavity, is prevalent in elderly individuals. The most common cause of xerostomia in aged individuals is their medications, but it can also result from systemic diseases such as diabetes, Sjogren's syndrome or AIDS, or from the effects associated with treatment of these disorders. Cancer of the head and neck and associated radiation and medications also play a role in decreased salivation.[28–31] The QoL can be affected by xerostomia as the disorder affects chewing, swallowing and speech.[32] Saliva provides many protective functions in the oral cavity (cleansing, lubricating, remineralizing, antibacterial, etc.). So hyposalivation can present difficult challenges to the sufferer and the dental practitioner. Xerostomia has been identified as one of the major risk factors associated with caries among elderly individuals. Studies of dental caries in the aged population have reported high incidences of coronal and root caries.[33–37] In studies by Papas et al.,[38,39] it was noted that patients with medication induced xerostomia tend to be more susceptible to root caries than healthy individuals. As recession occurs in older individuals, the root surfaces having less mineralization than the coronal surfaces, are far more susceptible to decay.

## *Oral bone and soft tissues*

Removable appliances often present a wide array of discomfort issues caused by dryness or loss of alveolar bone. Alveolar ridge resorption in both the mandible and/or maxilla occurs, leading to problems with retention of removable prostheses and associated irritation. As age increases, one often sees the development of hyperplastic tissues, denture stomatitis, angular chelitis, papillary hyperplasia, as well as ulcerations.

### Oral cancer and precancerous lesions

The risk of oral cancer increases as one ages. Cancerous lesions of the oral cavity and pharynx have higher mortality rates than other types of cancer. Elderly individuals are at greater risk for the development of precancerous lesions and oral cancer. Risk factors associated with development of these lesions are mainly smoking and alcohol consumption.[40,41] A study by Epstein, Lunn, and Le[42] noted that a decline in the elderly individuals' defensive mechanisms, combined with the presence of common risk factors related to oral and general health and to lower psychological and socio-economic status, had a great impact on cancer survival in that age group. Precancerous lesions such as leukoplakia are often seen occurring in the elderly, especially those within the lower socioeconomic level.[43]

Patients may be at risk for cancer, presently have it, or have been treated for various forms of it. The practitioner must assess for all risk factors, including those for oral cancers, as well as for the head and neck. This assessment is necessary so that modifications of the patient's behaviors can be instituted to reduce risks and attempt to prevent any occurrence of cancer. Before any cancer therapy is instituted, the patient should be instructed in the performance and maintenance of meticulous oral hygiene practices. During treatment, especially for head and neck tumors, continuous preventive practices must be maintained, as well as palliative treatment for mucositis and xerostomia. After treatment, maintenance of oral hygiene instruction and practices, salivary substitution agents, sialogogues, fluorides, diet modification suggestions should be implemented, together with assessment for depression, quality of life issues, function, pain and difficulty swallowing.

## Psychological and QoL risk factors associated with aging

Ettinger and Beck[44,45] classified older individuals into three categories according to psychosocial function:

(1)  the functionally independent older adult;
(2)  the frail older adult; and
(3)  the functionally dependent older adult.

Those individuals in the first group mostly remain independent even in the presence of chronic medical problems requiring continuing medical attention. Older individuals in the other two groups require aid in maintaining basic levels of personal care. The third group is composed mostly of those individuals requiring special care either in the home or in long-term facilities. Factors such as low income, low education, and reduced community support have been shown to be closely related to functional impairment. The more dependent a person is, the greater is the risk of burden by diseases such as:[45]

- mental disease, for example, depression, dementia;
- Alzheimer's or Parkinson's disease;
- visual and hearing impairments;
- osteoporosis;
- unintended weight loss, inadequate nutrition;
- dry mouth; and
- orofacial pain.

## Mental disease

Declines in mental health status can complicate other health issues in the elderly. With increased levels of dementia and memory loss, decision-making capacity is reduced. This may interfere with a person's ability to perform adequate oral hygiene procedures. Alzheimer's disease is the most common cause of dementia in the older person. Dementia may have a negative effect on the oral health of older individuals, and may result in higher levels of edentulism.[12,46–49] The demands of day-to-day care, changing family roles, and difficult decisions about placement in a long-term care facility place additional stress on the caregiver and family support structure.

## Depression, dementia, and paranoia

Elderly depressed patients are more likely to complain about physical problems as opposed to mood changes. They may also exhibit weight loss, complain of general aches and pains or difficulty sleeping, and shows evidence of impairment in physical, mental, and social functioning.[50,51] Dementia and paranoia are also psychiatric illnesses affecting the aged. Although not entirely inherent to aging, the aging process does increase the risk of such illnesses occurring. Dementia is a disorder characterized by deterioration in the intellect, cognitive abilities, behavior, and emotions. It may be due to any number of causes such as:

- malnutrition;
- tumors;
- decline in overall general health;
- depression;
- pharmacological agents; and
- Alzheimer's disease.

## Apathy

Apathy is increasingly recognized as a distinct psychiatric syndrome, and is associated with various neuropsychiatric disorders, including Alzheimer's disease. Apathy is associated with the reduction in daily functions, poor insight into one's own functional and cognitive impairment, and poor outcomes from rehabilitation treatment, and has a significant impact on the caregiver and relationship with the aged person.

## Effects of personal loss, such as death of a spouse

Many older individuals fear being forgotten by their loved ones. When individuals experience the loss of a loved one, they find their lifestyle changed, and, often, their income reduced. They tend to feel lonely and awkward attending social events where couples represent the majority of those present. They can become engulfed with:

- depression;
- loss of appetite;
- reduced ability to socialize;
- deteriorating health;
- feeling of being a burden to family;
- fear and anxiety about the future; and
- exaggerated complaints concerning well-being.

Frequently, the presence of poor health, ill-fitting dentures, and loneliness help maximize conditions in the elder individual, such as low esteem, hostility, and envy toward their family and friends, as well as their primary health and caregiver. They often try to impose guilt on family and friends as a means of keeping them close.

In 2008, Klieb and Wiseman[52] examined the prevalence of dental patient death and the dentist's role in the bereavement experience. They noted that consistent with a prior study in 1988,[53] a majority of dentists provided some degree of support to their patient's survivor. Such concern usually the by-product of a strong patient–doctor relationship. Many times, while the dental practitioner acknowledges the death of a patient's loved ones, he or she is seldom recognized as a source of support for survivors.[54] But in addition to expressing sympathy as a fundamental act of consideration, basic principles of ethics and professionalism demand that qualities of compassion, kindness, charity and integrity be a part the ethical practice of dentistry, and while these do not explicitly direct the practitioner to provide bereavement support, they do suggest that a dental practitioner's obligations extend beyond the mere performance of routine dentistry. Today, only a few dental schools provide information and training relating to death, dying, and bereavement. Many practitioners, however, study this subject on their own to gain information concerning the stress associated with death, dying, and bereavement and report a need for including such education in today's dental school curriculums.

## Elder abuse and neglect

Dentists are in an excellent position to identify elder abuse and neglect, yet they are, arguably, the least health professionals, likely to report or intervene in cases of suspected elder mistreatment. Elder abuse and neglect (EAN) is a widespread problem, and its harmful impact cannot be swept under the rug. A national awareness and concern about elder abuse and neglect has increased over the past 10–15 years. It crosses all racial, socioeconomic, and ethnic groups. Elder neglect is far more prevalent than abuse, and accounts for more than 60% of EAN.[55–58]

EAN may include physical, psychological, and financial or material forms of both abuse and neglect. Physical abuse is characterized by acts of violence, sexual abuse injury and pain. Psychological abuse is conduct resulting in mental anguish, depriving the aged individuals from needed stimulation and companionship. Financial abuse involves fraudulent and inappropriate use of the aged person's income and resources.

In the aged, it is often difficult to recognize abuse due to cognitive impairment, as well as the limited social contacts often associated with abused individuals. In long-term care (LTC) institutions, the recognition of EAN can be undetected and compromised by uncooperative and uneducated staff. Here dental care is often limited and only periodic, hindering the practitioner from recognizing abuse or neglect. Most abuser are related to or are the caregivers of the elderly. In many cases, they may be family members. Several characteristics common to abusers include:[57]

- social isolation;
- excessive caregiver burden;
- stress, inexperience, unrealistic expectations;
- abusive behavior acquired through childhood victimization;
- alcoholism; and
- substance abuse.

The ADA Principles of Ethics and Conduct emphasize dentists' obligation to educate themselves and report any instances of suspected abuse and neglect. Dental practitioners, because of increased utilization by older individuals, are in an excellent position to facilitate the early recognition and intervention of EAN. The dental practitioner must always be observant and look for signs and symptoms of maltreatment, however subtle, remembering that neglect occurs more frequently than abuse. Physical evaluation of the patient's appearance, especially exposed areas of skin, can reveal signs of abuse and neglect. Additional symptoms to be on the lookout for are:

- Signs of unclean and disheveled appearance;
- malnutrition;
- missing teeth; and
- bruises, scars, abrasions, burns, and wounds in varying stages of healing.

The dental practitioner must be careful not to associate physical signs of EAN as signs commonly associated with aging. But dental professionals, too, must be cautious so as to avoid inflicting EAN on their own patients by the use of inappropriate physical or pharmaceutical agents, embarrassment, omitting needed dental treatment, or failing to recognize symptoms of dental disease. Abandonment of the elderly patient because of inadequate funds, limited technical skills, or knowledge is unethical and should be avoided. The American Society of Geriatric Dentistry offers the following recommendations:

- Become familiar with the diagnostic criteria of EAN.
- Educate your staff on these criteria and signs.
- Identify local and state requirements for reporting EAN.
- Make identification, documentation and reporting of EAN an everyday part of your office procedure and training.

## General health considerations in the elderly

### Nutrition and the elderly and frail person

The relationship between oral health, adequate nutrition, and dietary intake needed for physiologic function are multifaceted.[59,60] Poor nutrition affects oral health, and diminished oral health influences dietary choices. A diet containing proper vitamins, minerals and adequate caloric intake can affect the operation of the immune system and have a direct impact on the oral health quality of the elderly individual. Diet issues, from starvation and malnutrition to obesity, are major issues for the geriatric population.

Adequate nutrition is extremely important for the maintenance of health and healing processes. Lack of appetite is prevalent among older adults, especially in individuals suffering from the side effects of various medications. Proper intake and quality of food is even of greater importance among individuals suffering from chronic diseases. Dental problems, such as esthetic issues or ill-fitting prostheses, can influence diet choices. The oral health and nutritional status of "frail" elderly adults are at risk of deterioration. The use of dentures tends to result in fragmented and restricted diets, low in nutritional value; difficult foods to chew or swallow are usually eliminated from the diet. The presence of chronic disease processes can alter energy intake, and the severity of these diseases can affect the individual's ability to carry out everyday activities. Increasing dependency in walking and transferring, difficulties with dressing, toileting, and even eating with family or friends can also impact the social aspect of the aged.[61]

Anorexia and malnutrition can occur due to a variety of factors. Both physical and psychological issues can impede the ability and desire to take in adequate calories and nutrition. Healthcare providers from dental practitioners to nurses, and the caregiver must maintain a close degree of cooperation between the dental office and home care, and within the entire healthcare system. Dental records must be integrated into the individual's medical records to assure that follow-up care, should it be needed, is implemented.

Older adults, especially frail, dependent persons, should be constantly evaluated for oral health conditions that may affect their nutritional status, because oral health in itself has a great impact on the individual's overall quality of life.

## Parkinson's disease

Nakayama, Washio, and Mori[62] reported in 2004 that patients with Parkinson's often complained of problems with chewing due to associated swollen and bleeding gums. Almost half of the patients failed to brush their teeth or clean their dentures. These patients were also at a high risk of losing their teeth because of the use of anticholinergic or momoamine inhibitor agents and accompanying xerostomia. Mental diseases and Parkinson's disease have both been shown to have links with:[12]

- high levels of caries;
- tooth loss;
- periodontal disease and impaired oral hygiene;
- experience of pain;
- chewing difficulties; and
- poor function of dentures.

## Frailty

Frailty has become an emerging geriatric syndrome.[63] A fairly common biological syndrome seen in the aged population, it is characterized by decreased reserves in various multiple organ systems. It may be brought on by disease, inactivity, malnutrition, stress, and/or normal physiological changes associated with aging. It develops slowly, in a stepwise manner, with increments of deterioration initiated by acute events. It is characterized by a loss of skeletal muscle mass, abnormal function in inflammatory and neuro-endocrine systems, and poor energy maintenance. There is in this group of the elderly a decreased ability in the body's physiologic response to maintain a state of equilibrium in times of acute stress. It is the result of excessive demand placed upon reduced capacity. That it is not found in all elderly persons, but associated with the elderly, suggest that it may be a preventable and treatable disorder.[64–67] The dental practitioner, as well as other caregivers, must work in concert with the patient's physician as part of a team providing all medical and dental management necessary to maintain homeostasis, as well as fostering a positive attitude, to prevent physical and mental decline.

# MANAGING THE RISK FACTORS ASSOCIATED WITH AGING

## Managing the psychological emotional and functional limitations of aging

According to Epstein, no dental practitioner should approach the geriatric patient without having empathy for him or her as a human being.[68] Success with the elder patient is more dependent on the dispensing of rapport and empathy than on the professional competence of the dental practitioner. Such treatment must not only pay attention to the physiological changes associated with aging, but must also include equal attention to the individual's psychological and emotional requirements. The behavior patterns of the elderly fearful and phobic patient have been established long before he or she was considered old. Dentistry was not as technically advanced in past years as it is today. Trauma, aversive, and negative experiences were far more prevalent, unpleasant, and uncomfortable than what one endures today. The behavior and attitude of an elderly patient may be governed by experiences that can be traced back to treatment received in childhood. Remembrance of a negative experience or the harsh attitude of an earlier practitioner may still linger. But an aged individual's attitude and emotions may also be the by-product of their environment, earlier treatment, or of a culture in which dentistry was not a priority.

Due to the change in the longevity of individuals, dentists must consider this increased variable: When treating children or young adults, they may well be treating their future elder population. In 2003, Nisizaki[69] suggested that older individuals and those accompanying them be made to perceive and feel that their physical and psychological needs are both understood. Physical needs can be accomplished by modifications in the physical elements of the dental office.

## Chairside clinical considerations

- Install ramps and hand rails.
- Widen doors and pathways.
- Include sturdier and taller chairs in reception rooms.
- Ensure that floors are not slippery.
- Train auxiliary staff to support and respect dignity of elders.

- Schedule appointments to accommodate patient's needs.
- Allow for periodic rest and toilet visits during treatment.
- Try to utilize shorter appointments.
- Offer, as disability increase, a home assistance program.
- Provide oral hygiene education to family and caregivers.

Emotional and psychological needs can be provided in the form of continuous reassurances of positive outcome of treatment and a abundance empathy.

In 2009, Brown, Goryakin, and Finlayson[70] demonstrated that women and men behave quite differently and emotionally with respect to their demand for dental care. Elderly women appear to be more vigilant about visiting the dentist than men, with or without insurance; however, in the presence of functional limitations, access to care is less with women than men. Women who have two or more functional limitations tend to have an increased need for special equipment, and this need may act as a crucial barrier that prevents them from obtaining needed dental service. These finding seem to coincide with the suggestions of Nisiyaki.[69]

## Managing pain

When it comes to the aged experiencing or reporting pain, studies suggest that that the various changes in sensory, cognitive, emotional, psychological, and behavioral systems may influence how the elderly perceive and express pain. With many individuals, the increase in age and increasing inability to execute certain activities may cause them to report pain less, accepting the natural aging process and decreasing overall general health as the cause. They still experience pain, but are less likely to report or complain about it. LeResche and Dworkin,[71] however, noted in 1985 that due to physical changes associated with aging (e.g., wrinkling of the skin, loss of muscle tone, less subcutaneous fat, hair loss, psychiatric disorders, and changes in emotions and attitudes), the facial expression of pain can be greatly modified. They note that the dental practitioner must constantly be able to recognize and react to these nonverbal cues, which may be the silent signs of anxiety and frustration on the part of the elderly patient.

## Challenges to providing effective preventive dental care for the elderly

Life expectancy for men and women continues to improve, lengthening due to slower progression of chronic diseases, in turn the result of newer and better methods of treatment. This translates into a significant increase in the number of significantly older individuals who will need special care and attention to maintain their overall general and oral-related quality of life in the face of increasing frailty and disability.[72,73] The use of LTC facilities will increase, requiring more specialized healthcare professionals, including dentists to staff these facilities. Concerns about oral hygiene must be maintained even in the face of other conditions that demand increased attention.

There are many changes that affect the QoL in older individuals, with impacts on self-esteem, daily life, and well-being. MacEntee et al in 1997 and 2005,[74,75] noted that there are three factors that are usually the most important for an older adult's oral health related quality of life:

- lack of pain;
- ability to maintain oral hygiene; and
- disease-free mouth.

General and associated oral health conditions directly influence the aged individual's quality of life and the manner in which they can perform and enjoy it. Appropriate care for the very aged and frail must be a mix of prevention and therapeutic care whose goal is to provide the very best to the least advantaged of our population.

The focus to prevent oral disease has increased importance in the elderly population that has or may develop barriers to receiving dental treatment. More frequent maintenance appointments may be indicated due to increased risk factors for oral diseases. Continuous motivation to comply with methods to prevent and control oral diseases must continue throughout life. Issues may arise, and a patient may discontinue daily oral hygiene practices after years of meticulous care or skip routine maintenance appointments after a lifetime of regular dental appointments. This is the result of many varying physical, psychological, emotional, and financial problems that have impacted and limited the activities of daily living. The quality of life and its concept requires the dental practitioner, as well as other healthcare providers, to expand their focus to not only include the effects of various disease processes, but to also include the broader psychosocial effects that aging and disease cause.

## Providing effective preventive dental care for the elderly

Preventive care for the elderly is of great importance for preventing the development of periodontal disease and dental caries. The delivery of dental care for the elderly and frail individual especially those who have to depend on others for support and care, should be founded on the premise that oral health greatly impacts the QoL, since it directly effects oral function, comfort, social image, and interaction. By understanding the various problems of elderly and aged individuals, especially the visually impaired and frail dependent person, the dental practitioner can directly improve their QoL. In 2007, Brondani, Bryant, and MacEntree[76] evaluated a model of oral health through focus groups among elders. The elders within these focus groups felt that components such as diet, personal expectations, economic priorities, and the influence of a person's personal and social environment were important elements, as well as general health and one's ability to cope and adapt. They also felt that to describe an individual's level of activity best, words like "activity and participation" should be utilized in place of other currently utilized descriptive terms to characterize an individual's functional ability as "restricted" or "limited" in defining a model of oral health.[77,78] The choice of words that imply failing or decreased abilities have a direct negative impact on an aged individual's attitude and feeling of well-being.

Here, the role of the care provider, family, and dental practitioner can be pivotal in the prevention and early detection of disease. The practitioner can be essential in helping the family to assist the individual by establishing a set of realistic goals via a step-by-step structured approach, utilizing oral hygiene aids, and seeing that the elderly person receives regular dental visits for scaling and cleanings. The family dentist plays an important role in educating the individual's family in the various methods of attaining good oral hygiene. Grundy et al. in 1985[79] recommended the use of disclosing tablets to aid caregivers in recognizing the timely need for brushing and dental service. He also recommended various principles of dental management for the impaired individual:

- dental interventions at early stages of oral disease;
- dental health education, preventative measures, and advice on environmental aids for independence;
- regular 3-monthly periodic review of the individual's need to avoid pain and minimize interventions; and
- reduction of fear, stress, and embarrassment for the patient.

Angerholm[80] in 1991 recommended the double-headed tooth brush to help achieve better lingual and palatal plague control. Other methods advocated as preventative measures are:[81–84]

- electric toothbrushes;
- large handled brushes with strap for compromised dexterity;
- wall-mounted holders for brushes, toothpaste and denture adhesives;
- verbal instructions printed in boldface;
- appropriate motivation enhancement by caregivers with visual and verbal demonstrations;
- training programs for nurses and caregivers;
- programs to increase awareness of importance of oral health; and
- constant surveillance by dentists rather than waiting for complaints and problems to arise.

In a study using a power toothbrush, and Papas et al.[85] and Kugel and Boghosian[86] found that the use of a Sonicare toothbrush was an important adjunct in combination with prescription-level fluorides for the prevention of caries. Continued education, and access to dental services, especially for the dependent elderly, serve to promote and maintain the oral health quality of life of this group of the population.

Petersen and Nortov[87] in 1989 stated that older individuals who led relatively inactive lifestyles combined with weak family support showed higher levels of poor oral hygiene and general and dental health care. Past studies[88,89] also, have shown a direct relationship between an individual's lessened capacity to function and care for oneself, namely brushing and detecting oral and gingival problems, demonstrating poorer oral health, as well as lessened use of dental treatment and a lower degree of quality of life.

## Clinical considerations for long-term care[90–92]

Concerns about the overall oral hygiene of residents in LTC results in increased stress to all involved in the care of the very aged individuals. Dentists and dental hygienists are often frustrated by the challenges involved in providing oral hygiene in these facilities. They find that often residents are without:

- toothbrushes;
- toothpaste;
- handles designed for those with hand impairments;
- mouthwashes;
- adequate vehicles to store and soak dentures; and
- lack of dental equipment to provide basic care.

The dental practitioner finds restorative procedures more difficult, and lacks confidence in implementing them without adequately equipped treatment rooms. Care and concern in these matters can differ from facility to facility. The variety of staff and the variations in socio-cultural and educational backgrounds, combined with the varying demands and expectations of some of the residents, add to the difficulties in implementing proper oral hygiene to such long-term individuals. Major considerations in long term care are that:

- Older individuals, whether in a nursing home, long-term facility are at risk of oro-dental problems.
- The responsibility of providing oral health care lies with those health professionals involved in the patient's care.
- A higher level of initial training for nurses, and healthcare professionals regarding oral care for the aged should be mandatory.
- Education and training in recognition of common oral conditions such as denture stomatitis, untreated caries and periodontal problems need to be provided to LTC caregivers.

## The future of dental care for the elderly

The world population is aging, and elders are increasingly maintaining their natural dentition. Ettinger[93] reported that when older individuals retain their teeth, they tend to utilize dental services to a similar extent as younger groups do. The oral health care of older individuals has become more challenging due to the fact that most no longer are willing to have their teeth extracted and to accept dentures as the solution to their restorative needs. The elderly individuals of today are better dentally educated and more aware of the importance of maintaining their dentition and the associated ramifications that can occur when teeth and oral diseases are not maintained.

Ettinger also concluded that dental schools need to rethink their curricula and to train dentist so that they have adequate skills to manage the complexities of restorative dentistry in the aged, including the care of the edentulous person. The present shortage of educationally trained dentists will exacerbate the lack of care that many older patients face, especially the edentulous frail individual. However, enticing students to treat the underserved elderly and disabled continues to be a challenge. Dentists see little value in treating this segment of the population due to low reimbursement and often having to provide care with the most minimal of equipment. Today's dental school challenge is to heighten awareness among dental students regarding the critical lack of adequate access to dental care, which many fear will only accelerate in years to come. In addition, the practicing dentist also must feel a sense of responsibility to provide some treatment regardless of ability to pay, while financial and state organizations must agree contribute increased subsidies to entice young professionals to serve this segment of our population.

# SUMMARY

The biomedical principles of aging that affect the elderly individual influences his or her emotional response to illness and therapy. Optimal care of the elderly requires a multidisciplinary approach of diagnosis, treatment, and prevention all geared to improving the overall general and oral-related quality of life of the aged individual. To treat elderly patients successfully, the practitioner must be aware of their concerns, attending to the following:

## Chairside clinical considerations[5,68,94]

- Identify the patient's specific needs and expectations.
- Identify the type and severity of the dental need.
- Assess the physical, medical status of the patient.
- Weigh the impact of treatment on the patient's quality of life.
- Assess the prognosis and probability of positive treatment.

- Identify and prioritize treatments.
- Evaluate the patient's social support network, emotional support, transportation, and motivation.
- Offer continuous support and reassurance.
- Assure the elderly patient that he or she will always be in control, and offer clear explanations, verbal and written.

Be empathetic and understanding, and remember your time is coming soon.

## REFERENCES

1.  United Nations. 2002. *World Population Ageing 19502050*. New York: United Nations.
2.  World Health Organization. 2002. *Active Ageing: A Policy Framework*. Geneva: World Health Organization.
3.  United nations Popular Division. 2003.*World Population Prospects: The 2002 Revision*. New York: United Nations.
4.  Peterson P. 2003. The World Health report: Continuous improvement of oral health in the 21st century—The approach of the WHO Global Oral Health Programme. *Community Dent Oral Epidemiol* 31(Suppl): 3–23.
5.  Weiner A. 1985. The psychophysiologic etiology of anxiety in the geriatric patient. *Spec Care Dentist* 5(4):174–7.
6.  Albert S. 2004. *Public Health and Aging; An Introduction to Maximizing Function and Well-Being*. New York: Springer Publishing Company.
7.  Birren J. 2007. *Cultural and Ethnic Influences on Aging in Encyclopedia of Gerontology*. Boston: Academic Press.
8.  Mahoney D, Cloutterbuck J, Neary S, et al. 2005. African-American, Chinese and Latino family care-givers impressions of the onset and diagnosis of dementia: Cross-cultural similarities and differences. *Gerontologist* 45:783–92.
9.  John MT, Koepsell TD, Hujoel P, et al. 2004. Demographic factors, denture status and oral health-related quality of life. *Community Dent Oral Epidemiol* 32:125–32.
10. John T, LeResche L, and Koepsell T. 2003. Oral health-related quality of life in Germany. *EurJ Oral Sci* 111:483–91.
11. McGrath C and Bedi R. An evaluation of a new measure of oral-related quality of life—OHQol-UK. *Community Dent Health* 18:138–43.
12. Kandelman D, Peterson P, and Ueda H. 2008. Oral health, general health, and quality of life in older people. *Spec Care Dentist* 28(6):224–36.
13. Belmin J, Chassagne O, Gonthier R, et al. 2003. *Gerodontologie. Collection pour le practicien*. Paris: Masson.
14. Berg N and Morgenstern N. 1997. Physiologic changes in the elderly. *Dent Clin North Am* 41:651–68.

15. Scully C and Ettinger R. 2007. The influence of systemic diseases on oral health care in older adults. *J Am Dent Assoc* 138(Sept):7S–14S.
16. Winkler S, Garg A, Mekayarajjanananth T, et al. 1999. Depressed taste and smell min geriatric patients. *J Am Dent Assoc* 130:1759–65.
17. Phillips P, Phil D, Rolls, B, et al. 1984. Reduced thirst after water deprivation in healthy elderly men. *N Engl J Med* 311:753–9.
18. Mentes J. 2006. Oral hydration in older adults: Greater awareness is needed in preventing, recognizing and treating dehydration. *Am J Nurs* 106:40–9.
19. Shembri A and Fiske J. 2001. The implications of visual impairment in an elderly population in recognizing oral disease and maintaining oral health. *Spec Care Dentist* 21:222–6.
20. Huttne E, Machado D, Belle de Olivera R, et al. 2009. Effects of human aging on periodontal tissues. *Spec Care Dentist* 29(4):149–55.
21. Beck J, Ekter J, Heiss G, et al. 2001. Relationship of periodontal disease to carotid artery intima-media wall thickness: The AtheroSclerosis Risk in Communities Study. *ArtheriosclerThrom Vasc Biol* 21:1816–22.
22. Mattila K, Valle M, Niemin MS, et al. 1993. Dental infections and coronary atherosclerosis. *Atherosclerosis* 103: 205–11.
23. Becj J, Garcia R, Heiss G, et al. 1996. Periodontal disease and cardiovascukar disease. *J Periodontol* 67(10 Suppl):1123–37.
24. Beck J and Offenbacher S. 2001. the association between periodontal disease and cardiovascular diseases: A state of-the-science review. *Ann Periodontol* 6:9–15.
25. Persson R, Hollender L, and Powell L. 2002. Assessment of periodontal conditions and systemnic disease in older subjects. *J Clin Periodontol* 29:796–802.
26. Lagervall M, Jansson L, and Bergstrom J. 2003. Systemic disorders in patients with periodontal disease. *J Clin Periodontol* 30:293–9.
27. Loesche W and Lopatin D. 1998. Interactions between periodontal disease, medical diseases and immunity in the older individual. *Periodontol* 2000 16:80–105.
28. Narhi T. 1994. Prevalence of subjective feelings of dry mouth in the elderly. *J Dent Res* 73:20–5.
29. Locker D. 1993.Subjective reports of oral dryness in an older adult population. *Community Dent Oral Epidemiol* 21:165–8.
30. Ship J, Pillemer S, and Baum B. 2002. Xerostomia and the geriatric patient. *J Am Soc Geriatr Dent* 50: 535–43.
31. Gerdin E, Einarson S, Jonsson M, et al. 2005. Impact of dry mouth conditions on oral health-related quality of life in older people. *Gerontology* 22:219–26.
32. Matear D, Locker D, Stephens M, et al. 2006. Associations between xerostomia and health status indicators in the elderly. *J R Soc Health* 126: 79–85.
33. Ravald N and Hamp S. 1981. Prediction of root surface caries in patients treated for advanced periodontal disease. *J Clin Periodontol* 8:400–14.

34. Griffin S, Griffin P, Swann J, et al. 2004. Estimating rates of new root caries in older adults. *J Dent Res* 83:634–8.
35. Takano N, Ando Y, Yoshihara A, et al. 2004. Factors associated with root caries incidence in an elderly population. *Community Dent Health* 20:217–22.
36. Papas A, Joshi A, Palmer C, et al. 1995. Relationship of diet to root caries. *Am J Clin Nutr* 61:423S–9S.
37. Sing M, Martuscelli G, Duguid Z et al. 2002. Prevalence of carious lesions in medicated patients (Abstract). *J Dent Res* 81(Special Issue A): 988.
38. Papas A, Joshi A, and MacDonald S. 1993. Caries prevalence in xerostomic individuals. *J Can Dent Assoc* 59:171–4.
39. Calvo J and Papas A. 2003. Do medication induced xerostomia subjects have more caries prevalence than non medicated subjects? (Abstract). *J Dent Res* 82(Special Issue A):985.
40. Greenlee R, Murray T, Bolden S, et al. 2000. Cancer statistics. *CA Cancer J Clin* 50:7–33.
41. Lewin F, Norell S, Johansson H, et al. 1998. Smoking tobacco, oral snuff, and alcohol in the etiology of squamous cell carcinoma of the head and neck: A population-based case-referent study in Sweden. *Cancer* 82:1367–75.
42. Epstein J, Lunn R, and Le N. 2005. Patients with oropharyngeal cancer: A comparison of adults living independently and patients in long term facilities. *Spec Care Dentist* 25:124–30.
43. Thomas G, Hashibe M, Jacob B, et al. 2003. Risk factors for multiple oral premalignant lesions. *Int J Cancer* 107:285–91.
44. Ettinger R and Beck J. 1983. Medical and psychosocial risk factors in the dental treatment of the elderly. *Int Dent J* 33:292–300.
45. Ettinger R. 2005. Oral health in aging societies. *Spec Care Dentist* 25(5):225–6.
46. Lewis S and Jagger R. 2001. The oral health of psychiatric in-patients in South Wales. *Spec Care Dentist* 21:182–6.
47. Persson G, Persson R, MacEntee C, et al. 2003. Periodontitis and perceived risk for periodontitis in elders with depression. *J Clin Periodontol* 30: 691–6.
48. Adam H and Preston A. 2006. The oral health of individuals with dementia in nursing homes. *Gerontology* 23:99–105.
49. Chalmers J, Carter K, and Spencer A. 2003. Oral diseases and conditions in community-living, older adults with and without dementia. *Spec Care Dentist* 23(1):7–17.
50. Little J. 2004. Dental implications of mood disorders. *Gen Dentist* 52:442–50.
51. Lautenschlarger N and Forsti H. 2007. Personality change in old age. *Curr Opin Psychiatry* 20:62–6.
52. Klieb H and Wiseman M. 2008. Death, dying and bereavement: A survey of dental practitioners. *Spec Care Dentist* 28(2):58–60.

53.  Chiodo G and Tolle S. 1988. Patient death and berveavement: What is the dentist's role? *Spec Care Dentist* 8:198–200.

54.  Chiodo G and Tolle S. 2000.The dentist's role in berveavement support. *Gen Dentist* 48:500–5.

55.  Fulmer T and Paveza G. 1998. Neglect in the elderly patient. *Nurs Clin North Am* 33:457–66.

56.  Jorgensen J. 1992. A dentist's social responsibility to diagnose elder abuse. *Spec Care Dentist* 12:112–5.

57.  Johnson T, Boccia A, and Strayer M. 2001. Elder abuse and neglect: Detection, reporting and intervention. *Spec Care Dentist* 21(4):141–6.

58.  Marshall C, Benton D, and Brazier J. 2000. Using clinical tools to identify clues of mistreatment. *Geriatrics* 55:42–4, 47–50.

59.  Walla A, Steele J, Sheinham A, et al. 2000. Oral health and nutriti on in older people. *J Public Health Dent* 60:304–7.

60.  Soini H, Routasalo P, Sirkka L, et al. 2003. Oral and nutritional status in frail elderly. *Spec Care Dentist* 23: 209–15.

61.  Sheiham A, Steele J, Marcenes W, et al. 2001. Prevalence of impacts of dental and oral disorders and their effect on eating among older people: A national survey in Great Britain. *Community Dent Oral Epidemiol* 29:195–203.

62.  Nakayama Y, Washio M, and Mori M. 2004. Oral health conditions in patients with Parkinson's disease. *J Epidemiol* 14:143–50.

63.  Ahmed N, Mandel R, and Fain M. 2007. Fraility: An emerging geriatric syndrome. *Am J Med* 120:748–53.

64.  Fried L. 2001. Frailty in older adults: Evidence for a phenotype. *J Gerontol* 56(Series A):M146–57.

65.  Klein B, Klein R, Knudtson M, et al. 2005. Frailty, morbidity and survival. *Arch Gerontol Geriatr* 41:141–9.

66.  Woo J, Goggins W, Sham A, et al. 2005. Social determinants of frailty. *Gerontology* 51:402–8.

67.  Woods N, LaCroix A, Gray S, et al. 2005. Frailty: Emergence and consequences in woman aged 65 and older in Woman's Health Initiative Observational Study. *J Am Geriatr Soc* 53:1321–30.

68.  Epstein S. 1988. Treatment of the geriatric phobic patient. *Dent Clin North Am* 32(4):715–21.

69.  Nisizaki S. 2003. Philosophical approach in old adults dental treatment. *Spec Care Dentist* 23(1):4–6.

70.  Brown T, Goryakin Y, and Finlayson T. 2009. The effect of functional limitations on the demand or dental care among adults 65 and older. *J Calif Dent Assoc* 37(8):549–57.

71.  LeResche L and Dworkin S. 1985. Evaluating orofacial pain in the elderly. *Gerodontics* 1:81–7.

72.  MacEntee M,Thorne S, and Kazanjiian S. 1999.Conflicting priorities: Oral health in long-term care. *Spec Care Dentist* 19(4):164–72.

73.  Thorne S, Kazanjjian A, and MacEntee M. 2001. Oral health in long-term care: The implications of organizational culture. *J Aging Stud* 15:271–83.

74. NacEntee M, Hole R, and Stolar E. 1997. The significance of the mouth in old age. *Soc Sci Med* 45:1449–58.

75. MacEntee M and Prosth D. 2005. Caring for elderly long-term care patients: Oral health-related concerns and issues. *Dent Clin North Am* 49:429–43.

76. Bronsani M, Bryant S, and MacEntee M. 2007. Elders assessment of an evolving model of oral health. *Gerontology* 24:189–95.

77. MacEntee M. 2006. An existential model of oral health from evolving views on health, function and disability. *Community Dent Health* 23: 5–14.

78. Avlund K, Holm-Pederson P, Morse D, et al. 2003. Social relations as determinants of oral health among persons over age 80 years. *Community Dent Oral Epidemiol* 31:454–62.

79. Grundy M, Shaw L, and Hamilton D. 1985. *Dental Care for the Medically Compromised Patient*. London: Wolfe Publishing.

80. Angerholm D. 1991. A clinical trial to evaluate plaque removal with a double-headed toothbrush. *Br Dent Journal* 170:411–3.

81. Tritten C and Armitage C. 1996. Comparison of a sonic and a manual tooth rush for efficacy in supraginigival plaque removal and reduction of gingivitis. *J Clin Periodontol* 23:641–8.

82. Dickinson C and Millwood J. 1999. Tooth handle adaptation using silicone impression putty. *Dent Updates* 26:288–9.

83. Warren K. 1990. Mouthsticks protheses and other gadgets. *Dent Update* 17: 428–30.

84. British Society for Disability and Oral Health. 2009. *Revised Guidelines for Oral Health Care and Long-Stay Patients and Residents*. Available at www.bsdh.org.uk (accessed July 10, 2010).

85. Papas A, Singh M, Harrington D, et al. 2007. Reduction in caries rate among patients with xerostomia using a power tooth brush. *Spec Care Dent* 27(2):46–51.

86. Kugel G and Boghosian A. 2002. Effects of the Sonicare toothbrush for specific indications. *Compend Contin Educ Dent* 23(7 Suppl 1):11–4.

87. Petersen P and Nortov B. 1989. General and dental health in relation to life-style and social network activity among 67 year old Danes. *Scand J Prim Health Care* 7:225–30.

88. Avlund K, Holm-Peterson P, and Schroll M. 2001. Functional ability and oral health among older people: A longitudinal study from age 75–80. *J Am Geriatr Soc* 49:954–62.

89. Chalmers J. 2003. Oral health promotions for our ageing Australian population. *Aust Dent J* 48:2–9.

90. Preston A, Kearns A, Barber M, et al. 2006. The knowledge of healthcare professionals regarding elderly persons' care. *Br Dent J* 201:293–5.

91. Isaksson R, Paulsson G, Fridlund B, et al. 2000. Evaluation of an oral health education programmne by nursing personnel in special housing facilities for the elderly. *Spec Care Dentist* 20: 109–13.

92. Peltola P, Vehkalahti M, and Simoila R. 2005. Oral health related well being of the long-term hospitalized elderly. *Gerontology* 22:17–23.

93. Ettinger R. 2004. Who is going to treat our older edentulous adults. *Spec Care Dentist* 24(6):281–2.

94. Mostofsky D, Forgione A, and Giddon D (eds.). 2006. *Behavioral Dentistry.* Oxford: Blackwell Munksgaard, pp. 215–27.

# 10

# Fear and anxiety management for the special needs patient

## Linda M. Maytan and Gina M. Terenzi

## INTRODUCTION

According to the Department of Human and Health Services Center for Disease Control, developmental disabilities are a diverse group of severe chronic conditions that are due to mental and/or physical impairments. People with developmental disabilities have problems with major life activities, such as language, mobility, learning, self-help, and independent living. Developmental disabilities begin anytime during development up to 22 years of age and usually last throughout a person's lifetime.

In 1994–1995, the National Health Interview Survey included a Disability Supplement to collect extensive information among individuals sampled as part of annual census-based household interview surveys. In our analysis, we estimate the prevalence of mental retardation in the non-institutionalized population of the United States to be 7.8 people per thousand (0.78%); of developmental disabilities, 11.3 people per thousand (1.13%); and the combined prevalence of mental retardation and/or developmental disabilities to be 14.9 per thousand (1.49%).

Mental retardation, a term that is falling out of favor in the United States, is diagnosed before age 18. Below average general intellectual functioning and lack of skills necessary for daily living are benchmarks. Generally speaking, a combination of well-below-average intellectual functioning plus significant limitations in two or more adaptive skill areas are reason for further testing. Mental retardation affects 1–3 % of the general

*The Fearful Dental Patient: A Guide to Understanding and Managing.* Edited by Arthur A. Weiner
© 2011 Blackwell Publishing Ltd.

population, with etiology determined in about 25% of the cases. The degree of impairment widely varies across a spectrum of mild to profound. Today, we focus less on the degree of retardation and more on what supports are necessary for the individual to successfully accomplish ADLs (activities of daily living). If the 1% estimate is true, then 2.5 million "retarded people" reside in the United States, with a male prevalence. Ten to 40% of patients with mental retardation also have mental health challenges. Over 25% of children with mental retardation also have a seizure disorder. These combinations can greatly increase communication and behavioral limitations for an affected person. WHO (World Health Organization) mimics these statistics in their findings; however, surveys are often very difficult to accomplish. It is known that disease burden worldwide is not well accounted for, and is increasing. Current trends include changing nomenclature from mental retardation to intellectual impairment, cognitive disability, or neurodevelopmental deficit.

Although there may be facilities in your community that specifically cater to the dental care of the special needs, it is well known that patients with disabilities have difficulties regarding access to care. Additionally, the special needs population is increasing. That said, dentists in the community at large will need to prepare themselves to include this population in their practice.

Management of anxiety and fear for special needs population in the dental setting is dependant on the patient diagnosis and not exclusive to common special care profiles. Not all special needs patients are necessarily fearful of the dentist specifically, but have behavioral characteristics due to their disability that limit completion of any task that is unfamiliar. This chapter will focus on those with intellectual developmental disabilities ranging from mild to moderate limitations, and those with autistic spectrum and pervasive developmental disorders, often referred to as a special needs population.

The literature for anxiety and fear management for special needs patients is historically limited, and more so for studies related to dentistry and special care management. Relaxation and anxiolyitic modalities using sensory perception techniques must be extrapolated for practical use from studies and observations in other behavioral patterns that may be similar to that of special care management and includes pediatrics, geriatrics, mental illness, and those with multiple severe medical comorbidities. The majority of articles written on this topic are by caregiver, healthcare provider observations, and surveys, and are anecdotal, because specific modalities and recommended treatments are limited. Oftentimes, a study will have an insufficient participant number and an inadequate study design that will not allow for placebo effects or control study groups. The exact science of special needs patients' perception is not well understood, studies are inconsistent with each other, and behavior traits are contradicting. What technique is good for one patient with a given diagnosis is not the same for another.

It is a hope that the authors can provide a collection of material and techniques for clinical management for patient care in the dental setting. This is not meant as an attempt to reiterate articles already written: rather, a practical guide for practitioners wishing to include this patient population into their practice. Time, patience, and realistic goal setting will allow providers, patients, caregivers, auxiliary staff, and others a successful and long-term relationship.

## LET US MEET AND EVALUATE YOUR PATIENTS

The special needs population we are generally referring to are those diagnosed with a developmental or acquired intellectual disability, and those diagnosed with autistic or developmental pervasive disorder. Patients with either of these disorders may be placed in the following categories in order to aid the provider determine the ability that the patient to demonstrates relative to accepted life skill needs. This includes aspects of communication skill and social interaction and not solely on IQ relativity. There is no true consensus to these definitions and they should be left to non-bias interpretation by the provider team for individual patient assessments on how the patient is able to tolerate procedures within the practice: They are:

- high functioning;
- mild;
- moderate;
- severe; and
- profound.

According to the DSM-IV,[1] the following criteria have been established as parameters for particular categories of mental retardation (Table 10.1).

Mental retardation is listed on the ICD-10 under Chapter 5, "Mental and Behavioral Disorders," as F70–F79.[2] This dissects numerous definitions and subdivisions. For the general dentist and dental team, it is simply useful to know that these levels of mental retardation, as each level indicates certain self-care functions and behavioral limitations.

**Table 10.1** Diagnostic criteria for mental retardation (MR): World Health Organization 2007, ICD-1 codes.

| MR | % of MR DX | IQ score range |
|----|------------|----------------|
| Mild | 85 | 50–75 |
| Moderate | 10 | 35–55 |
| Severe | 3–4 | 20–40 |
| Profound | 1–2 | Under 20–25 |

- F70 Mild Mental Retardation: Learning difficulties in school. Many adults will be able to work and maintain good social relationship and contribute to society at large.
- F71 Moderate Mental Retardation: Marked developmental delays in childhood but most can learn to develop some degree of independence in the area of self-care and acquire adequate communication and academic skills. Adults will need a varying degree of support to live and work in the community.
- F72 Severe Mental Retardation: Need continuous support for living.
- F73 Profound Mental Retardation: Severe/extreme limitation in self-care, continence, communication, and mobility.

The International Classification of Functioning, Disability, and Health, or ICF, is WHO's framework for measuring health and disability at both individual and population levels. This tool was endorsed by all 191 member states in May 2001 as the international standard to describe and measure health and disability. A goal of this standard is to recognize the "universal human experience" of experiencing a disability, considering the medical and social factors related to experiencing a disability. Additionally, this parameter focuses on the impact of the disability instead of etiology. This provides a functional assessment tool useful for goal setting, treatment planning, monitoring benchmarks, and outcomes. For the dental team, this type of information is important when considering realistic, attainable, and sustainable expectations.

It is important to remember that these measurement tools are indeed tools. These are not intended as punitive, but rather as a way to aid in the development of a life plan for the affected person. Likewise, it is essential that this information be transmitted on the health history with equal importance to medical comorbidities.

A general health history including the specific limitation is necessary, particularly to identify a specific syndrome. Additional research for a particular syndrome will help the provider to identify similar behavior characteristics. With the completion of the human genome project and the availability of genetic testing, it is likely that your patient will present with quite specific information regarding the genetic etiology of their developmental disability. This information will benefit the practitioner! Soft and hard tissue aberrations, salivary protein changes, dysmorphic odontogenic and osteogenic processes, and other related biologic systems may be coded for on the same DNA segment as the aberration causing the developmental delay.

In addition to a general history, these abbreviated questions from a sensory sensitivity[3,4] may be incorporated, as they are relative to sensitivities that are common to dental treatments. The patient, or in most cases, a patient representative, can answer in yes or no format. Personalize these questions as appropriate. Present yourself as a team member to the patient and staff. Both will be more willing to work with you to achieve a successful outcome.

- unusually sensitive to heat or cold;
- more sensitive to pain than other people;
- unusually insensitive to heat or cold;
- high pain tolerance;
- made uncomfortable by touch or texture of clothing;
- enjoys light brushing or touch;
- likes or seeks out deep pressure or squeezing;
- likes or seeks out gentle vibration;
- unusually sensitive to vibrations;
- unusually sensitive to light;
- bothered by sounds;
- unusually responsive to odor;
- unusually responsive to taste;
- covers ears in response to sound of "high-pitched," loud noises;
- becomes easily upset or overwhelmed in loud or crowded places;
- overall sensitivity to environment;
- bright lights: room or direct;
- bright colors;
- strong smells; and
- coarse fabrics.

Additionally, does the patient respond better to men or women? This is not unusual, and when possible, a patient with a gender preference should be accommodated. The systematic review of the above will help the provider to determine what may help the patient have a successful visit. For example if the questionnaire is significant for:

(1) *Bright light and general environmental sensitivity*: The treatment room should be dimmed if possible, and the patient given sunglasses prior to turning on the dental light. If the patient would not allow sunglasses, then direct intraoral lighting may be necessary yet effective for the dental provider, particularly for noninvasive treatments. For dental procedures, there are several products on the market for optimal intraoral visibility that allow the provider hands free illumination of the oral cavity, for example, Isolite Systems (www.isolite.com).

(2) *Sensitivity to "texture of clothing"*: A towel in place of a dental bib may be considered due to the course nature of the plastic-lined paper. In this case, if there are temperature sensitivity issues, a cold metal bib clip is best avoided, or warmed before use.

(3) *Loud noises*: General quiet room protocols should be followed, that is, closed operatory door if possible. In these cases, use of the dental drill can be difficult. Providing ear protectors or plugs will help if the

patient will allow their use. If not, the hand pieces can be started slowly for the patient to acclimate to the sound. With vibration, particularly for the slow speed hand piece, accommodation for touch may be needed.

The reader can see where we are going here: most events that occur in the dental office and operatory can have considerable impact on whether this patient population has a productive, comfortable visit versus a challenging visit for both the patient and dental team. The majority of actions on the providers' part need preparation, even those perceived insignificant and routine. With this in mind, the consideration of the sensory questionnaire is therefore an invaluable tool.

Social and communication evaluation questions the dental team should consider will help identify the individual likes and dislikes of the patient. Response to the following questions will give the dental team factors to use in positive reinforcement communication and preparation for visit events:

What are considered the patient's (your) favorite things? *Be specific!*

- music;
- people (celebrities, relatives, and friends);
- animals;
- hobbies;
- toys;
- colors;
- foods/flavors;
- activities: that is, bowling, organized sports like Special Olympics; and
- holidays.

The authors have found it useful to take all of these tools and combine them into a product that works in their own offices. Over time, this process of questioning and learning becomes second nature. Needs become clear quite often within the first few moments of meeting a patient and his or her staff/guardian. This will be expanded later in the chapter. Assessment of the patient is an ongoing, evolving process. It is important to develop a sixth sense about social, personal, medical, vocational, and other elements that make up who your patient is. Slight changes to a routine can greatly affect a special care patient for a protracted period of time. Engaging the patient, and secondarily, the direct care staff, during each appointment is a critically important function. The authors make it routine to meet all new patients for the first time in the waiting room. This is extremely effective and important in the journey of trust development. Meeting new people and coming in to an unfamiliar office can be insurmountable for many of these patients. Feeling welcomed into this strange setting by the doctor creates a sense of partnership from the outset, establishes a welcome, and validates the patient as an individual.

Depending on the patient and their ability to adapt, it may take several appointments before that patient feels comfortable entering into the treatment area when called by auxiliary staff (not the dentist). When possible, the initial waiting room meeting includes several intake questions, including dental/medical/social histories. If this would violate the privacy of the patient, then a simple introduction and warm welcome will do, with an invitation to join the author into the treatment room to continue getting to know each other. Many initial visits are conversational only, with a consequent appointment for the x-rays, dental exam, and prophylaxis. Talking to the patient directly, using eye contact, listening, shaking hands, and taking their concerns seriously (commonplace in treatment of your general population patients) is critical. Not only have you validated the patient and their needs to the patient, but also to yourself and your staff.

## General characteristics of this patient population in consideration of clinic behavioral management

There is no one therapy for predictable management for the fearful special needs patient but a multifaceted approach dependant on the patients likes and dislikes. Your own biases and the biases of your dental team greatly influence the success of the care for the special needs patient. Additionally, biases of the direct care staff, guardians, case managers, and others involved in the comprehensive needs of the patient will affect the outcomes. Values and beliefs of all parties can come into conflict. Working to dispel distrust and increase partnership for the sake of the oral and systemic health of the client is the core goal. If and when core goals are not in sync, then a referral to another provider is likely in order.

Recognize goals and objectives of visits and how to achieve them, as well as each technique necessary to achieve those goals: It is our experience that building your goals and objectives around a teamwork model is well-understood and accepted, and is usually more successful. Recognize the support and auxiliary staff roles to help with tasks associated with outcomes. Validate the difficulty each person may have completing their designated responsibility. This is especially true in high-functioning individuals who refuse help despite the reality that they are unable to adequately perform their own self-care, and in the most impaired patients who may be quite resistive to any ADLs, particularly those which involve the face/mouth. Outlining the oral healthcare plan in as much detail as is appropriate makes the plan concrete. Here are some examples which have worked for us.

The direct care staff will encourage excellent hygiene, perhaps using a point system for the client to accumulate enough for a reward. The authors prefer the reward is not Mountain Dew; rather, a noncaries-causing reward like an outing with a favorite staff, bowling, or the like. Informing the patient that the dentist, his or her mom, or another revered individual, will be privy to the results of points accumulated can serve as added incentive for the client who is "on the fence" about moving forward with oral care.

Home care plans should be as simple as possible, especially initially. Adding one adjunct as the previous adjunct is "mastered" will result in a longer-term success. The authors have historically suggested one implement at a time: first, a battery-operated toothbrush. If successful, then add on an antiseptic mouthwash swab. If accepted, add on floss picks. Patients with touch, sound, or motion sensitivities may not tolerate a battery or other mechanical toothbrush. Do not force the issue! Return to a traditional toothbrush and proceed with adding adjuncts as necessary and appropriate.

This process can take anywhere from months to years to reach its full potential. Remember to consider realistic expectations. Often, the dentist has to reevaluate their own biases to suit the patient. It is also important to recognize the value on oral health the direct care staff holds to be true. Remember, brushing someone else's teeth can be difficult! If the staff does not brush their own teeth regularly, it is unlikely they will be willing to struggle with a difficult client to attain that client's oral health goals. It is common for the authors to remind everyone that the oral care plan exists for the good of the client, and that everyone can do the best they can, but not more. When the oral care plan is viewed as a team effort, each person being assigned a role, the motivation and success increase.

We have chosen to discuss noninvasive behavior management techniques in this chapter, which can be used safely and effectively in most dental practices. As it is with the routine dental patient, a provider to patients with special needs will find it helpful to provide care in a calm setting. The authors believe using operatories with closeable doors aid in facilitating a sense of calm and privacy. In the event that the patient's claustrophobia or uncertainty supersedes privacy, the door would simply be left open. As treatment algorithms are case-by-case, it will be a process of discovery for all involved to determine the most appropriate treatment room setting. Allow patient to come into clinic with a care worker or parent they trust, or someone they have been known to take directive well from for daily tasks. It may prove very beneficial, or, it may soon be discovered that the patient will try to "use" his or her influence with their companion to the detriment of the appointment/treatment. In these events, it is reasonable to kindly dismiss the companion to the waiting room. Similar tactics are used in pediatrics when such an instance arises between a child and parent.

In conjunction with the evaluation tools mentioned, and in regard to the dental procedures attempted, it is helpful to select cooperation levels as a basic skill set for patients' abilities in the ambulatory setting. This approach helps even the playing field for all patient diagnosis and limitations both physically and psychologically. Over a period of time, it will allow the provider to document what procedures the patient does well with and under which conditions and therefore improve on patient management of fear and anxiety as the patient/provider relationship matures. Cooperation levels as follows will help the dental team discover what care can be delivered to each patient safely and effectively. Dental team safety should also be a consideration in regard to patients that may be extremely fearful and that need assistance for dental procedures.

- *Coop 6*: Allows all procedures without assistance.
- *Coop 5*: Allows all procedure with assistance more than 50% of the time.
- *Coop 4*: Allow all procedures with assistance the majority of the time.
- *Coop 3*: Allow limited procedures with assistance 50% of the time.
- *Coop 2*: Allow limited procedure with assistance all of the time.
- *Coop 1*: Will not allow procedures.

## SENSORY PERCEPTION MODALITIES FOR TREATMENT AND COMMUNICATION

Sensory perception, sensory processing, or sensory integration describes the way we receive and perceive sensory input through sight, sound, touch, tastes, sounds, and movement. Difficulty taking in or interpreting this input can lead to devastating consequences in daily functioning, social and family relationships, behavioral challenges, regulating emotions, self-esteem, and learning.

It is common for special needs patients to have a high significance of sensory perception disorder, and for the dental team, this can prove to be a challenging limitation to dental care. Most of the instruments we use in the operatory have a sensory component. We, as practitioners, forget! Attempting to think about the appointment in terms of the patient help, and you cannot overstate expectations. The author will repeat Tell–Show–Do to a client multiple times within one appointment, and usually repeat at each and every subsequent appointment. Surprising noises, lights, and vibrations can quickly terminate an appointment. Even for a prophylaxis appointment, validating the "scratching" of the scalers will alleviate tension for the patient and the dental team. Comparing dental treatment to nondental applications is well accepted. The author has frequently compared prepping and restoring a cavity with road workers fixing a pothole. This analogy to a familiar and nonpersonally threatening event makes the completion of the restoration less challenging. Other examples of this are demonstrating the curing light as a Light Saber, a scaler as a glorified toothpick, and the ultrasonic scaler as a power washer.

Sensory sensitivities may lead to significant behavior problems and may interfere with adaptive functioning across educational and social settings.[5] Additionally, although patients may crave the security of the lead apron or Rainbow Wrap (see later in the text), touching the patient shoulder with your hand may be intolerable and cause a cascade of behaviors. Some patients cannot tolerate the dental chair tipping back: for these patients, we make sure the dental chair is in the treatment position before the patient ever sits down. Knowing the touch threshold will help you have a more successful appointment!

## Counting methods

The author uses counting daily as a method of "understandable parameters" for patients, especially those in the moderate to severely retarded categories. Patients will respond to terms that are understood as finite. So, often, we count to 10, and then allow a break. It takes longer to complete treatment this way; however, it may allow the patient to accomplish restorative treatment in the offices and forego a trip to the OR. Counting is an additional method of developing the trust relationship: I stop working when I get to 10, and we take a break before resuming the next 10 count. Patients may not recognize how many times this is repeated, and it is often irrelevant. The point is doing what you say you are going to do: Simply counting to 10 and then stopping, even for a moment.

Honesty with your patient, regardless of their cognitive ability, is a foundational premise of practicing ethical dentistry. For a patient with cognitive limitations, it is even more important to be truthful: you will win trust, partnership, and loyalty, and the patient will be able to receive care. The author tells her patients from the outset, that the rule in the operatory is "no surprises." We agree that we like surprise birthday parties but not surprise medical procedures. I advise them when the materials are going to taste terrible, when something may be painful or unpleasant, or when they should expect their "brains to wiggle" from the use of the slow speed bur.

## Vision

Visual schedules, vision boards, and other visually based communication devices are particularly effective for any patient who functions on the Autism Spectrum. These can be for a specific task or activity, or, a variety of activities can be shown on one board. One example of a vision board is discussed later in the case presentation. The concept is simply this: autism spectrum disorders (ASD) folks intake information in a useful way through sight. Simply examining a picture, drawing, or photo of a specific object or activity, the learner is able to understand his or her interaction with it in a way that words or even experience cannot teach. These boards are used to introduce unfamiliar experiences, routine ADL's, teacher expectations, or about anything the user wishes. These tools can be homemade, to suit the exact need of the individual who requires supports. It is an effective communication device, allowing the patient on the autism spectrum to develop concrete life tools which are necessary for their brains to properly function.

## Role playing and show–tell–do techniques

- Demonstrate correct posture in the dental chair: hands on stomach feet out in front.
- Allow patient to show provider first, then allow provider to repeat.
- Allow care worker and/ or trained auxiliary staff to role play for patient to mimic.
- Echo learning for directives.
- Relate conversations to patient interests: that is, hobbies.
- Have patient observe trusted care taker or trained auxiliary undergo tasks: i.e. panoramic and regular radiograph taking. S
- Show pictures of the above prior to patient appointment.

## Other visual cues

### *The power of a smile*

It has been proven in many studies that the positive effects of smiling are endless.

Yes, it is as simple as a smile, and although it seems obvious that a smile offers a welcoming environment, a busy day at the office may leave the dental team short on this universal sign of happiness. It is important that the first welcoming team member is smiling as they greet the patient, looking directly at the patient—a behavior that all staff and providers should continue to do throughout the appointment to dismissal of the patient to the waiting room.

### *Visual participation*

Patient participation can be the key, so if a patient wants to watch or see what is happening, then allow it. The appointment 99% of the time will go better.

For example: Todd, a 28-year-old Asperger patient. He *needs* information to function and gets this by observing as much as possible. Allowing him to watch treatment has greatly increased treatment success, and has greatly decreased his treatment time. Even though Todd as a dental patient is difficult to treat overall, allowing him to use the hand mirror to observe treatments has greatly improved his cooperation; therefore, extensive operative procedures have been done using this method.

### *Time timer*

This clock-like appliance is an excellent treatment adjunct for particularly ASD patients. It addresses the linear thought process of an ASD brain, quantifying the abstract concept of time. The provider will place the timer in an obvious location in the operatory. The timer is then set to the number of minutes the appointment will take. This amount of "time" shows up as a red pie. The timer ticks away the minutes, reducing the red pie showing and increasing the clock face underneath. Patients know that when the red is gone, their appointment is over. If patients fail to cooperate (are naughty), red (time) is added to the timer. This introduces consequence of having to stay in the dental chair longer correlated to a specific inappropriate behavior.

## Sound

The study of auditory sensory perception integration for the special needs population is multifaceted and intense. It is not our intention to overcomplicate the use of music and sounds in the dental office for improved patient compliance, but to alert the team of its many powerful uses. Listening is a function of the entire brain and the whole body. The use of music or calming sounds for a means of relaxation for the special needs population has been shown to be a useful modality for general behavior management. Sound stimulation has been shown to have multiple areas of clinical outcomes, many of which are beneficial to the dental team:

- decreased tactile hypersensitivity or defensiveness;
- decreased oral hypersensitivity with increased exploration and acceptance of different foods;
- improved self-regulatory behavior, such as:
- more regulated sleep–wake cycle;
- more regulated hunger–thirst cycle;
- more regulated suck–swallow–breathe;
- more regulated respiratory control;
- decreased stress;
- improved balance and coordination of movement;
- increased postural organization;
- improved bilateral motor patterns;
- improved handwriting;
- increased visual–motor skills;
- increased and more elaborate social interactions, with better "timing";
- components of communication improved with greater range of non-verbal communication and improved/clearer articulation;
- greater emotional and verbal expression; and
- improvements in pragmatic language.

## Music

Delivery of music can be provided via head/earphones, which can help reduce background noise of office activities and equipment sound.

Adaptive speakers mount to dental chair headrest, but allow the dental care team to continue to interact with the patient during the procedure. General background music in the waiting and treatment rooms can also be considered to create a tranquil atmosphere. Again, it is important the provider use this modality as an individual approach for patient care, as not all patients can properly process auditory impulses, therefore the use of music can cause sensory overload.

### Music therapy

There are enormous volumes of literature on the effect of Music therapy as an anxiolytic approach to patient care, and the history goes as far back as observations made by Florence Nightingale in the early 1800s.[6] Music therapy can act as a nonpharmacologic adjunct to decrease pain perception and anxiety and increase patient comfort.[7-9]

Music is a safe, noninvasive, cost-effective measure to enhance patient relaxation both physically and psychologically.

Music selection should be based on patient preference whenever possible which may reflect cultural, age specific, social group backgrounds. With this in mind, characteristics of anxiety reducing music included simple repetitive rhythms, predictable melodies, low pitch, slow tempo, and low to no percussion.[10,11]

Singing directly to a patient or with the staff to accomplish procedures can be effective for cooperation and timing of a particular procedure. The "song" does not necessarily need to be a song, but a narration of what the dentist is doing in a sing-song voice. For example: While performing an exam, the provider, using a familiar tune like "Happy Birthday," would sing the words for the dental charting.

Singing a song to the patient during the procedure can also be a time stamp for the procedure start and finish, giving the patient a reference point for the treatment. If Sally knows that she needs to stay still until the doctor finishes the song, she may find it easier for her to understand that task than being told she needs to stay still "until the filling is done." Therefore, Sally's attention is focused on the song rather than the activity at hand.

### Voice control

Voice control for directives can be in the form of a sing-song, a low monotone, soft and coaxing voice, or close to the ear for focus. Allow the patient to see and touch sound-emitting instruments, that is, suction and hand pieces prior to introducing to the mouth. Start the sound slowly and softly, then increase as necessary. Use one voice: "I'm doing the talking." This is particularly important when either the dental assistant or the direct care staff are trying to "win" the conversation. I usually finally say, "I'm doing the talking. You need to listen to my voice, I will tell you everything that

I'm going to do, and I will let you know when we are done with this part." Most of the direct care staff eventually catch on (although there is always one who cannot)—the ones who have known me for a long time know that it is their cue to be quiet, and allow me to be the center of the patient's concentration.

## Smell[12–15]

### Aromatherapy

Use of aromatic oils has been used in many patient care settings in an attempt to decrease agitation and introduce a relaxing effect, the most popular being lavender and lemon balm, as well as neroli, cedarwood and sandalwood.[16] Literature reviews show both positive and inconclusive results for effectiveness involving a wide array of patient profiles, including those with dementia, autistic/pervasive disorders and varying levels of mental retardation. It has been noted that in some cases, the neuro-stimulation of aromatics on some patients with a diagnosed seizure disorder may actually cause a seizure in times of stress, therefore special attention to the sensory evaluation is important.

Aromatherapy is often used in conjunction with massage techniques with aromatic oils, and although the outcomes for anxiety reduction may be positive, the use of massage and oils in the dental setting may not prove realistic.

# ALTERNATIVE MODALITIES FOR ANXIETY MANAGEMENT

There are many cases in which attempts to manage fear and anxiety of the fearful Special needs patient in order to complete dental procedures safely and effectively are not possible due to the patients' inability to cooperate in regard to the ambulatory dental care setting and situational anxiety.

Providers should allow the patient a number of visits or several techniques with different modalities to attempt to achieve necessary treatments. If patient dental care is observed and documented to not be possible with sensory techniques, other modalities can be considered. The dental team training and experience level would need to be evaluated prior to safely proceeding to advanced levels of behavior management.

## Physical restraint methods and safety aids

- Direct care stabilization;
- papoose board; and
- Rainbow Wrap.

Use of medical stabilization and medical protective devices has fallen into contentious discussion in the modern day. Historic use of "restraints," particularly in institutional settings, has cast a shadow of disfavor upon stabilization use today. Each provider should be sensitive to the potential past experience each client may have had with such devices in their past. Additionally, the guardian may have heard of or seen unfavorable uses, and is now absolutely objectionable to stabilization devices. Training centers within the United States differ on their philosophies of use, so provider bias is also a strong consideration. The authors include this section both for completeness and to demonstrate how appropriate use in our own practices has allowed both patients and providers to receive necessary care safely. Informed consent for use of direct care and medical stabilization devices is recommended.

Sometimes the best version of stabilization is human contact. Caregivers or loved ones will simply be available to hold hands during a planned treatment. As in pediatric dentistry, a patient may sit on the lap of a loved one who is sitting in the dental chair. Mom may even hug the patient, as long as the provider is able to examine and diagnose the patient. Other instances include caregivers using touch to restrict movements in the dental chair to accomplish the appointment. Keeping in mind the potential strength and risk of harm to self or patient is important when implementing direct stabilization.

The slippery slope of medical stabilization devices runs the gamut from the use of mouth props (Molt, bite block) to the use of a Rainbow Wrap–type stabilizing modality. In some instances, patients are able to graduate to a lesser form of stabilization over time. This concept of least invasive treatment exists in all facets of care, and is certainly paramount to intent and treatment planning with regards to stabilizing devices. Stabilization is always used for the least possible amount of time, and is never a punishment.

Spasticity and other involuntary movements are challenging for both patient and provider, as these unexpected movements can easily result in injury to both the patient and the healthcare team. It is the experience of the author that use of the Rainbow Wrap in these cases is a welcome adjunct to the patient even more so than the provider. Spasticity increases as patients try harder to hold still. Use of the wrap takes the anxiety out of the equation. For example, a patient who has cerebral palsy may have constant involuntary movements. Use of medical stabilization devices allows the patient to relax knowing that his flailing arms and head will not pose a risk to himself or the dental team. This may be as simple as using wrist straps to help his arms and hands stay on the chair armrests, or it may be as advanced as using the wrap to "hug" his whole body into a cocoon.

In similar fashion, bite blocks, Molt mouth props, and other such devices are important elements of your armamentarium. Involuntary movements, unintentional closure, and simple fatigue or inability to keep ones mouth open independently are all reasons to make use of these items.

Often, patients desire to please the dental professional, but cannot cope with the actual treatment. Using "reminders" is a way to accomplish treatment, allow the patient to feel very proud that they "did it," and ensure that oral health is achieved. The author has one patient who uses only the leg strap around his feet and the end of the dental chair to remind him to stay sitting down: part of his deficit is the urge to unpredictably get up without any clear place to go. Use of the leg straps has allowed him to complete dental treatments in the office without incident. Some patients, particularly patients with ASD, are comforted simply by the weight of a lead apron. Placing this over their torso calms the patient, making no other protective devices necessary.

Considerations ought to be made regarding the risk of usage of medical protective devices versus the risk of general anesthesia to provide a similar level of treatment. While going to the operating room to provide comprehensive dental services under general anesthesia is an excellent care modality, use of the wrap allows frequent in-office assessments and debridements in the interim periods between OR visits.

## Oral sedatives

- Anxiolytic medications, such as benzodiazeprines and/or other mood stabilizers, as permitted by the patient's medical history.

Other sections of this book review anxiolysis and the use of oral medications. It is the experience of the authors that there is no one approach or drug regimen that works in every instance. Paradoxical reactions are common, unpredictable, and occur at any point in time, even in previous exposures have been effective.

The authors note that one of the most common reasons for less than optimal results of oral sedatives and behavior modification is the failure to identify the mechanism of action for the specific drug being used. When choosing a drug for its sedative powers, the provider is encouraged to be familiar with the drug's onset of action and the window of drug effectiveness at it relates to the dental procedure that is planned.

Usually, the drug is given to the patient by nursing or direct care staff at the patient's residence, and may not be the optimal window of time best for the dental provider to achieve a successful visit. If the medication is given to early, the window for effectiveness is long gone before the patient is seated. This may make the patient more irritable, as they are tired from the drug and want to be left alone. If the medication is give too late, the onset and window of therapy is not realized when the patient is seated. It is therefore important for the provider to be *very* specific in regard to drug administration protocols and patient support before, during, and after the dental visit (i.e., one-on-one patient monitoring). It is important that the direct care staff report to the dentist any lingering affects of the anxiolytic medications.

*Aging*, changes in systemic and mental health with related medication changes, behavioral responses, as well as nutritional and sleep variances, all play a role in the effectiveness of oral anxiolytic medications. It is wise to take a multispecialty approach, consulting with neurology, psychiatry, internal medicine, and others who know the patient well. Increases to routine drugs with or without additional benzodiazepines, addition of benzodiazepines only, use of Vistaril (and Phenergan) or Bendryl only, or some other combination are all potential therapies.

It is not uncommon for your patients to be on multiple medications for support of co-medical diagnosis, and the addition of oral sedatives should be used with caution. Monitoring of vital signs is required for patient safety. The authors recommend continuing education courses or advanced training experiences before administration of oral sedative medications. Please refer to your specific state dental board requirements for specific training in conscious sedation licensing.

## Inhalation sedation: nitrous oxide

Nitrous oxide can be a challenge in this patient population. While the drug is effective, administration of the drug is often not. Patients are facially defensive: that is, they do not like objects close to or on their face or mouth. Placing and keeping the mask in place can be nearly or completely impossible. Additionally, explaining to patients that they must breathe through their nose exclusively while their mouth is wide open can prove to be a concept impossible to communicate. Patient selection is critical. With the right patient, nitrous is a very effective adjunct.

## Intravenous sedation

Intravenous (IV) sedation may be an effective adjunct to dental treatments, particularly if the patient has a cooperation level that will allow most treatments with 50% support during the dental procedure *or* patients who need access to comprehensive dental care who are unable to be treated without pharmacological intervention due to either behavioral or medical issues.

The authors' use the following protocol for patient selection criteria to assure patient success outcomes under IV therapy:

- Patient must be able to cooperate at a reasonable level (Cooperation level 4 or above). The purpose of the conscious sedation is to reduce anxiety in a reasonably cooperative patient.
- Physical status 1 and 2 and selected physical status 3.
- Treatment under IV sedation is to be used for simple comprehensive dental cases. Proposed dental treatment should be able to be accomplished in 1 h per session, and the treatment plan should be completed in no more than two to three sessions.
- The patient should be able to have a panorex or PA radiographs taken without sedation. For the most part, all x-rays should be accomplished without sedation to complete the treatment plan effectively.

- Patients must have good IV access and be able to accept venipuncture with reasonable assistance
- All dentists who refer to the sedation program must have had training in how to refer the proper candidates for sedation.

## General anesthetic sedation: unconscious sedation in the operating room setting

The authors have worked in a myriad of settings (institutional, community-based, university-based, private). The age-old question is "who gets priority go the OR?" We have tried many models of queuing patients, with efforts for "fair" and "need" being considered. There is certainly no perfect system, but here are some guidelines that we have found useful: First and foremost, it is important to understand the risk–benefit continuum of dental rehabilitation and general anesthesia. While oral disease is systemic disease, the physical well-being of the patient may not be able to withstand general anesthesia. General anesthesia should not be taken for granted; while it is safe, untoward outcomes happen, including expiration. Exposures to general anesthesia are to be conservative, with regard that less is better. Additionally, and as previously stated in other sections of this chapter, philosophies regarding OR treatment vary greatly across North America. Bias of practitioner and patient/guardian will affect the success of the OR outcomes.

Criteria for treatment in the operating room under general anesthesia are based on behavior, level of dental and systemic disease, amount of dental rehabilitation necessary to achieve a base line level of health, patient preference, and a host of other consequential considerations. It is the belief of the authors that the concept of partnership extends to the patients who must utilize the OR for comprehensive dentistry. It is also important that expectations are clarified. This author expects a commitment for the patient to come to the office for routine visits (even if these are limited) every 3–4 months. The evidence supports fluoride varnish application even in the absence of scaling and prophylaxis and even the most contentious patients can usually tolerate fluoride varnish application ("Fluoride Varnish: An Evidence-Based Approach"). Often, guardians believe that one dental OR means stabilized oral health for the remaining lifetime of the patient; however, the guardian must understand that visits to the OR for comprehensive dental care may need to be considered periodically for optimal dental health over the patients lifetime.

It is common to incorporate more than one procedure into a dental OR case: eye exams, ear wax removal, gynecological exams, extensive blood draws, CT scans (when available in certain hospitals), and toenail clipping. It is important for the dentist practicing in the OR to develop a routine. This aids in maximizing efficiency with the goal of the shortest anesthesia time possible. This author proceeds as such.

Upon nasal intubation (whenever possible) and monitored anesthesia controls, the patient is prepped and draped in the usual manner and a throat pack placed. Once the mouth is isolated, dental treatment proceeds much as it would in the office. Full mouth radiographs and comprehensive dental and periodontal exams are completed. Diagnoses of hard and soft tissue disease processes are completed. Treatment proceeds with quad scaling and root planing, and prophylaxis. I then perform any necessary extractions, followed by gingival recontouring (when necessary) then restorations, irrigation and thorough suctioning of the oral cavity, application of fluoride varnish, removal of the throat pack, and subsequent extubation/ postanesthesia recovery. I perform extractions ahead of restorations for a number of reasons, the primary one being more successful control of bleeding earlier in the case.

Additionally, I use gel foam on all extractions (even in the clinic), and may suture depending on both the status of the soft tissues and the presence of patient habits (i.e., pica, picking, frequent inoculation of mouth with their own dirty fingers, etc.). Toradol is given via i.v. near the termination of the case often. Decodron is used if the case has been long or the patient is at risk of postoperation swelling. Anything I can do to decrease the postoperative risk of complications, the better for everyone, especially the patient. Remember, this patient is in the OR because they cannot tolerate treatment in the office. It is truly in your best interest to have bleeding and infection controlled in advance of the patient waking up! Cases requiring many hours may be "called" midway due to the length of the anesthesia. It is often safer for the patient to undergo two shorter GA's than one extremely long one. This author's longest single case was 6.5 h. Usually, if the case goes over 4 h, it will be terminated in favor of a second GA. Dental GA is considered elective surgery, so long cases are usually not justified compared to the risk of protracted anesthesia exposure.

# CASE MANAGEMENT PRESENTATION

## The story of Sondra

Sondra, a 22-year-old Asian-American female with pervasive developmental disorder—not otherwise specified (PDD-NOS), became a patient of the authors. She lived at home in a traditional family, including one younger unaffected sibling. Medically healthy, Sondra exhibited a range of behaviors that demonstrate the spectrum of PDD-NOS. Although intellectually moderately functioning, social responses were often unpredictable and varied. Sondra had attended dental office visits with her family members as an observer at their appointments. She understood the concepts of dental treatment, the purpose, and the expected behavior for the patient, as long as she was not the patient. Typical of ASD, dissociation occurs between self and the world in which one operates. Sarah would be able to report on another's appointment, but could not transfer that knowledge to a successful appointment for herself. Often she would see colleagues and friends from the special needs community when she was at our office. Gregariously (atypical of ASD), she would meet them, and even watch their dental treatment. She was also gregarious in her interactions with the dental staff, insisting on knowing where this assistant or that staff member might be on that day. She was always happy to see me, and willing to accompany me to the dental operatory. At this point, Sondra would be able to accomplish only minimal treatment despite exhaustive efforts on the part of her mom, the dental staff, and the dentist.

Sondra presented to the office every other Monday at precisely 9:30 a.m. for a desensitization appointment. In the very beginning, Sondra came to the office solely to see the space. Through her mom's own experienced suggestion, we repeatedly demonstrated only the panorex machine. Sondra stood in the machine, touched the bars, saw herself in the mirror and felt the chin rest, and watched the machine circle while she was standing nearby. Mom took a video of the panorex machine taking an x-ray of the dental assistant. Mom and Sondra would watch this homemade video over and over at home. On Sondra's seventh visit, a panorex was obtained. Although it was not a perfect radiograph, it contained useful information, including the presence of third molars. Our team and Sondra's mom defined this as success.

Mom wrote a handmade book for Sondra about each individual and collective dental office experience. In simple terms, it defines the reason for the visit, an emotional response, and the planned outcome. Using her own camera, Sondra's mom took pictures of each area, which she glued into a homemade book next to the story about it. Here are some examples:

*I am going to the Dentist today, I feel afraid, but I am safe.*
*I walk into the waiting room. It is full of people. I feel afraid, but I am safe.*
*I go into the dental chair. I sit down. I feel afraid, but I am safe.*
*There are a lot of machines around me. I am scared, but I am safe.*
*The polisher is noisy. I don't like it but it won't hurt me. I am afraid. I am safe.*

Sondra and her mom read this book at least once per week, usually the day before the next dental visit.

Additionally, the author and her dental assistant created and made a changeable story board (visual schedule), with suggestions from Sondra's mom. The story board itself was large and had Velcro on the face of it. Cartoon drawings of key points of a dental visit were created, and then laminated, and Velcro stuck on the back. A complement of teeth from a dental charting were "blown up," and two copies made—one set was left white and the other colored gray. These teeth were laminated, and then individually cut out. Velcro was applied to the back of each laminated tooth. The gray complement of teeth was attached to the board. When Sondra presented for the appointment, the storyboard was in a prominent place in the operatory. As each scene was accomplished, the cartoon drawing was stuck via Velcro to the board. As each tooth was polished, a gray tooth was taken off the board, and replaced with a white one. This helped Sondra understand quantitatively how many teeth had been polished and how many teeth were left.

Sondra had a mediocre response to all of these efforts. She knew what was expected of her. She watched and understood what was expected of other patients. No amount of information, however, would allow her to be able to successfully accomplish a prophylaxis. Some days she would simply get up a lot. Other days she would hit herself or her mom. Sometimes she would scream. She was not afraid of me or my staff or her mom. She was unable to communicate her fears, frustrations, and exhaustion through other mechanisms.

This is one of the great challenges of special care dentistry. It is often difficult to discern what the threshold of learning and growth is for a particular patient, when your efforts should be dialed back, or when you should insist on trying more. Sondra will always need to go to the OR for the accomplishment of comprehensive care. We were realistic from the outset about this. We did not realize that Sondra has a small threshold for desensitization, and after a handful of initial desensitization appointments, the effectiveness ended. Her gains early peaked, and no further gains were made. In this case, Sondra's excellent memory (ASD) would serve her well enough to accomplish a basic visit every 3 months with the aforementioned implements, and spare the staff and parents time, money, and energy.

If the reader prefers further familiarization with the topic of autism, the following sources are recommended for detailed, reliable information about autism spectrum disorder, or more simple autism.

(1)  http://www.nichd.nih.gov/health/topics/ash.cfm;
(2)  http://www.nimh.nih.gov/health/topics/autism-spectrum-disorders-pervasive-developmental-disorders/index.shtml;
(3)  http://www.nlm.nuh.gov/medlineplus/autism.html;
(4)  http://www.mayoclinic.com/health/autism/ds00348;
(5)  http://www.autism-society.org; and
(6)  http://www.autismspeaks.org.

## The story of Fred

Fred is a 42-year-old male with moderate MR and moderate to severe ASD. Fred has a happy disposition almost all of the time, and is very compliant for dental visits. Despite his 240 lbs and 6'2" frame, he is a pleasure to treat in the office. Some of my staff is afraid of him because his size and vocalizations feel intimidating; however, I have treated him for 12 years without incident. The keys for Fred are that he feels valued; he knows he has a right express himself, and he knows the expectations at each visit. He also can accommodate an appointment for about an hour. After that window of time, he loses many of his filters. He is able to successfully accomplish restorative in the office with very little coaching, perhaps with the exception of the injection for local anesthesia. Recently, Fred was in to see me for the restoration of no. 19. After the administration of local anesthetic, Fred announced that he wanted to lie on the floor. His staff said this was a new behavior that he was doing more of at home. I told him that would be fine with me. Fred lay on the floor. I went to perform an exam for the patient in the hygiene chair. When I returned about 10 minutes later, Fred, without any direction from me, immediately got up, returned to the dental chair, and the appointment proceeded and finished without incident.

# REFERENCES

1.  American Psychiatric Association. 2004. *Diagnostic and Statistical Manual of Mental Disorders: DSM IV TR. Guide Book*, 4th edn., text rev. Washington, DC: American Psychiatric Association.
2.  Ustun T, Chatterji S, Bickenbach J, et al. 2003. The International Classification of Functioning, Disability and Health. a new tool for understanding disability and health. *Disabil Rehabil* 25(11–12): 565–71.
3.  Minshew N and Hoson J. 2008. Sensory sensitivities and performance on sensory perceptual tasks in high-functioning individuals with autism. *J Autism Dev Disord* 38:1485–98.
4.  Baker A, Lane A, Angley MT, et al. 2008. The relationship between sensory processing patterns and behavioral responsiveness in autistic disorder: A pilot study. *J Autism Dev Disord* 38(5):867–75.
5.  Dawson G and Waitling R. 2000. Interventions to facilitate auditory, visual and motor integration in autism: A review of evidence. *J Autism Dev Disord* 30:415–21.
6.  Buckwalter K, Hartock J, and Gaffney J. 1985. *Nursing Intervention: Treatment for Nursing Diagnoses*. Philadelphia, PA: WB Saunters.
7.  Covington H and Crosby C. 1997. Music therapy as a nursing intervention. *J Psychosoc Nurs Ment Health Serv* 36:34–7.
8.  Brugnes M and Avigne G. 2003. Music therapy for reducing surgical anxiety. *AORN J* 78:816–8.
9.  McCaffrey R, Freeman E. 2003. Effect of music on chronic osteoarthritis pain in older people. *J Adv Nurs* 44:517–24.
10. Hendon C and Bohon L. 2007. Hospitalized children's mood differences during play and music therapy. *Child Care Health Dev* 34(2):141–4.
11. Lee OKA, Chung YFL, Chan MF, et al. 2004. Music and its effect on the physiological responses and anxiety levels of patient receiving mechanical ventilation. *J Clin Nurs* 14:609–20.
12. Price S and Price L. 1999. *Aromatherapy for Health Professionals*, 2nd edn. London: Churchill Livingstone.
13. Sanderson H, Harrison J, and Price S. 1991. *Aromatherapy and Massage for People with Learning Difficulties*. Birmingham, UK: Hands On Publishing Limited.

14. Harrison J and Ruddle J. 2009. An introduction to aromatherapy for people with learning disabilities. *Brit J Learning Disabilities* 23(1):37–40.
15. Williams T. 2006. Evaluation effects of aromatherapy massage on sleep in children with autism: A pilot study. *e-CAM* 3(3):373–7.
16. Fuji M, et al. 2008. Lavender aroma therapy for behavioral and psychological symptoms in dementia patients. *Geriatr Gerontol Int* 8:136–8.

# Index

Page numbers in *italics* refer to Figures; those with a "*t*" refer to Tables.

*The Fearful Dental Patient: A Guide to Understanding and Managing.* Edited by Arthur A. Weiner
© 2011 Blackwell Publishing Ltd.

**265**